PLATELETS IN BIOLOGY AND PATHOLOGY

Research monographs in cell and tissue physiology

Volume 1

General Editor

J. T. DINGLE

Cambridge

NORTH-HOLLAND PUBLISHING COMPANY
AMSTERDAM · NEW YORK · OXFORD

Platelets in biology and pathology

Editor

J. L. GORDON

Cambridge

1976

NORTH-HOLLAND PUBLISHING COMPANY
AMSTERDAM · NEW YORK · OXFORD

North-Holland ISBN: 0 7204 0601 3

Published by:

Elsevier/North-Holland Biomedical Press
335, Jan van Galenstraat, P.O. Box 1527
Amsterdam, The Netherlands

Sole distributors for the U.S.A. and Canada:

Elsevier/North-Holland Inc.
52 Vanderbilt Avenue
New York, N.Y. 10017

Library of Congress Cataloging in Publication Data

Main entry under title:

Platelets in biology and pathology.

   (Research monographs in cell and tissue physiol-
ogy ; v. 1)
   Bibliography: p.
   Includes index.
   1. Blood platelets. 2. Hemostasis. 3. Blood
platelet aggregation. 4. Thrombosis. I. Gordon,
J. L. II. Series. [DNLM: 1. Blood platelets--
Cytology. 2. Blood platelets--Physiology. W1
RE232GL v. 1 / WH300 P7185]
QP97.P58   591'.1'13   76-53005
ISBN 0-7204-0601-3

Printed in the Netherlands

Preface

Platelets are popular. Two years ago, Professor Dan Deykin commented in the New England Journal of Medicine, 'These are palmy days for platelet researchers', and this is even more true today. Why this latter-day research interest in the smallest circulating element of the blood, whose existence and basic functions were recognised a hundred years ago? The reasons are to be found in the chapters of this book, which illustrate the diverse biological roles of platelets, and emphasize the potential value of platelets as research tools in cell biology.

About fifteen years ago, platelet research began to move away from observational studies of thrombus formation and haemostasis towards an investigation of the intracellular reactions responsible for these processes, and progress in this field has been rapid, as evidenced by the number of monographs and reviews published in recent years. The purpose of this volume, however, is not merely to bring previous publications up-to-date: several of the topics covered are only peripherally related to haemostasis or thrombosis, and the book is primarily designed for readers who are not platelet specialists, and may therefore be unaware of the platelet's biological versatility and research potential.

The platelet's main function is initiating the haemostatic plug, and this topic is reviewed by Baumgartner and Muggli, in a most detailed account of the factors governing platelet deposition in vivo and in vitro. Also, Moore and Pepper describe how monitoring platelet secretion by radioimmunoassay of β-thromboglobulin could lead to more accurate clinical evaluation of haemostasis and thrombosis. Apart from these chapters, however, there is considerable emphasis elsewhere on the potential roles of platelets in biological processes other than haemostasis – such as atherogenesis, inflammation, immune reactions and cell proliferation.

Where relevant, platelet reactions and constituents are compared with those of other cells, as in MacIntyre's chapter on stimulated secretion and Crawford's review of microfilaments and microtubules. In addition, some of the most stimulating contributions are the reviews of current work on platelet membrane receptors for specific agents, and on the mechanisms regulating the responses of the cell, for such studies with platelets can help to elucidate reactions which occur in many other cells as well.

The choice of content in this book is my responsibility, and, although it may sometimes appear rather idiosyncratic, it reflects something of the variety of current platelet research. In order to reduce the overlap of content in some chapters I have reshaped several passages, and am therefore responsible for any resulting deficiencies of presentation. Special thanks are due to the publishers and to my family, who were both patient and helpful during the preparation of this book, and to my colleagues Carol Grainge, Euan MacIntyre and Jeremy Pearson, who helped prepare the index.

I hope that everyone with even a passing interest in platelets will find something of value here, and that some may be sufficiently stimulated to develop an active interest in platelet research.

John L. Gordon

Contents to Volume 1

Part II. Platelet constituents, cellular control mechanisms and biological significance

PART I

Outline of fundamental platelet reactions

CHAPTER 1

Blood platelets as multifunctional cells

J.L. GORDON and A.J. MILNER

University Department of Pathology, Tennis Court Road,
Cambridge CB2 1QP, England

1. Introduction

Blood platelets were overlooked in the early days of haematologic microscopy simply because they are small: the mammalian platelet is an anucleate body only about 2 μm in diameter, and was consequently much less easy to recognise than the larger red and white cells. In 1906, Buckmaster concluded that platelets were present in blood samples from healthy subjects only if the blood had been taken with insufficient care, but other work in the early years of this century soon made the concept of the platelet as a technical artefact untenable. Much of this work was concerned with the role of platelets in coagulation, and this may be partly responsible for the platelet being overlooked by research workers and pathologists today–the belief is still quite widely held that platelets are merely 'something to do with clotting'. In fact, although platelets are indeed important in coagulation, they have the capacity to participate in numerous other physiological and pathological processes, and also exhibit a wide variety of cellular reactions. This versatility, combined with the ready accessibility of platelets as a homogeneous population of intact cells, makes them valuable models for studying processes such as active transport, secretion, and cell adhesion. This point is emphasized by the diversity of topics covered by the other chapters in this volume: most of them deal with individual reactions of platelets in some detail, and the aim of this introductory chapter is to put the bulk of that information into perspective. The first part will deal briefly with platelet formation and structure, and we shall then consider platelets as multifunctional, both in terms of their intracellular reactions and their contribution to different biological processes.

Gordon (ed) Platelets in Biology and Pathology
© *Elsevier/North-Holland Biomedical Press, 1976*

2. Characteristics of platelets

2.1. Formation and turnover

Platelets are formed from megakaryocytes, which probably share a common precursor with myeloid and erythroid cells (Becker et al., 1963). Once the pluripotent stem cell becomes committed to become a megakaryocyte it undergoes a maturation period of about 70 h, and during this period the mass of a single megakaryocyte may measure sufficiently to produce several thousand platelets. This intense biosynthetic activity during maturation is accompanied by an increase in the ploidy of the cell. Once mature the megakaryocyte transforms from a spherical to a highly irregular shape (Behnke, 1969) and fragments of cytoplasm are pinched off to form platelets. As might be expected, newly-formed platelets often contain ribosomes and RNA from the parent cell cytoplasm, and elevated levels of platelets containing ribosomes and RNA are found during the recovery phases after bleeding (Ingram and Coopersmith, 1969). In general, however, platelets are incapable of synthesising proteins in biologically significant quantities.

The circulating platelet count varies with animal species, ranging from about 2×10^8/ml in man to about 10^9/ml in the rat. The normal turnover rate of platelets is about 3.5×10^7/ml/day in man (Harker and Finch, 1969) and their life span in the blood is about ten days, spent platelets being removed by sequestration in the spleen and liver. The mechanism by which the cells are recognised as being ready for removal from the circulation may, however, be unrelated to loss of functional capacity: Greenberg and coworkers (1975) found that removing 15% of the platelet sialic acid with neuraminidase results in the cells being immediately cleared from the circulation, whereas removal of up to 30% of the sialic acid failed to impair the platelet response to aggregating stimuli.

2.2. Structure

Considering that platelets are formed by fragmentation of megakaryocyte cytoplasm their uniformity in size is quite remarkable, although in some pathological conditions abnormally large platelets with deficient functions are found (see Tocantins, 1938). Microtubules may well play a critical role in platelet formation, and might help to regulate the cell's size: the equilibrium between monomer/polymer of microtubule protein is apparently far toward the monomer in the megakaryocyte, toward the polymer in the circulating platelet, and then is rapidly reversed toward the monomer again when platelets are activated and change in shape (see Chapter 6).

The general structural features of the platelet are indicated in Fig. 1 and the reader is referred to White (1971) for a detailed description of platelet morphology. Briefly, circulating platelets are discoid in shape with an equatorial bundle of microtubules running round the perimeter, close to the surface membrane, and supporting the platelet's asymmetric form. Within the microtubules is a complex canalicular system in direct continuity with the plasma membrane.

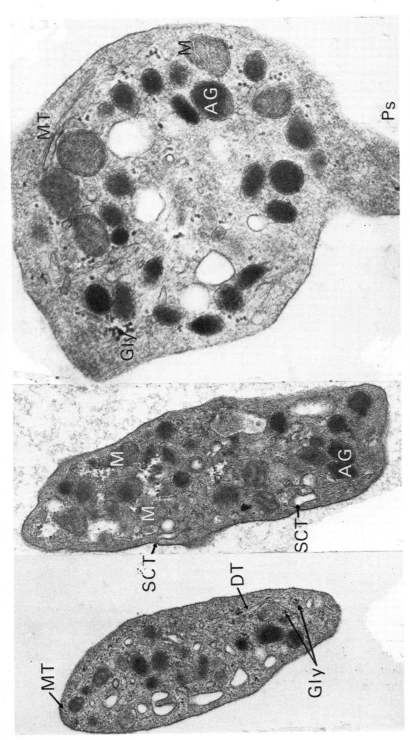

Fig. 1. Electron micrographs of blood platelets, kindly provided by Dr. G.R. Bullock of Ciba Laboratories, Horsham. Left: rabbit platelet, original magnification ×22,500. Centre: human, ×31,500. Right: guinea pig, ×37,500. Note the characteristic lenticular profile (left, centre) of discoid platelets sectioned sagitally, whereas the cell on the right, which is starting to undergo a shape change, has rounded up and extruded a pseudopod (Ps). This cell shows microtubules (MT) in longitudinal section, and these can also be seen in cross section at the poles of the cell on the left. Numerous alpha granules (AG) are present in all three platelets, together with mitochondria (M) and glycogen granules (Gly). Surface-connected tubules (SCT) are indicated in the centre cell, and the structures in the cell on the left which resemble vacuoles are probably invaginations from the SCT which do not show the point of surface contact. Dense tubules (DT) are also present in this cell.

It has been shown, using electron-dense vital stains, that plasma-borne sub-stances may enter the canalicular system and be transferred to platelet granules (White, 1968). At least two types of membrane-bound granules are present in the platelet: alpha granules and very dense bodies*. Alpha granules may exhibit an electron-dense nucleoid and at least some of these granules contain lysosomal enzymes (see Section 3.6) which are synthesised and packaged during megakaryo-cyte maturation (MacPherson, 1972; Young, 1973). In contrast, the very dense granules, which contain 5-hydroxytryptamine (5HT), are rarely seen in megakaryocytes (Pletscher et al., 1971; Silver and Gardner, 1968). We may therefore conclude that the 5HT granules are probably formed via uptake of 5HT from the plasma by the circulating platelet. Mitochondria and glycogen granules are also present in platelets, thus equipping the cells for glycolysis and for aerobic respiration. Finally, because platelets are apparently capable of phagocytosis both in vivo and in vitro (see Section 3.8), the platelet cytoplasm may contain ingested matter such as lipids, fibrin, and immune complexes.

3. Reactions of platelets

Platelets can be stimulated by many different biological agents (Table 1) and this capacity to respond to a range of stimuli is one reason why the platelet is such a fascinating cell to study. Also, paradoxically, the fact that it lacks a nucleus, DNA and protein-synthesising ability constitutes a positive advantage in the study of certain basic cellular reactions, such as those summarised in Table 1.

TABLE 1
Platelet stimulants

Adenosine 5′-diphosphate	Immune complexes
(Nor)adrenaline*	Collagen
5-hydroxytryptamine*	Thrombin
Calcium ionophores	Prostaglandins (and their metabolites)
Acetylcholine*	Vasopressin*

* Platelets from some animal species do not respond to these agents.

3.1. Active transport

Platelets possess the ability to accumulate by selective active transport proces-ses several substances including 5-hydroxytryptamine (5HT), dopamine, amino acids, adenine and adenosine. The amine uptake systems, discussed in Chapter 8, provide a striking example of the cell's ability to concentrate extracellular material – the platelet is capable of taking up 5HT against a concentration gradient of around four orders of magnitude. There is some debate about the function of

* See note added in proof, page 22.

TABLE 2
Main cellular reactions of blood platelets

Reaction		Probable biological role
Active transport	*Main substrates* (a) 5'-Hydroxytryptamine (b) Adenine, adenosine (c) Taurine	(a) 'Mopping up' free plasma 5HT (b) Substrates for conversion to metabolic nucleotides (c) Unknown
Adhesion	Vascular collagen	Primary step in formation of haemostatic plug
Aggregation	Platelet–platelet interaction	Growth of haemostatic plug
Unmasking membrane phospholipids	Exposure of 'platelet factor 3'	Promoting blood coagulation at sites of platelet aggregation
Active contraction	Activation of platelet contractile protein 'thrombosthenin' (actomyosin)	Clot retraction; ? aggregation; ? secretion
Secretion from storage granules	(a) *Dense bodies*: contain 5HT, ADP, Ca^{2+} (b) *Alpha granules*: contain fibrinogen, antiheparin factors, lysosomal enzymes	(a) Promoting growth of platelet aggregates (b) Promoting coagulation; enzymes may participate in atherogenesis, fibrinolysis, and inflammatory responses
Prostaglandin synthesis	PGE_2 and $PGF_{2\alpha}$ ultimately formed; larger quantities of short-lived intermediates also produced	PGE_2 and $PGF_{2\alpha}$ may participate in inflammation; some of the intermediates are potent platelet aggregating agents
Phagocytosis	Lipid, colloidal carbon, latex etc., can be ingested by platelets	Scavenging

the amine uptake mechanisms in platelets: the 5HT transport system certainly acts as a means of 'mopping up' any free 5HT which might be circulating in the plasma, but since platelets store this 5HT in granules from which it is readily released, it would seem likely that the 5HT stored in platelets also has an active role to play – and, indeed, the 5HT released from platelets does help to promote the continuing growth of platelet aggregates and thus improve the efficiency of haemostatic plug formation. In addition, the similarity between amine transport in platelets and in aminergic neurones has been the subject of considerable speculation (Bouillin and O'Brien, 1970; 1971), and this parallel has been extended to the platelet uptake processes for taurine, glycine and GABA – all putative central neurotransmitters (Bouillin and Green, 1972; Bouillin et al., 1973).

The adenine and adenosine which platelets take up are converted into nucleotides in a metabolic pool, thus helping to ensure a continuing supply of metabolic energy (see Chapter 3).

3.2. Adhesion

Platelets will adhere to certain biological polymers and to a variety of artificial surfaces. The most important physiological adhesion reaction is that which occurs betwen platelets and collagen in the vascular wall, as this can lead to platelet aggregation and the secretion of granule constituents. The morphological characteristics of these reactions are reviewed in Chapter 2 and the intracellular mechanisms are summarised in Chapter 3. Platelet–collagen adhesion is the primary step in the formation of a haemostatic plug, and as platelets do not adhere readily to other biological macromolecules such as elastin, gelatin and polymerised fibrin, there has been considerable interest recently in the specific mechanisms involved in the platelet–collagen adhesion reaction. This topic is discussed in Chapter 10.

3.3. Aggregation

Platelet aggregation (that is, platelet–platelet interactions leading to the formation of a multicellular mass or aggregate) can be induced by a variety of soluble physiological agents including ADP, adrenaline, noradrenaline, 5HT and thrombin (Table 1). Aggregation can also be induced by particulate stimuli such as collagen, antigen–antibody complexes and kaolin; in this situation, however, the aggregation reaction follows an initial adhesion between the platelet and the particulate agent, and depends on the secretion of certain platelet constituents. When aggregation is induced in the absence of any adhesion reaction, the first detectable response is usually an isovolemic shape-change in which the cells round up and put out pseudopodia. This shape-change occurs rapidly, and presumably facilitates the subsequent platelet–platelet contact because the pseudopods have a much smaller surface area at their tip than that of the parent cell. The catecholamines are unusual in causing platelet aggregation which is apparently not preceded by any shape-change, but the reasons for this difference are unknown. Platelet aggregation is calcium-dependent, and in the case of some agents (e.g., ADP) the presence of fibrinogen is necessary as well, although the precise manner in which this plasma protein acts as a cofactor for aggregation is not clear. Aggregation induced by thrombin and by high concentrations of ADP or catecholamines is usually associated with the secretion of constituents from platelet storage granules, and such aggregation is essentially irreversible (although the aggregates can be dispersed by treating them with agents such as EDTA and prostaglandin E_1). Reversible aggregation can be induced by low concentrations of ADP or 5HT, and when these aggregates disperse, the platelets thus released are then less responsive to aggregating stimuli.

Platelet aggregation is the process mainly responsible for the initial growth of a haemostatic plug, and is consequently of considerable biological importance. Although platelet aggregate formation is most obvious when a blood vessel is transected, aggregates also form at sites of microvascular damage and it is quite likely that some degree of platelet aggregation is taking place somewhere in the body almost all the time.

3.4. Unmasking membrane phospholipids

When platelets are stimulated by agents such as collagen or thrombin a phospholipid complex known as platelet factor 3 (PF_3) is exposed on the platelet membrane (see Chapter 5 for a discussion of platelet phospholipids). PF_3 plays an important role in the intrinsic coagulation system, being involved in the enzymic cascade at several stages including the activation of Factor VIII. Little PF_3 is actually released from platelets but large amounts are unmasked on the surface membrane and this promotes the coagulation process in the immediate vicinity of a platelet aggregate, thus helping to stabilise the haemostatic plug through the formation of fibrin strands. Considerable amounts of PF_3 activity can be extracted from the membrane of the platelet alpha granules, and it seems probable that at least part of the PF_3 activity which appears at the surface of a stimulated platelet is the result of fusion between the granule membrane and the plasma membrane during the secretion process. It is significant that the platelet alpha granule membrane fraction is also rich in acid phosphatase, for, like PF_3, there is not usually much acid phosphatase released from stimulated platelets, although the amount detectable at the cell membrane is increased. When some release of PF_3 and acid phosphatase does occur (e.g., during clotting of platelet-rich plasma), the two activities released from the cells can be sedimented together as lipoprotein complexes (Kubisz and Caen, 1972). This suggests that PF_3 and platelet acid phosphatase may be components of a lipoprotein complex on the alpha granule membrane.

3.5. Active contraction

Platelets contain large amounts of the structural protein *tubulin*, which is organised into an equatorial band of microtubules and appears to act as a cytoskeleton, maintaining the circulating platelet in a discoid shape. When platelets are stimulated to form aggregates or undergo a release reaction (see Chapter 3) the peripheral band of microtubules initially contracts with a concomitant centripetal movement of the platelet granules; subsequently, the microtubule band disperses. Platelets also contain large amounts of the contractile proteins actin and myosin, and these too are activated when platelets are stimulated. Biochemical studies of the platelet contractile proteins have demonstrated that their actin and myosin are very similar to those of smooth muscle, and that their activation may be regulated by a troponin–tropomyosin system (see Chapter 6).

The precise roles of contractile proteins in platelet reactions are not yet fully understood; it is generally accepted that clot retraction depends on the activation of platelet actomyosin, and Cohen and de Vries (1973) proposed an elegant model to explain how the process of clot retraction may be controlled by the platelet contractile proteins acting on inelastic fibrin strands in the clot. The part which contractile proteins play in other platelet reactions is, however, still controversial: the contraction wave resulting from actin-myosin activation presumably facilitates the release of granule contents from the platelet, and Booyse and his coworkers have suggested that rapid extrusion of contractile microfilaments in the very early stages of platelet aggregation is responsible for the formation of platelet–platelet bonds (Rafelson et al., 1973). This view is not, however, universally accepted and further work is needed to clarify this point.

3.6. Secretion from storage granules

When platelets are stimulated they may selectively release certain of their constituents stored in the dense bodies and the alpha granules. The dense bodies contain 5HT, ADP and ionised calcium, and stimulation of platelets by agents such as ADP or adrenaline can induce the release of most of the dense body contents with little concomitant secretion of alpha granule constituents (Mills et al., 1968). When the contents of the platelet dense bodies are released these can stimulate other platelets to aggregate in turn, and the main biological role of these platelet constituents is presumably to promote the growth of a haemostatic plug by this means, although they also have other biological effects – for example, the 5HT released from a platelet aggregate may cause a local increase in vascular permeability.

When platelets are stimulated by collagen or thrombin the constituents of the alpha granules as well as those of the dense bodies are usually released. Biologically active constituents of alpha granules which have so far been identified (listed in Table 3) include lysosomal enzymes (glycosidases and cathepsins), fibrinogen, and antiheparin factors – chief amongst which is platelet factor 4 (PF_4). The alpha granules also contain several cationic proteins with a range of biological activities which include increasing vascular permeability, releasing histamine from mast cells, and inducing chemotaxis of polymorphonuclear leucocytes. Therefore, although the primary biological role of constituents released from platelet alpha granules may be to promote coagulation through fibrinogen and the antiheparin factors, the other constituents (notably the degradative enzymes and the cationic proteins) could participate in both atherogenesis and inflammation (see Sections 4.1.5 and 4.2.2).

The biological mechanisms responsible for the platelet release reaction are still not fully understood: the reaction is initiated by the release-inducing agent binding to a specific recognition site on the cell membrane (see Chapters 7–9) and this probably then causes a local change in ionic distribution at the membrane. The cell's cyclic nucleotide balance (cyclic AMP/GMP ratio) is altered, and the contractile proteins are activated. These intracellular changes lead to the fusion of storage granules with the surface-connected tubular system, and the granule contents are then rapidly extruded through the tubules to the cell surface. This secretory process requires a considerable amount of metabolic ATP. In Chapter 3 D.E. MacIntyre reviews the platelet release reaction and compares it with secretory processes in other cells.

3.7. Prostaglandin synthesis

When platelets are stimulated by agents which induce the release reaction, the cells synthesise prostaglandin E_2 and prostaglandin $F_{2\alpha}$ (Smith et al., 1973). Since

TABLE 3
Constituents of human platelet alpha granules

Constituent	Characteristics	Reference
Fibrinogen	Accounts for virtually all platelet fibrinogen	Day and Solum, 1973
Platelet factor 4(PF4)	Antiheparin: mol. wt around 27,000	Moore et al., 1975
Proteinases	Cathepsin A Cathepsin D Cathepsin E (small amount)	Nachman and Ferris, 1968 Ehrlich and Gordon (see Chapter 14)
Glycosidases	Most prominent are β-glucuronidase and β-N-acetylglucosaminidase	Marcus et al., 1966 Day et al., 1969 Gordon, 1975
Cationic proteins	1. Mol. wt around 30,000; increases vascular permeability; releases histamine from mast cells 2. Generates leukocyte chemotactic factor by splitting C5	Nachman et al., 1972 Weksler and Coupal, 1973

these prostaglandins have little effect on platelets this observation appeared to be of limited significance, until it was discovered that, during this process of prostaglandin synthesis, short-lived endoperoxide intermediates were formed which were potent platelet stimulants (Willis and Kuhn, 1973). Samuelsson and his coworkers (Hamberg et al., 1975) showed that, in addition to these endoperoxides, there were other intermediates formed which were even more effective platelet stimulants. These intermediates are metabolised mainly to non-prostanoate derivatives, and therefore measuring the amounts of PGE_2 and $PGF_{2\alpha}$ produced gives no indication of the total amount of prostaglandin-related stimulatory products formed. It is likely that prostaglandin intermediates play a more important role in haemostasis and thrombosis than has hitherto been recognised, and we should also not overlook the fact that prostaglandins produced by platelets could play other biological roles – for example, in the inflammatory process (see Section 4.1.5). The subject of prostaglandin synthesis is discussed in considerable detail in Chapter 13.

3.8. Phagocytosis

Platelets can ingest several kinds of particles (e.g., carbon, latex, lipid, collagen) and the platelet membrane is also apparently capable of pinocytosis (Mustard and Packham, 1968; Behnke, 1967; White, 1972; Hovig, 1974). Although platelets can ingest only very small particles, they are capable of acting as scavengers in vivo: Van Aken and Vreeken (1969) showed that carbon particles are cleared from the blood stream to the reticulo-endothelial system largely by the actions of platelets. This phenomenon is largely unrecognised, and it ought to be further investigated to establish whether it is indeed true phagocytosis (rather than trapping of particles in the canalicular system) and whether it plays a biologically significant role.

4. Contributions of platelets to physiological and pathological processes

Although distinguishing between physiology and pathology is often difficult and sometimes meaningless, it is convenient for the purposes of this review to separate the functions of the blood platelets into these two classes. The criteria used for this subdivision are broadly that a physiological process contributes to the maintenance of a state which, under the conditions in question, we believe to be beneficial to the body, while a pathological process is deleterious. Having made this division, however, some anomalies still appear: for example, 'inflammation' appears in both categories and 'transplant rejection' appears under pathological processes, although the reactions involved are mainly those of the body's normal defence mechanism. Regardless of any eccentricities in the cataloguing, the primary purpose of this Section should remain clear: to summarise briefly the range of biological processes in which blood platelets can participate.

4.1. Physiological processes

4.1.1. Haemostasis

The one physiological contribution that platelets make which is of overriding importance is in the haemostatic process. The platelets' contribution to haemostasis takes two main forms: first, they initiate the formation of a haemostatic plug at the site of vascular injury; and secondly, they ensure efficient coagulation by virtue of factors which they release when stimulated or carry adsorbed on their surface.

The formation of a haemostatic plug depends almost exclusively on the platelet reactions of *adhesion, aggregation*, and *secretion*, (see Sections 2.2, 2.3, and 2.4). When the wall of a blood vessel is transected, the collagen in the vascular wall is exposed to the blood, and platelets immediately adhere to the exposed collagen fibres. These adherent platelets then release ADP, calcium, and 5HT from their dense bodies, and also synthesise and secrete prostaglandins and their intermediates – all these agents stimulate platelet aggregation and thus promote the formation of a haemostatic plug at the site of vascular damage. The processes involved in haemostatic plug formation are summarised diagramatically in Fig. 2, and ultrastructural details are shown in the elegant electronmicrographs of H.R. Baumgartner and R. Muggli in Chapter 2.

The ability of platelets to promote coagulation in the vicinity of a platelet aggregate depends on three reactions: first, the activation by collagen of coagula-

THE HAEMOSTATIC PROCESS

A. Initiation (duration: a few seconds)

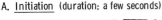
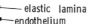
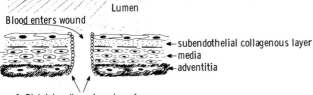

elastic lamina
endothelium
Lumen
Blood enters wound
subendothelial collagenous layer
media
adventitia

1. Platelets adhere to cut surfaces;
   release granule constituents, prostaglandins, procoagulants
2. Coagulation cascade initiated

B. Development (duration: a few minutes)

Released constituents induce more platelets to form aggregates
on the original adherent layer; wound is plugged; coagulation cascade proceeds

C. Consolidation (duration: several minutes)

Coagulation cascade completed; fibrin strands form around platelet plug,
trapping other blood cells; the fibrocellular mass retracts into the wound,
packing it tightly

D. Organisation (duration: a few days)

Macrophages invade the wound and clear the debris;
surrounding vascular cells proliferate and synthesize new connective tissue

tion Factor XI on the platelet membrane; secondly, the unmasking of the procoagulant phospholipid complex PF_3 at the surface of stimulated platelets; and thirdly, the release of platelet factor 4 (antiheparin) and fibrinogen from platelet storage granules. The role of platelet coagulant activities in the haemostatic process was the subject of a stimulating review by Walsh (1974).

4.1.2. Endothelial integrity

It has been well recognised for many years that thrombocytopenia is associated with an increase in capillary fragility. Johnson and her coworkers demonstrated that this was due not merely to platelets adhering to the capillary wall, but also to the platelets insinuating themselves into the junctions between the endothelial cells or actually becoming incorporated into the endothelial cytoplasm. When radiolabelled platelets were transfused into thrombocytopenic animals, ultrastructural studies revealed single platelets in close association with the endothelial membranes, and the radioactive label was deposited in the capillaries of numerous organs; labelled platelet-poor plasma did not result in a similar labelling of the capillary endothelial layers (Johnson, 1971). In support of this concept Gimbrone et al. (1969) investigated the factors responsible for the capillary permeability of isolated perfused organs maintained for transplantation and found that capillary integrity was better preserved when the perfusate contained whole, viable, platelets in addition to plasma proteins and the necessary ions.

4.1.3. Wound healing

When a wound is first made and blood flows into the cut, platelets adhere to the collagen exposed in the wound, and platelet plugs form at the ends of the transected blood vessels; consequently, when the blood has stopped flowing there are large numbers of platelets in the wound. There has been little consideration given to the possibility that the platelets could participate in the wound healing process after the flow of blood has been arrested, but when Simpson and Ross (1972) investigated wound healing in animals made severely leukopenic by anti-neutrophil serum they found that the wounds healed normally provided they were kept sterile – possibly because platelets were 'deputising' for the missing neutrophil leukocytes. Stimulated platelets secrete a factor which causes cells to proliferate (see Chapter 15) and fibroblast proliferation is important in the early stages of wound healing. Another characteristic of the early healing process is the secretion of collagen by these fibroblasts, and it may be more than coincidence that 5HT (which will be released in large amounts from platelets in a wound) is a fibrogenic agent – that is, it stimulates the secretion of collagen from fibroblasts (Aalto and Kulonen, 1972). In conclusion, platelets have the potential to participate in at least two aspects of the wound healing process, and although it is unlikely that they contribute significantly under normal conditions, further work is clearly necessary to determine whether they can, in unusual circumstances, assume a more important role.

4.1.4. Scavenging

As discussed above, the platelet membrane is apparently capable of both pinocytosis and phagocytosis. Platelets can play an important role in clearing particles from the blood (Van Aken and Vreeken, 1969), and may continue circulating in the blood stream with particles inside them (Vegge et al., 1968). Although platelets that have phagocytised particles may be more liable to form aggregates (Van Aken and Vreeken, 1969), Zir and his coworkers (1974) reported that after the injection of X-ray contrast media, platelet reactivity as measured in vitro was reduced; however, this could have been caused by the platelets having previously participated in aggregate formation in vivo, and hence being 'refractory' to later stimulation in vitro. Donald and Tennent (1975) emphasized that because platelets contribute significantly to the removal of particulate material from the bloodstream, it is often not valid to use particle clearance studies as a measure of reticuloendothelial function alone.

4.1.5. Inflammation

There has been increasing interest recently in the possibility that blood platelets play a significant role in the inflammatory process. It was recognised some years ago that platelets accumulate at sites of tissue damage (Cotran, 1965) and that they release constituents which increase vascular permeability (Mustard et al., 1965; Packham et al., 1968). Nachman and his coworkers (1972) found a platelet 'permeability factor' present in the alpha granules, which was a cationic protein with a molecular weight of approximately 30,000. The effect of this on permeability was biphasic: the immediate response (within 15 min of intradermal injection) was inhibited by pretreatment with antihistamine but the delayed effect (3 h after injection) was not mediated by histamine. The alpha granule factor caused degranulation of mouse or rat peritoneal mast cells, with concomitant histamine release, and it seems probable that the acute phase of increased vascular permeability was a consequence of mast cell degranulation.

The second phase of increased vascular permeability was characterised by clustering of leukocytes at the site of the injection of the factor, which suggested that this permeability response might be due to substances released from the leukocytes. Packham et al. (1968) had previously found that pig platelets contained a factor which was chemotactic for leukocytes, and Weksler and Coupal (1973) found that the cationic protein from human platelet alpha granules acted directly on the fifth component of complement (C5) to liberate a fragment with marked chemotactic activity for polymorphonuclear leukocytes. The properties of this leukocyte chemotactic factor from platelets were recently reviewed by Weksler (1974).

The effects of platelets on vascular permeability are not restricted to alpha granule constituents: when platelets are stimulated and the prostaglandin synthase complex is activated, the main product of the cyclo-oxygenase pathway (PGE_2) increases vascular permeability directly (Silver et al., 1974), and the lipoxygenase pathway produces a compound known as HETE (Nugteren, 1975) which has recently been shown to induce leukocyte chemotaxis (Turner et al., 1975; see Chapter 13). It should also be remembered that platelets normally contain all the 5HT circulating in the blood, and that since this is readily released when platelets are stimulated it could have a profound effect on vascular permeability. Rabbit platelets also contain and readily release relatively large amounts of histamine, although this is almost absent in the platelets of most other species.

Blood platelets from at least some animal species contain bactericidal proteins in their lysosomal granules – the bactericidal component of rabbit serum, active against gram positive organisms ('β-lysin'), which was first recognised last century is one such factor (Hirsch, 1960; Weksler and Nachman, 1971). This bactericidal protein is released when platelets are stimulated (e.g., by collagen or thrombin) and no plasma or serum cofactors are needed to produce its antibacterial reaction.

It is not certain yet whether human platelets also contain antibacterial activity (Clawson and White, 1970; Weksler and Nachman, 1971).

From the evidence cited above we can conclude that platelets have the capacity to cause a rapid increase in vascular permeability both directly (by virtue of their own constituents) and indirectly (e.g., by stimulating the release of histamine from mast cells). Also, by inducing leukocyte chemotaxis they can promote a further increase in vascular permeability, and ensure a concentration of bactericidal activity (from both platelets and neutrophils) at the site of tissue damage. The extent to which platelets participate in the early stages of the inflammatory response remains to be determined, but their potential contribution cannot be ignored. Platelets may also be involved in the destruction of connective tissue, which is a characteristic feature of many forms of chronic inflammatory disease, but since this more properly belongs in the realms of pathology it will be discussed in Section 4.2.3.

4.2. Pathological processes

4.2.1. Thrombosis

Thrombosis is the pathological counterpart of haemostasis – or, to put it another way, thrombosis represents an overactivity of the haemostatic process. The central role of blood platelets in arterial thrombosis is undisputed, and Walsh, (1975) has suggested that platelet coagulant activities may also play an essential role in triggering venous thrombosis. When thrombosis is initiated by frank vascular trauma, the sequence of events is the same as for haemostatic plug formation – adhesion of platelets to exposed collagen; secretion of ADP, 5HT, calcium, fibrinogen and PF_4; prostaglandin synthesis; platelet aggregation; activation of Factor XI and exposure of PF_3, leading to fibrin formation and stabilisation of the aggregate. Collagen is also exposed at ulcerations or fissures in atherosclerotic plaques, with the same consequences.

The role of platelets in thrombosis is not as simple as that outlined above, however, for in many cases thrombi form in the absence of gross vascular damage. In these situations thrombogenesis may be initiated by platelets interacting with endothelial cells, or forming aggregates without any vascular contact. There has been (and still is) considerable debate about the possible nature of platelet and endothelial changes which promote thrombogenesis, but regardless of any other factors involved, it seems clear that the pattern of blood flow plays a large part in determining the location and the ultimate size of thrombi: those which form at vessel branches or bifurcations where the blood flow is disturbed usually grow to cover more of the vessel lumen than thrombi in straight vessels where the flow is laminar, and thrombus formation is more frequent in areas of disturbed flow (see Chapter 2).

The pathological consequences of thrombosis are serious: the thrombus may grow to occlude the blood vessel, or parts of the thrombus may break off and embolise to occlude smaller vessels downstream from the original site. In either case, the tissue supplied is deprived of its oxygen supply unless there is a collateral circulation available, and if the tissue in question is the brain or myocardium the consequences are often fatal. Vascular occlusion is a major cause of morbidity and mortality, and it is only right that there should be an increasing research interest in thrombogenesis.

4.2.2. Atherosclerosis

Atherosclerosis is a process characterised by localised lesions of the arterial intima. These lesions consist of plaques containing variable amounts of fibrous tissue and lipid, which result in focal thickening of the intima with a consequent narrowing of the vascular lumen. Atherogenesis seems to involve localised increases in the permeability of the endothelial lining, resulting in an accumulation of plasma constituents (notably lipids) in the inner layers of the arterial wall and a proliferation of the smooth muscle cells at that point, with concomitant increased synthesis of connective tissue proteins by these cells. The role of blood platelets in atherosclerosis has not yet been unequivocably established, but there is increasing evidence that platelets can participate in three main ways:

1. By forming mural thrombi which become covered by endothelium and thus incorporated into the arterial wall.
2. By releasing constituents which injure the endothelial cells (thus increasing the permeability of the endothelial lining) and stimulate the vascular smooth muscle cells to proliferate and synthesise more connective tissue proteins.
3. By forming thrombi on pre-existing atherosclerotic lesions and thus contributing to the morbidity and mortality associated with advanced atherosclerotic disease.

When a mural thrombus persists, the endothelial cells surrounding it eventually grow over the top and the thrombus becomes incorporated into the intimal layer of the arterial wall. The thrombotic material apparently stimulates the proliferation of arterial smooth muscle cells and in due course the organised thrombus comes to resemble the intimal thickenings known as atherosclerotic plaques. Schwartz and his coworkers (Craig et al., 1973) have shown that although the histological resemblance between these two types of intimal thickening is close, the lipid composition of thickenings derived from organised thrombi is clearly different from that of atherosclerotic plaques occurring 'spontaneously', or produced experimentally by feeding a lipid-rich diet to laboratory animals. It therefore appears that although the incorporation of thrombi into an arterial wall (with subsequent intimal thickening) can certainly occur, it is apparently an infrequent event; consequently, the contribution made by blood platelets to atherosclerosis through this mechanism is limited. Of much greater pathological importance, however, is the effect of platelet constituents on the cells of the arterial wall.

The orifices and bifurcations of blood vessels are sites of predilection for the development of atherosclerotic lesions (Murphy et al., 1962; Caro et al., 1971), apparently because the blood flow is disturbed at these points. This disturbance of blood flow can also lead to the formation of small platelet aggregates and the release of platelet constituents in close proximity to the endothelium (Goldsmith, 1972; Jorgensen et al., 1972). Endothelial injury could be caused by 5HT released from the platelet dense bodies – Constantinides and Robinson (1969) showed that infusion of 5HT induces endothelial contraction – and constituents released from the platelet alpha granules can also increase vascular permeability (Packham et al., 1968; Nachman et al., 1972). Other constituents released from platelets (e.g., ADP, ATP and prostaglandins) may also affect endothelial cells, but this has not yet been investigated.

Such changes in the vascular endothelium not only facilitate entry of plasma proteins into the arterial wall but also make it easier for platelet constituents themselves to diffuse into the inner layers. This will result in the smooth muscle cells of the arterial media being exposed to two potent proliferative stimuli – a factor from platelets and a low density lipoprotein fraction of plasma – the effects of which are additive (Ross and Glomset, 1973; Ross et al., 1974; see Chapter 15). Localised proliferation of smooth muscle cells is a characteristic feature of the atherosclerotic plaque.

In conclusion, evidence at present available indicates that local endothelial injury plays an important part in the genesis of the atherosclerotic lesion, and that the subsequent development of the lesion involves the arterial smooth muscle cells. Since platelets are now known to have specific and potent effects on both these cell types, the contribution of platelets to atherogenesis appears to be much greater than was generally accepted a decade ago.

4.2.3. Inflammation

In Section 3.1.4, the potential role of the blood platelet in the inflammatory process was discussed, with respect to those aspects of inflammation which could, broadly speaking, be considered beneficial to the body as a whole. When this aspect of platelet function is considered, one point which emerges is the close similarity between the blood platelet and the polymorphonuclear leukocyte. Although platelets can be justifiably regarded as the specialised haemostatic cells while leukocytes are cells primarily designed to deal with infection and injury, both cell types accumulate at sites of tissue injury and they are also alike in many of their constituents and reactions. Both can apparently release constituents which are chemotactic and bactericidal as well as others which are capable of degranulating mast cells and directly increasing vascular permeability. The similarity may also extend to the pathological aspect of the inflammatory process related to the destruction of connective tissue: neutrophils contain and release several lysosomal enzymes capable of degrading elastin, proteoglycan and collagen; and platelets contain lysosomal glycosidases (Gordon, 1975), cathepsins (Chapter 14), and also possibly elastase and collagenase (Robert et al., 1970; Chesney et al., 1974). Before concluding that blood platelets could play an important part in the degradation of connective tissue, however, the following points should be considered.

First, the amount of the enzymes contained in platelets and readily released must be calculated, in order to determine how many platelets would need to accumulate at a site of injury to provide a biologically significant amount of enzyme activity; secondly, before embarking on such a calculation it is important to take account of the numbers of contaminating leukocytes (and their enzyme content) in the preparations from which 'platelet' proteinase activities were extracted; and finally, even if platelets do secrete significant amounts of degradative enzymes, their biological effects will depend on the amount of proteinase inhibitors present.

Studies in our own laboratory and others have established that platelets contain and release numerous glycosidases (for review, see Gordon, 1975) and we have also characterised the acid proteinases present in human and rabbit platelets, but we were unable to detect significant amounts of elastase or collagenase in human platelet preparations from which leucocytes were rigorously excluded (Chapter 14). In addition, recent work has shown that human platelets contain inhibitors which affect trypsin and other neutral proteolytic enzymes (A.J. Barrett, H.P. Ehrlich and J.L. Gordon, unpublished). Therefore, although we would support the view expressed in several recent reviews (Weksler and Nachman, 1973; Zucker, 1974; Silver et al., 1974) that the potential role of blood platelets in the inflammatory process ought to be investigated more fully, the biological importance of neutral proteinases from platelets seems open to question.

4.2.4. Transplant rejection

Rejection of a transplanted organ is associated with occlusion of blood vessels and extensive damage to the vascular walls. Platelet aggregates are largely responsible for this vascular occlusion and may also contribute to the vascular damage. The formation of antigen–antibody complexes precedes the rejection of an organ transplant, and immune complexes interact with platelets and induce the release reaction (Packham et al., 1968; Pfueller and Lüscher, 1972). Haft and his colleagues (1972) found that when small blood vessels were occluded by platelet aggregates showing morphological signs of degranulation then there was vascular damage, whereas the endothelium remained intact in vessels containing platelets that had not degranulated. When platelets are pretreated to deplete their granules of 5HT the extent of vascular injury in response to intravascular immune complex formation is reduced (Kniker and Cochrane, 1968) and treatment with drugs which inhibit platelet aggregation and the release reaction prolongs the survival time of transplanted organs (Kincaid-Smith, 1975; Mowbray, 1975).

Since there is little doubt that platelets play an important role in the clinical complications of transplant rejection, the possibility of treating patients routinely in the immediate post-transplant period with agents which interfere with adhesion, aggregation, or the platelet release reaction ought to be seriously considered. The selection of anti-platelet agents for long-term clinical trials as prophylactics against thrombosis has been dictated largely by considerations of drug safety and lack of toxicity; however, since treatment of patients undergoing organ transplantation is relatively short-term, and a higher degree of anti-platelet activity than in long-term thrombosis trials would be desirable, a critical evaluation of the newer, more potent inhibitors of platelet aggregation for use in this situation would seem to be indicated.

4. Conclusions

In this chapter we have reviewed the evidence implicating blood platelets in a wide range of biological processes. The role of the platelet in thrombosis and haemostasis is accepted without question, and the fundamental platelet reactions of adhesion, aggregation and secretion are primarily responsible. As we have discussed, however, the same reactions may be involved in other processes such as atherosclerosis, inflammation, wound healing, and transplant rejection. This alone would justify the description 'multifunctional cell', but more important than this is the spectrum of cellular reactions which the platelet exhibits and which can be readily studied: platelets are well suited for investigations of membrane recognition sites, intracellular control processes, active transport, and cell–cell interactions (to give but a few examples). If some of the findings summarised in the preceding pages are instrumental in stimulating research with platelets in these or in allied fields, then the main purpose of this chapter – and, indeed, of this volume, will have been fulfilled.

Acknowledgement

We thank the Arthritis and Rheumatism Council for financial support during the preparation of this review.

References

Aalto, M. and Kulonen, E. (1972) Biochem. Pharmacol., 21, 2835.
Aken, W.G. Van and Vreeken, J. (1969) Thromb. Diath. Haemorrh., 22, 496.
Becker, A.J., McCullogh, E.A. and Till, J.E. (1963) Nature, 197, 452.
Behnke, O. (1967) Anat. Rev., 158, 121.
Behnke, O. (1969) J. Ultrastruct. Res., 26, 111.
Bouillin, D.J. and Green, A.R. (1972) Br. J. Pharmac., 45, 83.
Bouillin, D.J. and O'Brien, R.A. (1970) Br. J. Pharmac., 39, 779.
Bouillin, D.J. and O'Brien, R.A. (1971) J. Physiol., 212, 287.
Bouillin, D.J., Ahtee, L., Airaksinen, E. and Paasonen, M.K. (1973) The Pharmacologist, 15, 166.
Buckmaster, G.A. (1906) Sci. Progress, 1, 73.
Caro, C.G., Fitz-Gerald, J.M. and Schroter, R.C. (1971) Proc. Roy. Soc. Lond. (B), 177, 109.
Chesney, C.M., Harper, E. and Colman R.W. (1974) J. Clin. Invest., 53, 1647.
Clawson, C.C. and White, J.G. (1970) Blood, 36, 843.
Cohen, I. and de Vries, A. (1973) Nature, 246, 36.
Constantinides, P. and Robinson, M. (1969) Arch. Path., 88, 108.

Cotran, R.S. (1965) Am. J. Path., *46*, 589.
Craig, I.H., Bell, F.P., Goldsmith, C.H. and Schwartz, C.J. (1973) Atherosclerosis, *18*, 277.
Day, H.J., Holmsen, H. and Hovig, T. (1969) Scand. J. Haemat., Suppl. 7.
Day, H.J. and Solum, N.O. (1973) Scand. J. Haematol., *10*, 136.
Donald, K.J. and Tennent, R.J. (1975) J. Path., *117*, 235.
Gimbrone, M.A., Aster, R.H., Cotran, R.S., Corkery, J., Jandl, J.H. and Folkman, J. (1969) Nature, *222*, 33.
Goldsmith, H.L. (1972) in Progress in Haemostasis and Thrombosis (Spaet, T.H., ed.), Vol. 1, p. 97, Grune and Stratton, New York.
Gordon, J.L. (1975) in Lysosomes in Biology and Pathology (Dingle, J.T. and Dean, R.T., eds), Vol. 4, p. 3. North-Holland, Amsterdam.
Greenberg, J., Packham, M.A., Cazenave, J.-P., Reimers, H.-J. and Mustard, J.F. (1975) Lab. Invest., *32*, 476.
Haft, J.I., Kranz, P.D., Albert, F.J., and Fani, K. (1972) Circulation, *46*, 698.
Hamberg, M., Svensson, J. and Samuelsson, B., (1975) Proc. Natl. Acad. Sci. U.S.A., *72*, 2994.
Harker, L.A. and Finch, C.A. (1969) J. Clin. Invest., *48*, 963.
Hirsch, J.G. (1960) J. Exp. Med., *112*, 15.
Hovig, T. (1974) in Platelets: production, function, transfusion and storage (Baldini, M.G. and Ebbe, S. eds), p. 221, Grune and Stratton, London.
Ingram, M. and Coopersmith, A. (1969) Brit. J. Haematol., *17*, 225.
Johnson, S.A. (1971) in The circulating platelet (Johnson, S.A., ed) p. 284. Academic Press, New York.
Jørgensen, L., Packham, M.A., Rowsell, H.C., and Mustard, J.F. (1972) Lab. Invest., *27*, 341.
Kincaid-Smith, P. (1975) in Platelets, drugs and thrombosis (Hirsh, J., Cade, J.F., Gallus, A.S. and Schonbaum, E., eds), p. 301, Karger, Basel.
Kniker, W.T. and Cochrane, C.G. (1968) J. Exp. Med., *127*, 119.
Kubisz, P. and Caen, J. (1972) Path. Biol., *20*, 34.
MacPherson, G.G. (1972) J. Cell Sci., *10*, 705.
Marcus, A.J., Zucker-Franklin, D., Safier, L.B. and Ullman, H.L. (1966) J. Clin. Invest., *45*, 14.
Mills, D.C.B., Robb, I.A. and Roberts, G.C.K. (1968) J. Physiol., *195*, 715.
Moore, S., Pepper, D.S. and Cash, J.D. (1975) Biochim. Biophys. Acta, *379*, 370.
Mowbray, J.F. (1975) in Platelets, drugs and thrombosis (Hirsh, J., Cade, J.F., Gallus, A.S. and Schonbaum, E., eds), p. 200. Karger, Basel.
Murphy, E.A., Rowsell, H.C., Downie, H.G., Robinson G.A. and Mustard J.F. (1962) Canad. Med. Assoc. J., *87*, 259.
Mustard, J.F., Movat, H.Z., MacMorine, D.R.L. and Senyi, A. (1965) Proc. Soc. Exp. Biol. Med., *119*, 988.
Mustard, J.F. and Packham, M.A. (1968) Ser. Haematol., *2*, 168.
Nachman, R.L., Weksler, B. and Ferris, B. (1972) J. Clin. Invest., *51*, 549.
Nugteren, D.H. (1975) Biochim. Biophys. Acta, *380*, 299.
Packham, M.A., Nishizawa, E.E., and Mustard, J.F. (1968) Biochem. Pharmacol. Suppl. *17*, 171.
Pfueller, S.L. and Lüscher, E.F. (1972) Immunochemistry, *9*, 1151.
Pletscher, A., Da Prada, M., Berneis, K.H. and Tranzer, J.P. (1971) Experientia, *27*, 993.
Rafelson, M.E., Noveke, T.P. and Booyse, F.M. (1973) Ser. Haemat. VI, *3*, 351.
Robert, B., Szigeti, M., Robert, L., Legrand, Y., Pignaud, G. and Caen, J. (1970) Nature, *227*, 1248.
Ross, R. and Glomset, J.A. (1973) Science, *180*, 1332.
Ross, R., Glomset, J., Kariya, B., and Harker, L. (1974) Proc. Natl. Acad. Sci., U.S.A., *71*, 1207.
Silver, M.D. and Gardner, H.A. (1968) J. Ultrastruct. Res., *23*, 366.
Silver, M.J., Smith, J.B. and Ingerman, C.M. (1974) Agents and Actions, *4*, 233.
Simpson, D.M. and Ross, R. (1972) J. Clin. Invest., *51*, 2009.
Smith, J.B., Ingerman, C., Kocsis, J.J. and Silver, M.J. (1973) J. Clin. Invest., *52*, 965.
Tocantins, L.M. (1938) Medicine, *17*, 155.
Turner, S.R., Tainer, J.A. and Lynn, W.S. (1975) Nature, *257*, 680.
Vegge, T., Mann, E. and Hjort, P.F. (1968) Thrombos. Diath, Haemorrh., *20*, 354.
Walsh, P.N. (1974) Blood, *43*, 597.
Walsh, P.N. (1975) Thrombos. Diathes. Haemorrh., *33*, 435.
Weksler, B.B. and Coupal C.D. (1973) J. Exp. Med., *137*, 1419.
Weksler, B.B. (1974) in Platelets: production, function, transfusion and storage (Baldini, M.G. and Ebbe, S., eds) p. 277. Grune and Stratton, New York.
Weksler, B.B. and Nachman, R.L. (1971) J. Exp. Med., *134*, 1114.
White, J.G. (1968) Am. J. Path., *58*, 31.

White, J.G. (1971) in The Platelet, p. 83, Williams and Wilkins, Baltimore.
White, J.G. (1972) Am. J. Path., 69, 439.
Willis, A.L. and Kuhn, D.C. (1973) Prostaglandins, 4, 127.
Young, R.W. (1973) J. Cell Biol., 57, 175.
Zir, L.M., Carvalho, A.C., Harthorne, J.W., Colman, R.W. and Lees, R.S. (1974) New Engl. J. Med., 291, 134.
Zucker, M.B. (1974) in The Inflammatory Process (Zweifach, B.W., Grant, L. and McCluskey, R.T., eds) 2nd edn, Vol. I, p. 511.

Note added in proof

Another platelet organelle has recently been described by Bentfield and Bainton (1975), but until this is more fully characterised we shall include it in the general term 'alpha granules', recognising that this represents a heterogeneous population of organelles.

CHAPTER 2

Adhesion and aggregation: morphological demonstration and quantitation in vivo and in vitro

H.R. BAUMGARTNER and R. MUGGLI

Department of Experimental Medicine, F. Hoffmann-La Roche & Co.,
CH-4002 Basle, Switzerland

1. Introduction

Bizzozero and Hayem independently observed for the first time in 1882 that small formed elements of the circulating blood adhere to a damaged vessel wall and subsequently to each other, building up a mural thrombus or a hemostatic plug. This was the discovery of the blood platelet and its basic functions. Bounameaux (1959) and Hugues (1960), by directly investigating the hemostatic process in mesenteric blood vessels with the light microscope, realized that platelets primarily adhere to subendothelial connective tissue. Their finding was confirmed by later electron microscopic observations: platelets were shown to fill the gaps between endothelial cells (Majno and Palade, 1961, Tranzer and Baumgartner, 1968, Fig. 1) and to form a continuous 'platelet carpet' at sites of endothelial denudation (Kjaerheim and Hovig, 1962, French et al., 1964, Baumgartner et al., 1967). Several structural components of the subendothelial tissue were considered as reactive substrates for platelet adhesion. These included collagen fibrils (Hugues, 1960, Kjaerheim and Hovig, 1962), elastin (Hugues, 1960, French et al., 1964), fine fibrillar elements (French et al., 1964), basement membrane (Baumgartner et al., 1967, Tranzer and Baumgartner, 1968) and microfibrils of elastin (Stemerman et al., 1971). Of these structural connective tissue components only fibrillar collagen was found to induce platelet aggregation in vitro (Zucker and Borelli, 1962, Hovig, 1963). In vivo platelet adhesion to subendothelium is usually followed by platelet–platelet cohesion leading to the formation of mural platelet thrombi or hemostatic plugs. Electron microscopy revealed that this process is accompanied by the disappearance of α-granules and serotonin storage organelles (Kjaerheim and Hovig, 1962). Extensive studies in vitro demonstrated that the morphologic phenomenon of degranulation corresponds to the 'platelet release reaction' (Grette, 1962, Holmsen et al., 1969), a phenomenon which will be covered in detail elsewhere in this volume.

In order to investigate the kinetics of platelet adhesion and aggregation and to define the relative importance of physiologic factors which influence these

Gordon (ed) Platelets in Biology and Pathology
© *Elsevier/North-Holland Biomedical Press, 1976*

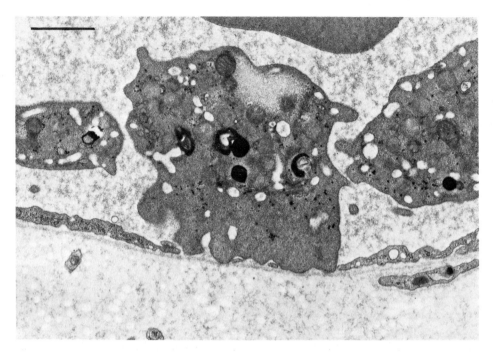

Fig. 1. A platelet fills the gap between two endothelial cells and is seen in close association with the endothelial basement membrane. The platelet cytoplasm close to the site of adhesion appears devoid of subcellular organelles. Profiles of two additional platelets and an erythrocyte are seen in the lumen of the capillary. In this and the following electron micrographs the black bar indicates 1 μm.

reactions, qualitative morphology was insufficient. Turbidimetric measurement of platelet aggregation in stirred platelet suspensions, which was introduced by Born in 1962, soon became the most widely used method for the study of platelet aggregation induced by different agents and yielded important new information about this reaction. However, platelet 'aggregometry' yields only indirect information about adhesion. In addition, the possible effects of blood flow, the presence of other blood cells, and other factors operating in vivo are not taken into account in this artificial system. Therefore, systems have been devised which allow the exposure of artificial surfaces (Friedman et al., 1970) and natural vascular surfaces (Baumgartner and Haudenschild, 1972, Baumgartner, 1973) to blood in a controlled fluid dynamic environment, and the measurement of platelet adhesion by direct morphometric techniques. In such systems, platelet–surface adhesion and aggregation can be reproduced in vitro using appropriate blood flow conditions. The discussion below is mainly based on quantitative morphology of platelet–surface interaction and subsequent platelet–platelet interaction in in vivo and in vitro systems with controlled blood flow.

2. Morphometric quantitation of platelet–surface and platelet–platelet interactions

A number of techniques have been described for assessing the amount of platelet material adhering to a surface after exposure to blood or platelet-rich plasma. Either (1) the drop in platelet count after exposure of the surface is recorded (Hellem, 1960, Salzman, 1963, Stormorken et al., 1965, Mason et al., 1974, and others), (2) the amount of radioactivity associated with the surface after its exposure to labelled platelets is equated with the mass of adhering platelets (Hirsh et al., 1968, Hovig et al., 1968, Cazenave et al., 1973, Lagergren et al., 1974) or (3) the surface under investigation is evaluated by direct microscopic examination.

While the first two methods lead rapidly to an estimate of the average mass of platelets deposited per unit area, only the third can also provide information on the three-dimensional distribution of platelets on the surface; that is, on the type and extent of platelet–surface and platelet–platelet interactions.

2.1. Evaluation from 'en face' preparations

This method has the advantage of being technically simple, and large surfaces can be scanned easily (Breddin, 1964, D.J. Lyman et al., 1970, B. Lyman et al., 1971, Friedman and Leonard, 1971, Mason and Gilkey, 1971, George, 1972). One disadvantage, however, is that for transmission light microscopy the surface under investigation must be translucent. Surface coverage with platelets is evaluated with the aid of an eyepiece net micrometer and expressed as the number of platelets per unit area or percent surface covered with platelets. Precise quantitation of platelet–platelet interaction is difficult with this technique.

2.2. Evaluation from cross-sections

The additional labor involved in embedding and sectioning the specimens is offset by the additional information which can be obtained: for example, cross-sections can reveal multiple layering of platelets, and give information on how intimate the interaction between a surface and a platelet is. However, conventional paraffin embedding and sectioning is inadequate for this, but sufficient resolution is obtained when approximately 0.8 μm thick Epon sections are stained with toluidine blue and basic fuchsin (Haudenschild and Studer, 1972) and viewed through a Zeiss microscope (Planapochromat 100/1.30, oil). The percent surface covered with platelets can then be determined with an eyepiece micrometer (Baumgartner and Haudenschild, 1972) (Fig. 2).

The determination of platelet interactions in semithin sections leads to a systematic error due to the thickness of the section: when the ratio of section thickness to structural dimension is finite, the surface occupied by the opaque structures (in our case, the platelets), is overestimated (Weibel, 1969), but with increasing surface coverage this error is progressively reduced due to overlapping

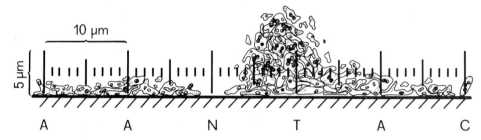

Fig. 2. Morphometric evaluation of platelet–surface and platelet–platelet interactions from cross-section. The surface fraction covered with platelets is determined at a total magnification of ×1000 by shifting the calibrated scale of a 10:100 eyepiece micrometer parallel to the surface. The intersection points of the surface profile with the principal bars of the micrometer scale at 10 μm intervals are evaluated according to the classification: naked (N), contact (C), 'adhesion' (A) and thrombi (T).

of the structures. The extent of overestimation is greatest at about 50% surface coverage, and although for comparative purposes the apparent surface coverage from cross-section is adequate, in some cases it may have to be corrected for overestimation due to section thickness. True surface coverage of 50% is overestimated by about 15% when the cross-section thickness is 0.8 μm and the average platelet diameter is 2 μm (Turitto and Baumgartner, 1975a).

2.3. Classification of platelet adhesion and aggregation as revealed in cross-sections

The percent surface covered with platelets incompletely characterizes platelet–surface interaction. A more detailed description is obtained by subdividing platelet–surface interaction into classes. Apart from making loose contacts, platelets have the capability of subsequently interacting more intimately with certain surfaces, by extruding pseudopods and spreading out, thus increasing the area of contact between their membranes and the underlying substrate. This shape-change provides a basis for classifying platelet–surface interaction according to platelet shape. As platelets also interact with each other, leading to multiple layering, the height of platelet accumulations provides a further basis for subdivision. The following classification proved valuable in the description of platelet–surface interaction and will be used throughout this chapter. Surface coverage with a specific class of platelet–surface interaction is expressed as a percentage of the total surface examined.

Symbol	Definition
Primary quantities	
N	Surface devoid of platelets (naked).
C	Surface covered with platelets which are not spread out (contact).

A	Surface covered with platelets which are spread out and whose multiple layering does not exceed 5 μm in height ('adhesion').
T	Surface covered with aggregates of more than 5 μm in height (thrombi).

Secondary quantities

$S = A + T$	Surface covered with platelets which are spread out (spread).
$C + A + T$	Surface covered with platelets.
$\dfrac{100\,T}{S}$	Percentage of spread platelets covered with platelet aggregates of more than 5 μm in height.
$\dfrac{100\,C}{C + S}$	Percentage of contact platelets on the surface.

3. Morphologic sequence of platelet interaction with subendothelium in vivo

3.1. Experimental techniques for the removal of endothelium

Many experimental procedures have been described for inducing desquamation of vascular endothelium and subsequent platelet accumulation in vivo. These include mechanical, chemical and thermal injuries. The most interesting and widely used techniques are ballooning of arteries (Baumgartner and Studer, 1966, Baumgartner et al., 1971, Stemerman and Ross, 1972, Nam et al., 1973), brief air drying (Fishman et al., 1975), homocystine infusion (Harker et al., 1974), focal thermal injury by a laser beam (Arfors et al., 1968) or electrically-induced damage (Reber, 1966). Thermal injuries are not suitable for the study of platelet interaction with subendothelium since burned red and endothelial cells are the main site of platelet adhesion and subendothelium is usually not exposed (Hovig et al., 1974). Homocystine infusion causes patchy desquamation of endothelium and, in addition, the time of endothelial detachment is undetermined. Only ballooning or air drying allows the removal of the entire endothelium from a defined area and the establishment of a proper baseline for kinetic studies in vivo.

3.2. Platelet adhesion to subendothelium and loss of platelet organelles

In rabbits (Baumgartner, 1963, Baumgartner and Studer, 1966, Baumgartner and Spaet, 1970), monkeys (Stemerman and Ross, 1972) and swine (Nam et al., 1973) the subendothelial surface is covered with platelets within minutes after removal of the endothelium with a balloon catheter (Fig. 3). In specimens fixed by perfusion with buffered glutaraldehyde approximately 30 sec after removal of

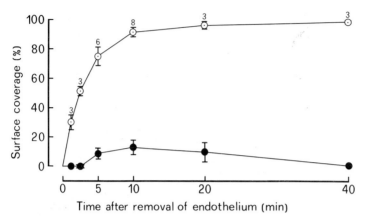

Fig. 3. Platelet adhesion and aggregation on the subendothelial surface of rabbit iliac artery in vivo. Surface coverage with platelets (○–○) and platelet thrombi (●–●) at different time intervals after the removal of the endothelial lining by means of a balloon catheter. Similar results were observed on aortic subendothelium of the same rabbits (Baumgartner, 1973). Means ± S.E.

endothelium a few single platelets are seen at the surface. Most of these platelets have changed their shape and are apparently attached at the surface through some of their pseudopods. They still contain their subcellular organelles. Surface coverage then rapidly increases (Fig. 3). The platelets spread out on the surface and partially overlap each other. By 10 min they form a virtually complete carpet (Baumgartner, 1973), a 'pseudoendothelium' (Fig. 4a). The platelets associated with the subendothelial surface have lost approximately 70% of their α-granules and serotonin storage organelles as revealed by quantitative electron microscopy (Table 1). However, their plasma membrane appears intact and the number of mitochondria per platelet profile is unchanged. At 40 min the platelets associated with the subendothelium are even more spread out (Fig. 4b) than at 10 min and have lost 97% of their α-granules and 81% of their serotonin storage organelles. These platelets form a very thin monolayer which is apparently 'unattractive' to circulating platelets and is barely visible with the light microscope.

3.3. Platelet aggregation

Formation of platelet thrombi (i.e., aggregates of more than 5 μm in height) on the subendothelial surface after removal of the endothelium from an iliac artery of rabbits is a transient process (Fig. 3). Platelet cohesion is already apparent in specimens fixed 1.25 min after ballooning. The platelets at the base of mural platelet thrombi have usually lost their α-granules and serotonin storage organelles, whereas many of the platelets which form the platelet mass (aggregate) still contain most of their organelles (Fig. 5). By 40 min after removal of the endothelium virtually all the platelet thrombi have disappeared (Fig. 3) leaving only a thin monolayer of platelets behind. The observation that platelets associated with the subendothelial surface progressively lose their granules (Table 1)

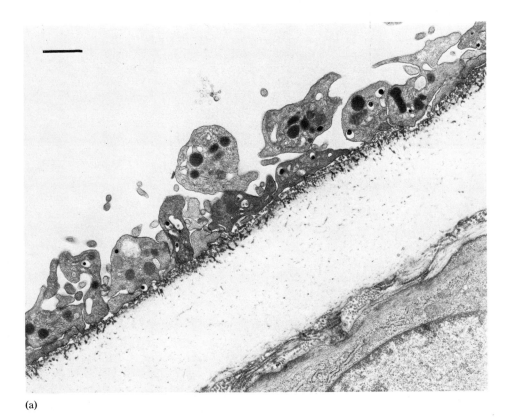

(a)

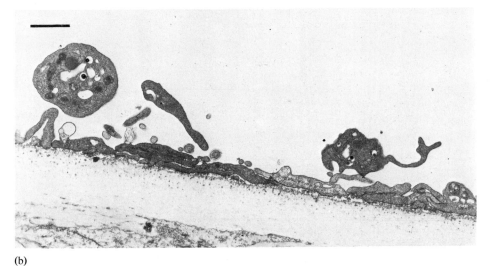

(b)

Fig. 4. Electron micrographs of platelets adhering at the subendothelial surface of rabbit aorta in vivo. (a): Ten minutes after removal of the endothelium. Platelets are spread out and form a continuous 'carpet'. They still contain some of their α-granules and serotonin storage organelles. (b): Forty minutes after removal of the endothelium. Platelets at the subendothelial surface are even more spread out and have lost virtually all their α-granules.

TABLE 1
Disappearance of subcellular organelles from rabbit platelets adherent to subendothelium in vivo and in vitro as revealed by quantitative electron microscopy

Exposure	Number of organelles counted	Distribution (%)			Disappearance (%)*	
		Mitochondria	α-Granules	Serotonin storage organelles	α-Granules	Serotonin storage organelles
10 min in vivo	1183	36.8	39.3	23.9	79	64
40 min in vivo	268	66.0	10.8	23.2	97	81
10 min in vitro	539	65.2	25.8	9.0	92	92
40 min in vitro	290	86.2	10.4	3.4	98	98
Isolated platelets	2467	12.5	65.0	22.5	–	–

* The number of α-granules and serotonin storage organelles per mitochondrion in isolated platelets was set as 100%.

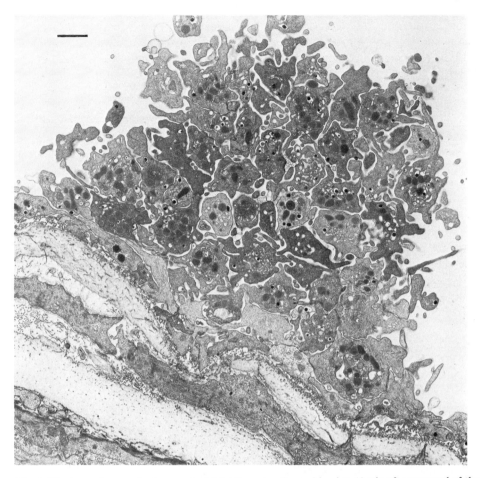

Fig. 5. Electron micrograph of a mural platelet thrombus formed in vivo 10 min after removal of the endothelium from an iliac artery in a rabbit. The platelets close to the subendothelial surface contain their mitochondria but have lost most of their α-granules and serotonin storage organelles. The more peripheral platelets still contain most of these granules.

and that the resulting monolayer of degranulated platelets appears non-thrombogenic indicates that thrombi usually do not break off at the subendothelial surface itself but one or more platelet layers away from it. This concept is supported by the results of in vitro studies which showed that platelet thrombus formation is more easily reversible than platelet adhesion at a surface (Baumgartner et al., 1976). The formation and fate of mural thrombi have been directly observed in arterioles or venules by light microscopy (Honour and Russell, 1962, Reber, 1966, Arfors et al., 1968, and others). Frequently, the platelet thrombus breaks off and can be seen as a 'white body' being carried downstream by the flowing blood. The platelets of these 'white bodies' may disaggregate in the bloodstream without causing any harm, but in some cases they can cause vascular damage and occlude vessels of the microvasculature. Myocardial infarction, stroke and nephrosclerosis are among the severe consequences which can follow multiple embolization from mural platelet thrombi (for review see Mustard et al., 1974).

3.4. Long-term consequences of endothelial desquamation

In vivo, the initial adhesion and accumulation of platelets is followed by adhesion of neutrophils and monocytes to the degranulated platelets. Within days after removal of endothelium the smooth muscle cells of the inner media proliferate and migrate through the fenestrations of the internal elastic lamina to the luminal side of this membrane where they continue to proliferate for approximately 4 weeks (Baumgartner, 1975). These processes of smooth muscle cell proliferation and migration lead to a marked intimal thickening, and the possible relationship between platelet adhesion and smooth muscle cell proliferation is discussed elsewhere in this volume. Concomitantly with smooth muscle cell proliferation, new endothelium grows in from branches of the denuded artery. What eventually inhibits the proliferative process, and which cells finally form the new endothelium, are important but still unanswered questions (Spaet et al., 1975).

4. Reproduction in vitro of platelet reactions observed in vivo: a perfusion system

4.1. Original annular perfusion chamber and standard perfusion conditions

Associated with the perfusion in situ of isolated vessel segments denuded of endothelium were technical problems such as leakage of the perfusate and changes in the lumen diameter caused by spontaneous contraction or dilation. These caused considerable variability in the results (Baumgartner et al., 1971, Stemerman et al., 1971), and therefore, an annular perfusion chamber was constructed (Baumgartner, 1973) in which everted vessel segments or other surfaces positioned on a central rod (Fig. 6) could be exposed to flowing blood. Leakage is avoided by the rod which supports the exposed surface, and the annular space – corresponding to the vessel lumen – between surface and outer cylinder of the chamber remains constant. Thus, rheologic parameters such as average flow velocity and wall shear rate can be calculated fairly accurately from the flow rate of the perfusate and the dimensions of the chamber. The physical parameters of the original annular chamber which was used for most of the studies described in this paper are shown in Table 2. Turitto (1975) has analysed the flow parameters of this chamber by measuring the dissolution rates of benzoic acid in water.

In this perfusion system the perfusate (for example, anticoagulated blood) is

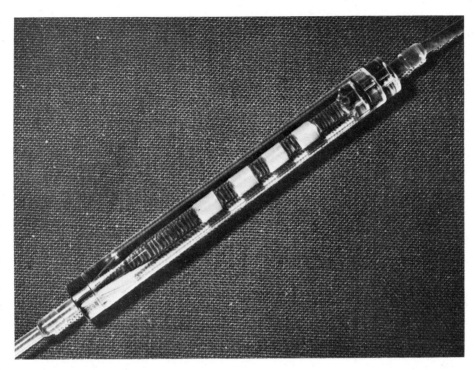

Fig. 6. Photograph of the original annular perfusion chamber with four segments of everted rabbit aorta mounted on the rod. See text for further explanations.

TABLE 2
Dimensions and physical parameters of the original and a modified annular perfusion chamber at three blood flow rates

Flow rate ml/min	Effective annular width*	Average flow velocity mm/sec	Reynolds number	Vessel wall shear stress dynes/cm²
Original chamber	1.2 mm			
10		9	6.1	1.8
40		36	24.5	7.2
160		144	97.5	28.8
Small chamber	0.35 mm			
10		37.5	6.9	32.9
40		150	27.8	131
160		600	111.2	526

* The nominal annular width of the chambers were 1.3 and 0.45 mm respectively (effective annular width plus thickness of aortic wall). The other dimensions are identical for the two chambers: 3.5 mm rod diameter, 75 mm chamber length.

circulated from a reservoir into the annular chamber (prefilled with phosphate buffered saline) and back into the reservoir by a roller pump. Chamber, reservoir and buffer are all immersed in a waterbath maintained at the desired temperature by an electronic controller. Standard conditions were: Perfusion with rabbit blood, anticoagulated with approximately 14 mM citrate in plasma, for 10 min at 37°C in the original perfusion chamber; for further parameters see Table 2. Whenever any of these conditions are varied for a specific experiment, this is stated explicitly.

4.2. *Platelet adhesion to subendothelium and subsequent platelet aggregation*

When the subendothelium of rabbit aorta was exposed to flowing blood under standard perfusion conditions, the kinetics of platelet interaction with the subendothelial surface (Fig. 7) were qualitatively and quantitatively similar to those observed in vivo (Fig. 3); the platelets attached to the surface, spread out on it and concomitantly lost most of their α-granules and serotonin storage organelles. The rate of disappearance of these subcellular organelles was somewhat more rapid in vitro than in vivo (Table 1), and more mural thrombi (Figs. 3, 5, 7 and 8) were observed in vitro than in vivo after 10 min exposure, but again the mural thrombi had virtually disappeared from the subendothelium after 40 min perfusion (Fig. 7), leaving a non-thrombogenic monolayer of spread and degranulated platelets behind.

To investigate further the concept that the platelet monolayer remaining at the subendothelial surface is unattractive for circulating platelets, specimens which had been exposed to circulating blood for 40 min were briefly rinsed in buffer and re-exposed to fresh citrated blood for 10 min. No thrombi developed on such

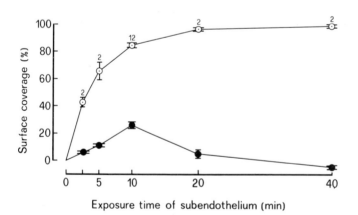

Fig. 7. Platelet adhesion and aggregation on the subendothelial surface of rabbit aorta in vitro. Time dependence of surface coverage with platelets (O–O) and platelet thrombi (●–●) after exposure to whole blood anticoagulated with citrate and perfused through the original perfusion chamber at a flow rate of 160 ml/min. Means ± S.E.

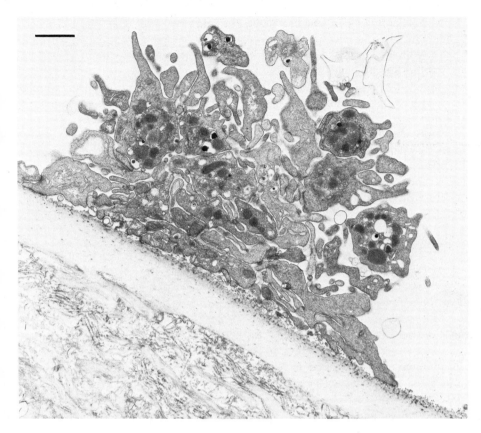

Fig. 8. Electron micrograph of a mural platelet thrombus produced on subendothelium in vitro by exposing it to anticoagulated blood in the original perfusion chamber under controlled flow conditions. As in vivo (Fig. 5), the platelets close to the surface have lost most of their α-granules and serotonin storage organelles, whereas those at the periphery still contain most of their granules.

specimens, whereas mural thrombi were always present on control specimens (untreated subendothelium) exposed to the same blood sample (Baumgartner, unpublished). It seems, therefore, that spread, degranulated platelets protect the subendothelial surface from further platelet deposition.

4.3. Modified annular perfusion chambers

The original annular perfusion chamber used in most of the studies summarized in this paper has several disadvantages. The blood volume which must be circulated through the chamber to obtain substantial platelet deposition is large (160 ml/min) and therefore recirculation of a blood sample is necessary unless substantial blood volumes are available. Prolonged recirculation of blood reduces the ability of platelets to form mural platelet thrombi, although their ability to adhere remains unchanged (Baumgartner, unpublished). In addition, the wall shear stresses obtained with the original chamber are relatively low (Table 2) when compared to the peak wall shear stresses of about 400 dynes/cm^2 which occur in vivo (Fry, 1968, Schmid-Schönbein et al., 1975).

An improved chamber (Turitto and Baumgartner, 1974a) with reduced annular width (Table 2) gave deposition rates at 10 ml/min similar to those obtained at 160 ml/min in the original chamber. This makes it possible to perfuse anticoagulated blood without recirculation, to draw native blood directly from a vessel through the chamber (Baumgartner et al., 1976), and to reproduce in vitro the peak wall shear stresses encountered in vivo. Furthermore, perfusion chambers with different characteristics facilitate the systematic study of the influence of flow parameters on platelet adhesion, and the comparison of rates of platelet deposition obtained experimentally with those predicted from mass transfer theory.

5. Factors affecting platelet adhesion and aggregation

Platelet adhesion to subendothelium is the earliest observable response of the blood to vascular injury and it is therefore not surprising that great efforts are being directed towards investigating the nature of platelet–surface adhesion. A better understanding of the factors involved will aid the prevention and treatment of thromboembolic disorders, as well as the development of blood-compatible materials for vascular prostheses.

The annular perfusion chamber offered us the opportunity to investigate variables such as rheologic factors, the presence of other blood cells, and changes in plasma constituents, surface properties, and platelet function which might influence platelet–surface interaction in flowing blood. These investigations are still continuing. To facilitate the discussion, adhesion and adhesion-induced aggregation will be considered separately, but the reader must keep in mind that apart from the obvious relation between adhesion, release, and aggregation, the presence of mural platelet thrombi can either inhibit platelet adhesion ('lee effect': see 5.1.6) or enhance it (translocation of platelets from thrombi: see 5.4.2).

5.1. Fluid dynamics

The rate at which platelets adhere to surfaces depends on physical variables which must be studied under controlled fluid dynamic conditions (Petschek and Weiss, 1970, Dutton et al., 1968, Friedman et al., 1970, Baumgartner, 1973). In such defined systems a number of investigators have been able to correlate rates of platelet deposition, predicted from theoretical equations for mass transport of molecular species, with those experimentally obtained on *artificial surfaces* (Grabowski et al., 1972, Turitto and Leonard, 1972, Turitto, 1975) and on *natural surfaces* (Turitto and Baumgartner, 1974a, 1975a and b).

For molecules in Newtonian fluids, flowing laminarly within an annulus, mass transport theory predicts that the diffusional flux (J) to the walls will be:

$$J = K_1 \left(\frac{V_{av}D^2}{d_e z} \right)^{1/3}. \tag{1}$$

where K_1 is dependent on the physical constants of the system and on the concentration of the molecular species, V_{av} is the average flow velocity, D is the diffusivity, d_e the effective diameter of the system and z is the axial distance (Turitto, 1975, Turitto and Baumgartner, 1975b).

By introducing the vessel wall shear rate γ_w, Eq. (1) can be transformed to:

$$J = K_2 \left(\frac{\gamma_w D^2}{z} \right)^{1/3} \tag{2}$$

where K_2 is a factor proportional to the concentration but independent of the physical dimensions of the system.

As a first approximation, these relations also hold for the diffusional flux of platelets; this can be equated to platelet deposition rate, provided that the reaction between platelets and surface is fast compared to the radial diffusion of platelets. That platelet deposition is a diffusion-controlled reaction is indicated by its strong dependence on flow and dimensional parameters both on *artificial surfaces* (Friedman et al., 1970, 1971) and on *natural surfaces* (Baumgartner, 1973, Turitto and Baumgartner, 1974a, 1975a).

The parameters of Eqs. (1) and (2) will be discussed in turn, and the theoretical predictions of platelet deposition compared to experimental findings.

5.1.1. Blood flow velocity (V_{av})

Equation (1) predicts an increase in the rate of platelet deposition with average blood flow velocity. Platelets are carried in streamlines parallel to the surface, and must diffuse perpendicularly to these streamlines in order to reach the surface. The steady deposition of platelets at the surface and the continuous supply of platelets by convection creates a concentration gradient perpendicular to the streamlines. The higher the average blood flow velocity, the faster the supply of new platelets and, therefore, the steeper the radial concentration gradient which provides the driving force for the rate of platelet diffusion towards the surface.

An increase in platelet deposition with blood flow velocity has been reported on *artificial surfaces* exposed to heparinized blood in a tubular flow chamber (Friedman et al., 1970, Friedman and Leonard, 1971, Grabowski et al., 1972) and on *natural surfaces* (Baumgartner, 1973, Turitto and Baumgartner, 1975b). Figure 9 shows that surface coverage with platelets increases as a function of average flow velocity after exposure of subendothelium to citrated blood under standard perfusion conditions, until the subendothelium is completely covered. When initial rates of surface coverage versus average blood flow rate were plotted on logarithmic coordinates, the slope of the best straight line, with 95% confidence limits, was $m(V_{av}) = 0.61 \pm 0.06$ (Turitto and Baumgartner, 1975b). This slope is

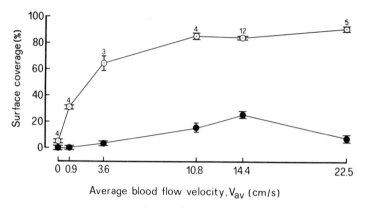

Fig. 9. Coverage of the subendothelial surface with platelets (O–O) and platelet thrombi (●–●) in vitro as a function of the average blood flow velocity in the original perfusion chamber. Exposure time was 10 min in all experiments.

significantly greater than that predicted by Eq. (1) where $m(V_{av})$ equals 0.33. A similar difference was found with the other parameters investigated (q.v.), and this may be due to the dependence of platelet diffusivity on blood shear rate. This point is discussed below.

Formation of platelet thrombi was also flow-dependent (Fig. 9). Surface coverage with thrombi increased up to an average flow velocity of 14.4 cm/sec and then declined at higher flow rates. Current data do not allow a clear interpretation of this finding.

5.1.2. Vessel geometry (d_e)

According to Eq. (1) the rate of surface coverage with platelets is inversely related to the effective diameter d_e. Hence, the smaller the effective diameter (i.e., the width of the annular gap) at constant average flow velocity, the greater should be the rate of supply of platelets from the free stream to the depleted boundary layer.

An experiment designed to investigate this effect (Turitto and Baumgartner, 1974a) showed that surface coverage with platelets on subendothelium decreased markedly with the effective diameter of the perfusion chamber. A logarithmic plot gave the slope of the best straight line, with 95% confidence limits, as $m(d_e) = -0.60 \pm 0.20$. As above, the significant difference from the slope predicted by Eq. (1), $m(d_e) = -0.33$, has been attributed to the fact that the shear rate dependence of platelet diffusion (see below) is not taken into account by Eq. (1) (Turitto and Baumgartner, 1975b).

5.1.3. Wall shear rate (γ_w)

Wall shear rate γ_w relates flow velocity V_{av} and effective diameter d_e:

$$\gamma_w = f(k) \left(\frac{V_{av}}{d_e} \right) \tag{3}$$

where $f(k)$ is a function of the physical parameters of the system. It enables rates of surface coverage in perfusion chambers of different dimensions to be compared. According to Eq. (2) the slope of the logarithmic plot relating initial rate of surface coverage to average wall shear rate is $m(\gamma_w) = 0.33$. The experimentally determined value, with 95% confidence limits, was $m(\gamma_w) = 0.48 \pm 0.09$ (Turitto and Baumgartner, 1975b). This again suggests that platelet diffusion increases with wall shear rate (see below).

5.1.4. Platelet diffusivity (D)

Platelet diffusivity is a measure of the rapidity with which platelets move perpendicular to flow streamlines along the concentration gradient of the boundary layer supplying it with new platelets from the free stream. The rate of platelet deposition should therefore increase with platelet diffusivity. Goldsmith (1971, 1972) proposed that platelet diffusion in whole blood is not determined by Brownian movement, but rather by local movements of fluid induced by rotation and oscillation of erythrocytes in shear fields. He observed cinematographically that the mean square radial excursions of latex microspheres (2 μm in diameter) increased when red cell membranes (ghosts) were present. Platelet diffusivity should similarly depend on red blood cell concentration and shear rate.

The only direct experimental evidence showing that platelet diffusivity is greater in whole blood than in platelet-rich plasma was obtained by Turitto et al. (1972) who found a 100-fold increase in platelet diffusivity when red cells were present. There is no direct experimental evidence showing that the increased platelet diffusivity in whole blood is dependent on shear rate, but such dependence has been inferred by a number of investigators (Friedman and Leonard, 1971, Grabowski et al., 1972, Turitto and Baumgartner, 1975b) from the increased shear rate dependence of surface coverage with platelets (see above) compared with that predicted from classical mass transfer theory, assuming constant platelet diffusivity. These authors have also calculated values for platelet diffusivity in whole blood for the range of shear rates investigated which are about two orders of magnitude greater than those predicted by Brownian movement alone.

Additionally it has been observed that when subendothelium was perfused with platelet-rich plasma in situ and in a perfusion chamber very few platelets adhered to the subendothelial surface as compared to perfusion with anticoagulated whole blood (Baumgartner and Haudenschild, 1972). In a series of experiments in vitro Turitto and Baumgartner (1975a) exposed subendothelium for various periods in the original perfusion chamber to platelet-rich plasma or whole blood. A 54-fold difference in initial rates of surface coverage with platelets between whole blood and platelet-rich plasma experiments was found and this was calculated to correspond to a 400-fold difference in platelet diffusivity.

Because platelet diffusivity depends on red cell concentration and flow, experiments in vitro designed to reproduce or investigate situations of thrombosis or hemostasis in vivo should be carried out with whole blood under controlled conditions of flow.

From the foregoing one should expect the rate of platelet deposition to increase with red blood cell concentration, and, indeed, when subendothelium was exposed to flowing blood under standard perfusion conditions, surface coverage with platelets increased markedly with red cell concentration (Fig. 10). Whether the dramatic increase in surface coverage at about 10^9 red blood cells per ml reflects a critical blood cell concentration is an open question at present.

The effect of red blood cell count on thrombus formation is more complex (Fig. 10): surface coverage with thrombi initially paralleled coverage with platelets, reaching a maximum at about 4×10^9 red blood cells per ml, but decreased to about 5% at 7×10^9 red blood cells per ml.

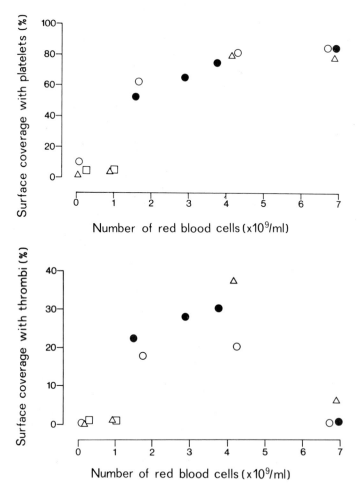

Fig. 10. Effect of red blood cell concentration on surface coverage with platelets (top) and platelet thrombi (bottom). Subendothelium was exposed for 10 min in the original perfusion chamber to anticoagulated blood flowing at an average rate of 160 ml/min. Identical symbols are used for surface coverage with platelets from blood of the same rabbit.

5.1.5. Axial position (z)

As indicated by Eq. (1) the rate of platelet deposition is inversely related to the axial position of the reaction site. In an experiment where 2 cm long vessel segments, exposed under standard perfusion conditions for 1, 2, 3 and 4 min, were evaluated at 7 axial positions, surface coverage with platelets decreased as axial position increased at all positions except the first, which may be influenced by its nearness to the proximal edge of the vessel (Turitto and Baumgartner, 1975b). Initial rates of surface coverage with platelets (excluding position 1) plotted on logarithmic coordinates versus axial distance, yielded a best straight line whose slope, with 95% confidence limits, was $m(z) = -0.17 \pm 0.10$. This slope was significantly lower than predicted from Eq. (1), where $m(z) = -0.33$. Friedman and Leonard (1971) in a study investigating the effect of axial position on platelet adhesion to glass reported a value of $m(z) = -0.41$.

5.1.6. Separated flow (vortices)

Equation (1) describes the rate of platelet transport in the annular chamber only under conditions of laminar flow. This is the case when smooth surfaces are exposed, but obstructions will disturb the laminar flow pattern, since proximal and distal to an obstruction regions of separated flow (vortices) may be created. Unlike simple laminar flow, where streamlines never touch, in a vortex the streamlines form closed areas. Platelets entrapped in such regions have a long residence time – that is, they cannot readily escape or enter these regions save by the relatively slow process of diffusion.

The effect of separated flow on platelet deposition may be considered in two situations: (1) Macroscopic observations have shown that platelets tend to aggregate downstream from sites where laminar flow is disturbed. This has been observed in vivo at bifurcations (Geissinger et al., 1962, Kwaan et al., 1967) and in implanted vena cava rings (Gott et al., 1969), and in vitro in extra-corporeal shunts of plastic (Murphy et al., 1962) and glass (Fry et al., 1965). (2) Microscopically separated flow may occur around platelet thrombi, and in valleys between thrombi, leading to spacing of aggregates (Monsler et al., 1970). We have observed spacing of platelet thrombi when collagen-coated gelatine segments were exposed to flowing blood in the original perfusion chamber (Fig. 11). This pattern of platelet thrombus formation may result from the initial rapid growth of thrombi causing different flow conditions at the proximal, distal (lee-side) and top of platelet thrombi. The term 'lee-effect' is proposed for such phenomena.

Due to the complex motions of fluid and particles, an analytical description of mass transfer in situations of separated flow is well-nigh impossible. The behaviour of platelets in non-laminar flow may, however, be studied by direct observation of model particles or blood cells (Yu and Goldsmith, 1973). These authors microscopically observed particles flowing past a spherical obstruction and reported the following findings: (1) Shear rates were greatly reduced in all vortex regions compared to those at the tube wall without any obstruction. (2) The

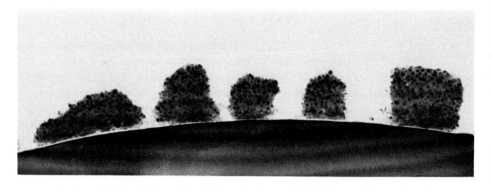

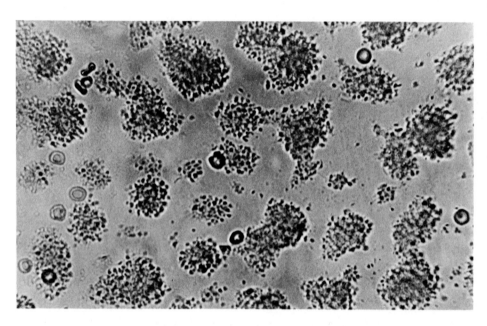

Fig. 11. Spacing of platelet thrombi on collagen coated gelatine segments exposed to blood under standard perfusion conditions. (Top): 0.8 μm thick cross-section after 20 min exposure. (Bottom): 'en face' view after 10 min exposure. ×660.

relative concentration of platelets within a vortex was greater than in the bulk of the suspension. (3) Latex spheres 4 μm in diameter adhered to the downstream edge of the spherical obstacle close to the tube wall, but not elsewhere in the region of separated flow. The magnitude of all these effects depends, of course, on the physical and dimensional characteristics of any particular system, and therefore their importance in vivo remains to be established.

5.2. Blood composition

5.2.1. Red blood cells

Hellem (1960) showed that red cells greatly enhanced the retention of platelets in a glass bead column through which anticoagulated blood was circulated at a constant flow rate. He proposed that a Factor R from red cells was responsible for the increased 'adhesiveness' of platelets. This 'Factor R' was later identified as adenosine diphosphate (ADP) by Gaarder et al. (1961) and was shown to induce platelet aggregation in platelet-rich plasma at very low concentrations (Born, 1962). Zucker et al. (1972) and others confirmed Hellem's observation that platelets are not retained when platelet-rich plasma is circulated through a glass bead column, and showed that adding red cell ghosts to platelet-rich plasma improved retention, although not as effectively as intact erythrocytes. They therefore concluded that red cell ghosts (which contain virtually no ADP) must act by altering hemodynamics. Salzman (1963) showed that large platelet aggregates form and are trapped within a glass bead column, but the sequence and relative importance of platelet–glass and platelet–platelet interaction in this system is unknown.

As shown above, red cells greatly enhance platelet adhesion to subendothelium either in arteries perfused in situ (Baumgartner et al., 1971) or in the perfusion chamber (Baumgartner and Haudenschild, 1972), and since this effect can be explained physically (Turitto and Baumgartner, 1975a) it was discussed in Section 5.1.4. Supporting the concept of a primarily physical role for red cells is the observation that adding ADP to perfused platelet-rich plasma does not increase adhesion unless marked aggregation has occurred (Baumgartner and Haudenschild, 1972). However, these findings by no means exclude the possibility that humoral factors derived from red cells could play a significant role in platelet adhesion and aggregation under certain pathological or experimental conditions, such as in laser-induced microthrombosis (Hovig et al., 1974).

5.2.2. White blood cells

White blood cells are regularly observed in association with platelet thrombi (Bizzozero, 1882, French et al., 1964, Hovig, 1963) and in association with the platelet monolayer on the subendothelial surface an hour or so after removal of endothelium in vivo (Fig. 12). Direct adhesion of white cells at the subendothelial surface was encountered in vivo but very rarely at early times after endothelial denudation. Therefore, white cell adhesion appears to be secondary to platelet adhesion and is probably related to the generation of chemotactic substances by adhering platelets. Indeed, when platelets react with release-inducing stimuli, they release a factor which interacts with the fifth component of complement to produce a chemotactic activity (Weksler and Nachman, 1973). No positive evidence is available at present showing direct involvement of white cells in the initial platelet adhesion reaction, but morphologic evidence indicates that they are

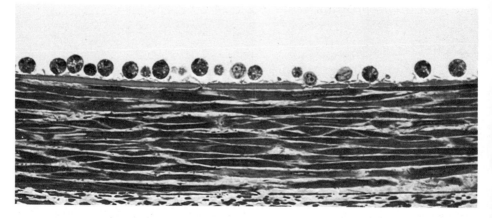

Fig. 12. Adhesion of leucocytes in vivo to the monolayer of platelets on subendothelium of rabbit iliac artery 3 h after removal of the endothelium. ×700.

involved in the removal of adherent platelets by phagocytosis (Baumgartner, unpublished).

5.2.3. Plasma constituents

The methods for separating platelets from blood and plasma have been critically reviewed by Day et al. (1975). So far, adhesion of washed platelets has only been studied with artificial surfaces (mainly glass) under conditions of uncontrolled flow. Packham et al. (1969) who used an indirect method for assessing platelet interaction with surfaces, and George (1972) found that the suspension medium has a profound influence on platelet adhesion to artificial surfaces. Washed platelets were markedly adhesive to glass and other artificial surfaces when suspended in saline or Tyrode's solution, but the same platelets showed a significantly reduced tendency to adhere to these surfaces when suspended in plasma or serum. Similarly, precoating artificial surfaces with plasma or certain plasma proteins such as albumin resulted in decreased platelet surface interaction (Packham et al., 1969, Lyman et al., 1971) although precoating glass with other plasma components, such as fibrinogen or γ-globulin, enhanced platelet adhesion (Packham et al., 1969, Zucker and Vroman, 1969, Mason et al., 1973). These results therefore suggest that platelets in media devoid of protein will attach to most artificial surfaces upon contact, but that precoating a surface with protein (or the presence of protein in the suspension fluid) may profoundly influence the adhesion reaction. The relevance of these observations (which were made in highly artificial systems) to the situation in vivo is not clear at present.

Tschopp et al. (1974) observed that platelets in the blood of patients with Von Willebrand's disease were less adhesive to subendothelium in the annular perfusion chamber than were platelets of normal volunteers. Studies with a specific antibody against human Factor VIII complex (Meyer et al., 1973) indicate that the inhibitory effect of Von Willebrand factor deficiency on platelet adhesion increases with increasing wall shear stress (Baumgartner et al., unpublished). Hence, the Von Willebrand factor, i.e., the high molecular weight portion of Factor VIII (Weiss, 1975), appears to be an essential co-factor for platelet adhesion to natural surfaces such as subendothelium or fibrillar collagen, at least under conditions of high vessel wall shear stresses, such as those observed in arteries and small vessels. Impaired platelet adhesion, a consequence of Von Willebrand factor deficiency, appears to be responsible for the bleeding disorder in the patients with Von Willebrand's disease.

The effects of plasma constituents on *platelet aggregation* has been studied extensively in stirred suspensions of washed platelets and will not be discussed here. Most investigators agree that fibrinogen and calcium are necessary for optimal ADP-induced aggregation (Day et al., 1975).

5.2.4. Effect of anticoagulation

Studies on platelets in vitro require the inhibition of the coagulation system, at least during the initial isolation procedure. The most widely used approach is chelation of Ca^{2+} ions by sodium citrate. Experiments with platelets suspended in plasma are based on the observation that these cells still adhere and aggregate at concentrations of citrate which prevent the formation of fibrin. However, higher citrate concentrations (>25 mM) strongly inhibit platelet aggregation. Studies with platelets suspended in artificial media indicate that ADP induces the platelet release reaction (in the presence of Mg^{2+}) only when Ca^{2+} is well below the physiological level (Mustard et al., 1975). Therefore, low citrate concentrations in plasma may enhance release induced by ADP and possibly other agents and surfaces. Heparin – another widely used anticoagulant – which acts mainly by its antithrombin activity enhances primary aggregation and induces aggregation by causing the release reaction (Zucker, 1974). Thus anticoagulation may introduce artefacts and therefore the data obtained in vitro are not necessarily relevant to the situation in vivo.

Platelet adhesion to subendothelium is also affected by chelation of Ca^{2+} when studied under controlled blood flow conditions in the annular perfusion chamber (Baumgartner, 1974a). Up to a plasma concentration of 25 mM sodium citrate, surface coverage with platelets on subendothelium was unaffected, but at higher concentrations spreading was strongly inhibited, and surface coverage declined from 80% to below 20% at 80 mM citrate. The initial rate of surface coverage with platelets on subendothelium was slightly higher in citrated (14 mM) blood as compared with native blood under identical flow conditions (Baumgartner et al., 1976).

The release of constituents from platelets adherent to subendothelium or fibrillar collagen as revealed by the disappearance of subcellular organelles (α-granules and serotonin storage organelles) was more rapid in the presence of 14 mM citrate than in vivo (Table 1), and the extent of platelet thrombi was greater in the perfusion chamber (Fig. 7) than in vivo (Fig. 3) after 10 min exposure.

However, at high citrate concentrations (80 mM) or with EDTA (3 mM) present, the disappearance of α-granules and serotonin storage organelles was inhibited (Baumgartner et al., 1976).

5.3. Surface properties

Platelets adhere to a variety of surfaces and attempts have been made to correlate physical and chemical properties of surfaces with their attractiveness towards platelets. It should be borne in mind, however, that probably all surfaces exposed to blood will be coated with plasma proteins a few seconds after the initial contact (Scarborough et al., 1969, Baier and Dutton, 1969). It follows that the quality of a surface with respect to adhesion is modified by the composition and pattern of this coating. Vroman et al. (1971) showed that if fibrinogen is adsorbed on foreign surfaces platelet adhesion is promoted. This initial adsorption process (and, consequently, the subsequent platelet adhesion) is influenced by a combination of factors including surface smoothness, surface charge, wettability and surface tension. However, none of these factors alone can explain why one material differs from another. Some insight has been gained by studying the adhesion prototype, platelet–collagen interaction, and although the picture is far from clear, current concepts suggest the involvement of rigidly spaced polar groups on the collagen molecule, in particular the ϵ-amino groups of lysine (Wilner et al., 1968, Nossel et al., 1969, Wilner et al., 1971). Further details on platelet–collagen interaction are given in Chapter 9 of this volume. The relative paucity of information on the fundamental principles operating in platelet–surface interaction makes it difficult to explain satisfactorily the morphological and quantitative differences observed with the various substrates.

5.3.1. Components of connective tissue

Adhesion of platelets to vascular structures is important because it represents the earliest observable blood response in both normal hemostasis and thrombosis. In the intact vessel these structures are protected by the endothelial lining and do not come into contact with blood. The affinity of platelets for exposed subendothelium is much greater than for intact or damaged endothelial cells (for references see Introduction).

Collagen fibrils, microfibrils associated with elastin, basement membrane-like amorphous material and elastin represent the morphologically identifiable connective tissue elements of subendothelium (Fig. 13). Their proportion and proximity to the luminal surface differs in the various parts of the circulatory system. For example, in capillaries and small vessels the subendothelium is a continuous basement membrane which covers underlying connective tissue structures (Fig. 1), whereas in intermediate and large vessels all four components are present and exposed after endothelial detachment.

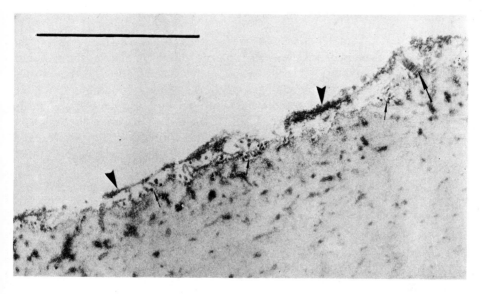

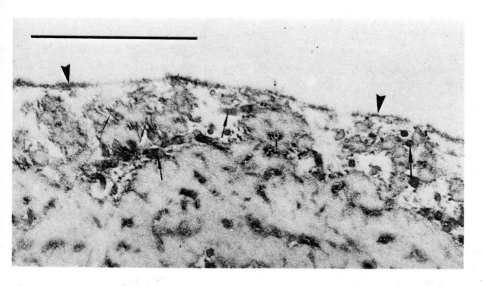

Fig. 13. Electron micrographs of the subendothelial region of rabbit aorta. The vessel segments were routinely prepared but fixed without previous exposure to blood. Amorphous basement membrane-like material (▶) is the main connective tissue component exposed at this surface. Profiles of collagen fibrils (—), microfibrils associated with elastin (—▬) and the internal elastic lamina are seen underneath the amorphous material.

5.3.2. Surfaces investigated in the annular perfusion chamber

The fine structural characteristics of the surfaces investigated so far in the original annular perfusion chamber are shown in Table 3. Table 4 summarizes the extent of platelet–surface interaction and subsequent platelet aggregation on the various surfaces exposed to flowing blood under identical perfusion conditions and Table 5 summarizes the extent of α-granule and serotonin storage organelle disappearance. It is clear that the surfaces differ in their capacity to induce platelet attachment, spreading, release and mural thrombus formation. The chemical and physical properties of the surfaces apparently determine to what extent these reactions take place.

TABLE 3

Fine structural components of surfaces exposed to blood in the annular perfusion chamber

| Surface exposed | Material present at exposed surface as revealed by electron microscopy | | | | |
	Basement membrane-like amorphous material	Collagen fibrils	Microfibrils	Elastin	Deposition of plasma protein
Subendothelium	+++	+	+	+	*
Collagenase-digested subendothelium	0	0	++	++	*
α-chymotrypsin-digested subendothelium	0	++	0	++	*
Collagen-coated gelatine	+++§	0	0	0	*
Gelatine	0	0	0	0	+
Epon	0	0	0	0	++

0 Material absent.
+ Material present in various amounts.
* Electron dense proteinaceous layer not detectable.
§ Neutral salt soluble collagen of guinea pig skin precipitated in amorphous form by air drying.

On all six surfaces investigated the first observable form of attachment were platelets in *contact*, indicating that this reaction is of little surface specificity. On two of the surfaces, namely collagenase-digested subendothelium and Epon, contact was the only form of platelet attachment after 10 min exposure and total surface coverage did not exceed 25% after 40 min. Whether this incomplete saturation is due to a mosaic structure of the surfaces, a purely physical effect (such as the 'lee effect'; see 5.1.6), or an inhibitory effect of attached platelets on deposition of additional platelets (e.g., by their negative charge, which might disappear only after spreading and release) is at present an open question. Three of the surfaces investigated, namely subendothelium, α-chymotrypsin-digested subendothelium, and collagen-coated gelatine segments, stimulated rapid *spreading* of platelets, indicating that collagen fibrils and basement membrane-like amorphous material are substrates which strongly induce this reaction. Disappear-

TABLE 4
Platelet interaction with different surfaces exposed under standard perfusion conditions for 10 and 40 min respectively

Surface coverage (%)

Exposure time	Subendothelium (SE) (mainly basement membrane)		Collagenase digested SE (elastin + microfibrils)		α-chymotrypsin digested SE (elastin + collagen fibrils)		Collagen coated gelatine		Gelatine		Epon	
	10 min	40 min	10 min	40 min	10 min	40 min	10 min	40 min	10 min	40 min	10 min	40 min
Spread (S)	80	100	0	2	30	90	60	90	9	20	0	2
Contact (C)	2	0	3	5	4	4	2	1	20	30	16	18
Thrombi (T)	20	2	0	0	20	60	20	5	0	0	0	0
Surface coverage with platelets (S+C)	80	100	3	7	30	90	60	90	30	50	16	20
$\frac{100T}{S}$	25	2	0	0	70	60	50	5	0	0	0	0

Values above 20% are rounded to the nearest 10%.

TABLE 5
Disappearance of platelet organelles from adhering platelets as revealed by quantitative electron microscopy

Surface exposed	Number of organelles counted	Distribution (%)			Disappearance (%)*	
		Mitochondria	α-granules	Serotonin storage organelles	α-granules	Serotonin storage organelles
Subendothelium	539	65.2	25.8	9.0	92	92
Collagenase digested subendothelium	866	12.8	67.2	20.0	−1	13
α-Chymotrypsin digested subendothelium	252	87.7	6.4	5.9	99	96
Epon	794	15.0	60.5	24.5	22	9
Isolated platelets	2467	12.5	65.0	22.5	–	–

* The number of α-granules and serotonin storage organelles per mitochondrion in isolated platelets was set as 100%. Standard perfusion conditions and an exposure time of 10 min were used in all experiments.

ance of α-granules and serotonin storage organelles was almost complete on subendothelium and α-chymotrypsin digested subendothelium (Table 5), suggesting that spreading and release are intimately related. However, since platelet constituents are also released by collagen in the presence of 3 mM EDTA (Brass and Bensusan, 1974) and since α-granules disappear from platelets attached to, but not spread on, fibrillar collagen after perfusion of blood anticoagulated with 3 mM EDTA (Baumgartner, unpublished), spreading and release appear to be governed by at least partially different mechanisms. Gelatine (denatured collagen) seems to range in between the non-triggering and fast-triggering surfaces of spreading and release. One possible explanation would be that some of the gelatine molecules have partially renatured, forming submicroscopic areas of segments with triple-helix conformation and thus creating a surface of mosaic structure with regions of collagen-like characteristics.

Only subendothelium, α-chymotrypsin digested subendothelium, and collagen-coated gelatine segments induced *platelet aggregation*. Aggregation is therefore surface-specific in the sense that platelet spreading and release are a prerequisite for it to occur. In addition, the surface texture may determine whether platelet thrombi are removed under critical shear stress. Ultrastructural investigations revealed that collagen fibrils protruding from the surface of α-chymotrypsin-digested subendothelium are incorporated into the platelet mass (Fig. 14). We believe that the fibrils anchor the platelet mass to the surface and thus prevent it from being pulled away by the blood stream. On subendothelium which has very few of these protruding collagen fibrils, formation and removal of platelet thrombi are in a state of dynamic equilibrium, resulting in a much lower surface coverage with thrombi (100 T/S) then would be expected from the virtually complete coverage with spread platelets.

Interaction between platelets and synthetic materials is clearly of low affinity as compared to basement membrane or collagen. The initial rate of platelet attachment to a variety of artificial surfaces under controlled flow conditions is similar (Friedman and Leonard, 1971), indicating a comparatively unspecific reaction. In contrast, interaction of platelets with basement membrane and collagen fibrils appears specific in the sense that after initial contact these substrates induce rapid platelet spreading and release.

5.4. Platelet reactivity

The investigation of hereditary defects or experimentally induced alterations of platelet function represents an important approach for evaluating the basic mechanisms involved in platelet adhesion and the subsequent reactions. The current knowledge about platelet pharmacology and functional defects of platelets in hereditary bleeding disorders, as revealed by conventional test systems and biochemical evaluation, are extensively discussed in a number of recent review articles (Dodds, 1974, Weiss, 1975, Mustard and Packham, 1975). The present section focusses on the interaction of abnormal or experimentally altered platelets with subendothelium and α-chymotrypsin digested suben-

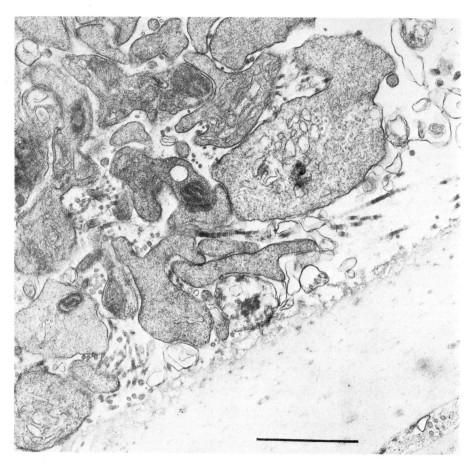

Fig. 14. Electron micrograph of part of a mural platelet thrombus on α-chymotrypsin digested subendothelium. Profiles of collagen fibrils are seen within the aggregates. The platelets contain mitochondria only; their α-granules and serotonin storage organelles have disappeared.

dothelium in the annular perfusion chamber. It is proposed that the initial attachment of platelets to a surface, their subsequent spreading, the release reaction, and the formation of mural platelet thrombi, involve mechanisms which are at least partially different and independent from each other.

5.4.1. Relation between platelet spreading and surface coverage

Surface coverage with platelets does not reach 100% unless spreading occurs (Baumgartner, 1974b). Surfaces such as Epon or collagenase-digested subendothelium, which do not trigger the spreading of platelets, appear to be saturated with platelets below 25% surface coverage, a value which corresponds to less than 5×10^4 platelets per mm^2 of surface (Leonard and Friedman, 1970, Baumgartner, 1974b). These platelets adhere singly with a platelet-free area around them (Fig.

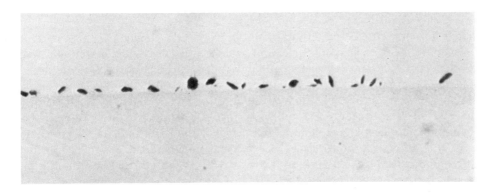

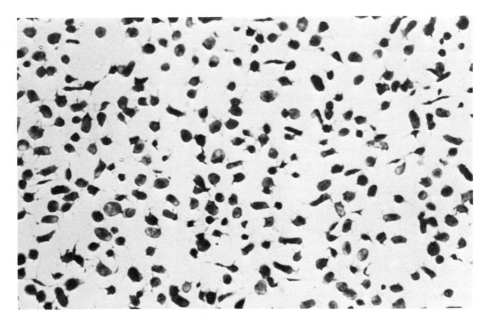

Fig. 15. Platelet interaction with Epon. An Epon surface was exposed to anticoagulated blood flowing at 160 ml/min in the original perfusion chamber for 10 min. The platelets adhere singly and are virtually not spread out on the surface: (top) 0.8 μm thick cross-section; (bottom) surface of the same specimen viewed 'en face'.

15) and are not removed by perfusion with platelet-free blood or plasma (Baumgartner et al., 1976). Similarly, platelets which are unable to spread (see below) adhere singly and cover only part of the surfaces which otherwise induce rapid spreading of normal platelets. Therefore, low values of surface coverage with platelets may reflect a defect of the initial attachment reaction and/or inhibition of platelet spreading. The ratio between contact (C) and adhering (C + S) platelets indicates which one of the two mechanisms is predominantly affected. Low ratios (≪1) suggest a defect only in the initial attachment reaction, higher ratios indicate inhibition of spreading as well.

5.4.2. Activation of platelets by upstream thrombi

Platelets from circulating citrated blood have little tendency to adhere to collagenase-digested subendothelium (Table 4). However, when platelet thrombi develop on a surface exposed upstream from the collagenase-digested subendothelium, more platelets and platelet thrombi adhere at the latter surface (Baumgartner et al., 1976). Such a situation can be created in the perfusion chamber by exposing on the rod a surface known to produce thrombi (α-chymotrypsin-digested subendothelium, for example) adjacent to and upstream from a segment of collagenase-digested subendothelium. A strong positive correlation between the extent of surface coverage with thrombi on the 'thrombogenic' upstream surface and the extent of surface coverage with platelets and platelet thrombi on collagenase digested subendothelium was found (Fig. 16). In addition, the ultrastructural appearance of thrombi on the two surfaces was strikingly different. On 'thrombogenic' surfaces the platelets are spread out, tightly attached and have lost most of their α-granules and serotonin storage organelles (Fig. 8, Fig. 14), but on collagenase-digested subendothelium the thrombi are loosely attached, the platelets associated with the surface are not spread out, and they often still contain their granules (Fig. 17).

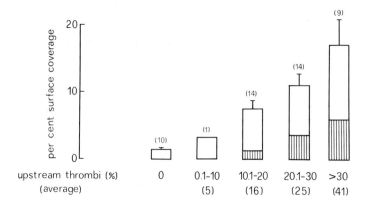

Fig. 16. Effect of upstream thrombi on surface coverage with platelets (whole column) and platelet thrombi (hatched part of column) on collagenase-digested subendothelium. Upstream thrombi were produced on a surface exposed on the rod of the perfusion chamber adjacent to and upstream from collagenase-digested subendothelium.

These observations suggest that single platelets or aggregates derived from platelet thrombi and translocated by the flowing blood are more 'sticky' than platelets from the circulation. Therefore, these platelets and aggregates are more likely to adhere, even to a surface which is 'unattractive' for unstimulated platelets.

Additional experiments demonstrated that surface coverage with platelets and platelet thrombi on collagenase-digested subendothelium decreased with increasing distance from the source of thrombi (Baumgartner et al., 1976), indicating that

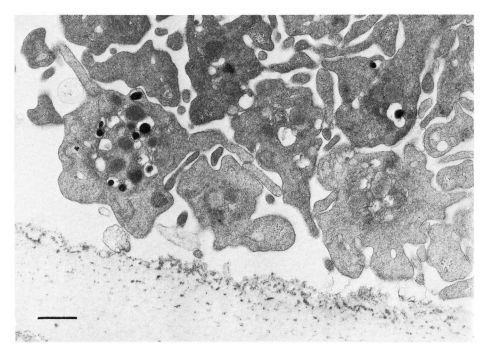

Fig. 17. Electron micrograph of part of a mural platelet thrombus attached to collagenase digested subendothelium. The platelets associated with the surface are not spread out and still contain part of their subcellular organelles.

platelets or aggregates which detach from a 'thrombogenic' surface either lose their increased stickiness shortly after they have broken off, or are removed from the boundary layer by the flowing blood a few millimeters downstream from the site of detachment.

5.4.3. Functional defects of platelets associated with decreased adhesion

Conditions associated with decreased platelet–surface interaction are listed in Table 6. Since surface coverage with platelets is also dependent on platelet spreading, inhibition of the initial attachment and inhibition of spreading will be considered separately.

Surface coverage with platelets from patients with Von Willebrand's disease or the Bernard-Soulier syndrome is decreased without a substantial increase in the percentage of platelets merely 'in contact' (Table 6), indicating that spreading occurs at a normal rate once a platelet has attached to the surface, and that only the initial attachment reaction appears to be altered in these conditions. In Von Willebrand's disease, there is deficiency of a plasma factor essential for normal adhesion (Weiss, 1975). It remains to be established whether the Von Willebrand factor must be present in plasma, on the exposed surface, or on the platelet membrane. Platelets of patients with the Bernard-Soulier syndrome have normal

TABLE 6
Inhibition of platelet adhesion to subendothelium

	n	$C + S^a$	C^a	$\dfrac{100\,T^a}{S}$	Reference
Human platelets					
Controls	27	83.5 ± 1.0	1.5 ± 0.2	17.3 ± 2.3	Baumgartner et al., 1976
Von Willebrand's disease	9	58.1 ± 3.5^b	1.9 ± 0.4	16.6 ± 3.1	Tschopp et al., 1974
Bernard-Soulier syndrome	2	39.7 ± 9.4^b	2.3 ± 0.4	12.3 ± 10.1	Weiss et al., 1974
Storage pool disease	6	60.3 ± 3.7^b	1.8 ± 0.4	0^b	Weiss et al., 1975
Rabbit platelets					
Controls	44	82.5 ± 1.2	2.2 ± 1.9	25.0 ± 1.9	Baumgartner et al., 1976
Low temperature (20°C)	6	44.3 ± 6.0^b	22.8 ± 3.6^b	0.6 ± 0.2	Turitto and Baumgartner, 1974b
EDTA (3 mM)^c	6	24.3 ± 3.0^b	16.6 ± 2.2^b	0^b	
Prostaglandin E$_1$(1 μM)^c	3	46.7 ± 13.8^b	17.2 ± 3.8^b	0^b	Baumgartner et al., 1976
Dipyridamole (1 mM)^c	3	48.4 ± 8.1^b	1.8 ± 1.0	0^b	

Unless otherwise stated, blood anticoagulated with citrate (14 mM–20 mM in plasma) was circulated through the original perfusion chamber at 160 ml/min for 10 min. The results are means ± S.E.
[a] For explanation see Section 2.3, and Fig. 2.
[b] $2P < 0.05$ as compared with the corresponding control group (Student's t-test).
[c] Concentrations in whole blood.

Von Willebrand factor activity in their plasma, but their platelet membrane glycoproteins, especially glycoprotein I, are drastically reduced–whereas the glycoprotein pattern is normal in platelets from patients with Von Willebrand's disease (Nurden and Caen, 1975, Jenkins et al., 1975). Therefore, glycoprotein I of the platelet membrane and its interaction with von Willebrand factor may be essential for the initial attachment of a platelet at the subendothelial surface and at fibrillar collagen.

When experimental conditions are altered in certain ways (e.g. by low temperature, chelation of Ca^{2+} ions, or the addition of low concentrations of prostaglandin E$_1$) surface coverage with platelets is decreased and there is an increase in the percentage of 'contact' platelets (Table 6). These results indicate inhibition of spreading, but it is not clear at present whether this is solely responsible for the decrease in surface coverage with platelets. Inhibition of spreading was always associated with a substantial reduction in the formation of platelet thrombi (Tables 4 and 6), although in the presence of EDTA platelet degranulation was only slightly inhibited (Baumgartner et al., 1976). We conclude from these results that although initial attachment, spreading, release, and aggregation are interrelated, the mechanisms involved in these reactions are not identical.

5.4.4. Functional defects of platelets associated with decreased aggregation

Clinical and experimental conditions associated with normal platelet adhesion but decreased formation of mural platelet thrombi (platelet aggregates) on suben-

TABLE 7
Inhibition of platelet aggregation (mural platelet thrombi) on subendothelium

	n	$C + S^a$	C^a	$\dfrac{100\,T^a}{S}$	Reference
Human platelets					
Controls	27	83.5 ± 1.0	1.5 ± 0.2	17.3 ± 2.3	Baumgartner et al., 1976
Storage pool disease	6	60.3 ± 3.7^b	1.8 ± 0.4	0^b	Weiss et al., 1975
Thrombasthenia	2	69.6 ± 2.7	0.7 ± 0.4	0^b	Tschopp et al., 1975
Ingestion of acetyl-salicylic acid (1 g)	7	90.0 ± 4.5	0.3 ± 0.1	0.1 ± 0.006^b	Weiss et al., 1975
Rabbit platelets					
Controls	44	82.5 ± 1.2	2.2 ± 1.9	25.0 ± 1.9	Baumgartner et al., 1976
Ingestion of acetyl-salicylic acid (18 mg/kg)	6	90.0 ± 2.1^b	0.9 ± 0.2	7.1 ± 4.5^b	
Ingestion of sulfin-pyrazone (40 mg/kg)	7	87.7 ± 2.8^b	1.4 ± 0.6	0.7 ± 0.3^b	

Only those conditions were included in this table in which inhibition of platelet thrombi was not explained by inhibition of adhesion.
For further explanation see Table 6.

dothelium under standard perfusion conditions are listed in Table 7. The results are in agreement with findings obtained using other test systems (such as the aggregometer) and are consistent with the following interpretation. The interaction of platelets with collagen triggers the release of platelet granule constituents (Grette, 1962, Holmsen et al., 1969) and activates platelet prostaglandin synthesis (Smith and Willis, 1971, Willis, 1974); both these reactions promote aggregation. Deficiency of releasable aggregation-inducing substances (e.g., in storage pool disease), or inhibition of prostaglandin synthesis (e.g., after ingestion of Aspirin), or an intrinsic inability of platelets to aggregate (e.g., in thrombasthenia (Caen, 1972)) can all reduce or abolish platelet thrombus formation. The observation that platelet adhesion to subendothelium (Table 7) is not significantly impaired in any of these conditions indicates that adhesion can occur independently of the release reaction and aggregation, but the release of platelet constituents may well influence platelet adhesion by activating platelets and rendering them more 'sticky' (q.v.).

6. *Reversibility of adhesion and aggregation*

The formation of a mural platelet thrombus is a transient event (Figs. 3 and 7) as long as the exposed surface is smooth; thrombi which persisted for longer periods of time (>30 min)–for example on the α-chymotrypsin-digested subendothelium (Table 4)–always had collagen fibrils incorporated (Fig. 14) which presumably anchor the mural thrombi to the surface.

To investigate further the question of reversibility, additional experiments were performed in which perfusion of anticoagulated whole blood was followed by perfusion of platelet-free plasma or platelet-poor blood. Under standard perfusion conditions the platelet-free perfusates caused (1) disappearance of platelet thrombi and increased surface coverage with platelets on subendothelium; (2) a decrease in the average height of platelet thrombi and increased surface coverage with platelets on α-chymotrypsin-digested subendothelium; but (3) no significant change of surface coverage with platelets on Epon (Baumgartner et al., 1976). These findings indicate that platelets (and possibly small aggregates) are translocated by the stream of platelet-free plasma or platelet-poor blood from the mural thrombi to the surface. In contrast, platelets adhering to a surface (either as 'contact' or spread platelets) are *not* removed under flow conditions which remove platelet thrombi. Further studies are required to determine whether very high wall shear rates will remove adhering platelets as well, but the present data suggest that platelet adhesion is virtually irreversible compared with mural platelet thrombus formation (aggregation) under similar flow conditions.

References

Arfors, K.E., Dhall, D.P., Engeset, J., Hint, H., Matheson, N.A. and Tangen, O. (1968) Nature (London), *218*, 887.
Baier, R.E. and Dutton, R.C. (1969) J. Biomed. Mater. Res., *3*, 191.
Baumgartner, H.R. (1963) Z. Ges. Exp. Med., *137*, 227.
Baumgartner, H.R. (1973) Microvasc. Res., *5*, 167.
Baumgartner, H.R. (1974a) Thromb. Diath. Haemorrh. (Stuttg.) Suppl., *59*, 91.
Baumgartner, H.R. (1974b) Thromb. Diath. Haemorrh. (Stuttg.) Suppl., *60*, 39.
Baumgartner, H.R. (1975) Blutplättchen und Gefässwand. Verhandlungen der Deutschen Gesellschaft für innere Medizin. In press.
Baumgartner, H.R. and Haudenschild, C. (1972) Ann. N.Y. Acad. Sci., *201*, 22.
Baumgartner, H.R., Muggli, R., Tschopp, Th.B. and Turitto, V.T. (1976) Thromb. Diath. Haemorrh. (Stuttg.), In press.
Baumgartner, H.R. and Spaet, T.H. (1970) Fed. Proc., *29*, 710.
Baumgartner, H.R., Stemerman, M.B. and Spaet, T.H. (1971) Experientia, *27*, 283.
Baumgartner, H.R. and Studer, A. (1966) Path. Microbiol., *29*, 393.
Baumgartner, H.R., Tranzer, J.P. and Studer, A. (1967) Thromb. Diath. Haemorrh. (Stuttg.), *18*, 592.
Bizzozero, J. (1882) Virchows Arch., *90*, 261.
Born, G.V.R. (1962) Nature (London), *194*, 927.
Bounameaux, Y. (1959) C. R. Soc. Biol., *153*, 865.
Brass, L.F. and Bensusan, H.B. (1974) J. Clin. Invest., *54*, 1480.
Breddin, K. (1964) Thromb. Diath. Haemorrh. (Stuttg.), *12*, 269.
Caen, J.P. (1972) in Clinics in Haematology (O'Brien, J.R., ed), Vol. 1, p. 383, W.B. Saunders Company, Philadelphia.
Cazenave, J.-P., Packham, M.A. and Mustard, J.F. (1973) J. Lab. Clin. Med., *82*, 978.
Day, H.J., Holmsen, H. and Zucker, M.B. (1975) Thromb. Diath. Haemorrh. (Stuttg.), *33*, 648.
Dodds, W.J. (1974) in Progress in Hemostasis and Thrombosis (Spaet, T.H., ed), Vol. 2, p. 226. Grune and Stratton, New York.
Dutton, R.C., Baier, R.E., Dedrick, R.L. and Bowman, R.L. (1968) Trans. Amer. Soc. Artif. Int. Organs, *14*, 57.
Fishman, J.A., Ryan, G.B. and Karnovsky, M.J. (1975) Lab. Invest., *32*, 339.
French, J.E., MacFarlane, R.G. and Sanders, A.G. (1964) Brit. J. Exp. Path., *45*, 467.
Friedman, L.I. and Leonard, E.F. (1971) Fed. Proc., *30*, 1641.

Friedman, L.I., Liem, H., Grabowski, E.F., Leonard, E.F. and McCord, C.W. (1970) Trans. Amer. Soc. Artif. Int. Organs, *16*, 63.
Fry, D.L. (1968) Circulation Res., *22*, 165.
Fry, F.J., Eggleton, R.C., Kelly, E. and Fry, W.J. (1965) Trans. Amer. Soc. Artif. Int. Organs, *11*, 307.
Gaarder, A., Jonsen, J., Laland, S., Hellem, A. and Owren, P.A. (1961) Nature (London), *192*, 531.
Geissinger, H.D., Mustard, J.F. and Rowsell, H.C. (1962) Can. Med. Assn. J., *87*, 405.
George, J.N. (1972) Blood, *40*, 862.
Goldsmith, H.L. (1971) Fed. Proc., *30*, 1578.
Goldsmith, H.L. (1972) In: Progress in Hemostasis and Thrombosis (Spaet, T.H., ed), Vol. 1, p. 97. Grune and Stratton, New York.
Gott, V.L., Ramos, M.D., Najjar, F.B., Allen, J.L. and Bekker, K.E. (1969) In: Artificial Heart Program Conference (Hegyeli, R.J., ed), p. 181. U.S. Govt. Printing Office, Washington D.C.
Grabowski, E.F., Friedman, L.I. and Leonard, E.F. (1972) I&EC Fundamentals, *11*, 224.
Grette, K. (1962) Acta Physiol. Scand., *56* (Suppl. 195).
Harker, L.A., Slichter, S.J., Scott, G.R. and Ross, R. (1974) New Engl. J. Med., *291*, 537.
Haudenschild, C. and Studer, A. (1971) Eur. J. Clin. Invest., *2*, 1.
Hellem, A.J. (1960) Scand. J. Clin. Lab. Invest., *12* (Suppl. 51).
Hirsh, J., Glynn, M.F. and Mustard, J.F. (1968) J. Clin. Invest., *47*, 466.
Holmsen, H., Day, H.J. and Stormorken, H. (1969) Scand. J. Haemat. Suppl., *8*, 1.
Honour, A.J. and Russell, R.W.R. (1962) Brit. J. Exp. Path., *43*, 350.
Hovig, T. (1963) Thromb. Diath. Haemorrh. (Stuttg.), *9*, 248.
Hovig, T., McKenzie, F.N. and Arfors, K.-E. (1974) Thromb. Diath. Haemorrh. (Stuttg.), *32*, 695.
Hovig, T., Jørgensen, L., Packham, M.A. and Mustard, J.F. (1968) J. Lab. Clin. Med., *71*, 29.
Hugues, J. (1960) C.R. Soc. Biol., *154*, 866.
Jenkins, C.S.P., Phillips, D.R., Clemetson, K.J., Meyer, D. and Larrieu, M.J. (1975) Thromb. Diath. Haemorrh. (Stuttg.), in press.
Kjaerheim, A. and Hovig, T. (1962) Thromb. Diath. Haemorrh. (Stuttg.), *7*, 1.
Kwaan, H.C., Harding, F. and Astrup, T. (1967) Thromb. Diath. Haemorrh. (Stuttg.) Suppl., *26*, 208.
Lagergren, H., Olsson, P. and Swedenborg, J. (1974) Surgery, *75*, 643.
Leonard, E.F. and Friedman, L.I. (1970) Chem. Eng. Progr. Symp. Ser., *66*, 59.
Lyman, B., Rosenberg, L. and Karpatkin, S. (1971) J. Clin. Invest., *50*, 1854.
Lyman, D.J., Klein, G.K., Brash, J.L. and Fritzinger, B.K. (1970) Thromb. Diath. Haemorrh. (Stuttg.), *23*, 120.
Majno, G. and Palade, G.E. (1961) J. Biophys. Biochem. Cytol., *11*, 571.
Mason, R.G. and Gilkey, J.M. (1971) Thromb. Diath. Haemorrh. (Stuttg.), *25*, 21.
Mason, R.G., Shermer, R.W. and Zucker, W.H. (1973) Am. J. Path., *73*, 183.
Mason, R.G., Zucker, W.H., Shinoda, B.A., Chuang, H.Y., Kingdon, H.S. and Clark, H.G. (1974) Lab. Invest., *31*, 143.
Meyer, D., Jenkins, C.S.P., Dreyfus, M.D. and Larrieu, M.J. (1973) Nature (London), *243*, 293.
Monsler, M., Morton, W. and Weiss, R. (1970) Am. Inst. Aeronautics and Astronautics Paper *70–787*, 1.
Murphy, E.A., Rowsell, H.C., Downie, H.G., Robinson, G.A. and Mustard, J.F. (1962) Can. Med. Assn. J., *87*, 259.
Mustard, J.F., Kinlough-Rathbone, R.L. and Packham, M.A. (1974) Thromb. Diath. Haemorrh. (Stuttg.) Suppl., *59*, 157.
Mustard, J.F. and Packham, M.A. (1975) Drugs, *9*, 19.
Mustard, J.F., Perry, D.W., Kinlough-Rathbone, R.L. and Packham, M.A. (1975) Amer. J. Physiol., *228*, 1757.
Nam, S.C., Lee, W.M., Jarmolych, J., Lee, K.T. and Thomas, W.A. (1973) Exp. Mol. Pathol., *18*, 369.
Nossel, H.L., Wilner, G.D. and LeRoy, E.C. (1969) Nature (London), *221*, 75.
Nurden, A.T. and Caen, J.P. (1975) Nature (London), *225*, 720.
Packham, M.A., Evans, G., Glynn, M.F. and Mustard, J.F. (1969) J. Lab. Clin. Med., *73*, 686.
Petschek, H.E. and Weiss, R.F. (1970) Amer. Inst. Aeronautics and Astronautics, Paper *70–143*, 1.
Reber, K. (1966) Thromb. Diath. Haemorrh. (Stuttg.), *15*, 471.
Salzman, E.W. (1963) J. Lab. Clin. Med., *62*, 724.
Scarborough, D.E., Mason, R.G., Dalldorf, F.G. and Brinkhous, K.M. (1969) Lab. Invest., *20*, 164.
Schmid-Schoenbein, B.W., Fung, Y.C. and Zweifach, B.W. (1975) Circulation Res., *36*, 173.
Smith, J.B. and Willis, A.L. (1971) Nature New Biol. *231*, 235.
Spaet, T.H., Stemerman, M.B., Veith, F.J. and Lejnieks, I. (1975) Circulation Res., *36*, 58.
Stemerman, M.B., Baumgartner, H.R. and Spaet, T.H. (1971) Lab. Invest., *24*, 179.

Stemerman, M.B. and Ross, R. (1972) J. Exp. Med., *136*, 769.
Stormorken, H., Lund-Riise, Å. and Rørvik, T.O. (1965) Scand. J. Clin. Lab. Invest., *17* (Suppl. 84), 183.
Tranzer, J.P. and Baumgartner, H.R. (1967) Nature (London), *216*, 1126.
Tschopp, T.B., Weiss, H.J. and Baumgartner, H.R. (1974) J. Lab. Clin. Med., *83*, 296.
Tschopp, T.B., Weiss, H.J. and Baumgartner, H.R. (1975) Experientia, *31*, 113.
Turitto, V.T. (1975) Chem. Eng. Sci., *30*, 503.
Turitto, V.T. and Baumgartner, H.R. (1974a) Thromb. Diath. Haemorrh. (Stuttg.) Suppl., *60*, 17.
Turitto, V.T. and Baumgartner, H.R. (1974b) Haemostasis, *3*, 224.
Turitto, V.T. and Baumgartner, H.R. (1975a) Microvasc. Res., *9*, 335.
Turitto, V.T. and Baumgartner, H.R. (1975b) Trans. Amer. Soc. Artif. Int. Organs, *21*, 593.
Turitto, V.T., Benis, A.M. and Leonard, E.F. (1972) I&EC Fundamentals, *11*, 216.
Turitto, V.T. and Leonard, E.F. (1972) Trans. Amer. Soc. Artif. Int. Organs, *18*, 348.
Vroman, L., Adams, A.L. and Klings, M. (1971) Fed. Proc., *30*, 1494.
Weibel, E.R. (1969) in International Review of Cytology (Bourne, G.H., Danielli, J.F., and Jeon, K.W., eds), Vol. 26, p. 235. Academic Press, New York–London.
Weiss, H.J. (1975) New Engl. J. Med., *293*, 531–541 and 580–588.
Weiss, H.J., Tschopp, T.B. and Baumgartner, H.R. (1975) New Engl. J. Med., *293*, 619.
Weiss, H.J., Tschopp, T.B., Baumgartner, H.R., Sussman, I.I., Johnson, M.M. and Egan, J.J. (1974) Amer. J. Med., *57*, 920.
Willis, A.L. (1974) Prostaglandins *5*, 1.
Wilner, G.D., Nossel, H.L. and LeRoy, E.C. (1968) J. Clin. Invest., *47*, 2616.
Wilner, G.D., Nossel, H.L. and Procupez, T.L. (1971) Amer. J. Physiol. *220*, 1074.
Yu, S.K. and Goldsmith, H.L. (1973) Microvasc. Res., *6*, 5.
Zucker, M.B. (1974) Thromb. Diath. Haemorrh. (Stuttg.), *33*, 63.
Zucker, M.B. and Borrelli, J. (1962) Proc. Soc. Exp. Biol. Med., *109*, 779.
Zucker, M.B., Rifkin, P.L., Friedberg, N.M. and Coller, B.S. (1972) Ann. N.Y. Acad. Sci., *201*, 138.
Zucker, M.B. and Vroman, L. (1969) Proc. Soc. Exp. Biol. Med., *131*, 318.

CHAPTER 3

The platelet release reaction: association with adhesion and aggregation, and comparison with secretory responses in other cells

D.E. MACINTYRE

Department of Pathology, University of Cambridge, Tennis Court Road, Cambridge, CB2 1QP, England

1. Introduction

Cell secretion reactions are vital in many biological processes: for example, all hormones and neurotransmitters are secretory products, and the selective release of cellular constituents is an important component of the inflammatory response.

Stimulated secretion could be broadly defined as 'the selective exportation of cell contents to the cell exterior in response to a specific stimulus', and the secreting cell remains viable after it has selectively released some of its constituents.

Two types of selective release processes can be distinguished:

(1) *Merocrine Secretion* – defined as 'the output from cells of products that have been produced and packaged and that can be released in response to a stimulus in a specific release reaction' (Stormorken, 1969). This is also known as 'degranulation'.

(2) *Secretion Without Degranulation* – cell constituents are exported by active transport across the cell membrane, or by orientation of the biosynthetic apparatus towards the cell exterior – e.g., prostaglandins (Bito, 1975).

Merocrine secretion occurs in a variety of tissues including exocrine glands and endocrine glands, and also in isolated cells. The precise sequence of events in degranulation reactions has been the subject of debate since the early 1950s. Bennett (1956) speculated that if cells could perform pinocytosis, then the reverse might also occur, and the membrane of cytoplasmic droplets (granules) could be incorporated into the cell surface. This process was termed 'reverse micro-pinocytosis', 'emiocytosis' and later 'exocytosis' (de Duve, 1963)–the term in use today.

Electron microscopy facilitated the investigation of the secretory process, and Palade (1958) demonstrated the direct discharge of material from the zymogen granule of the pancreatic acinar cell to the cell exterior by a process involving fusion of granule membrane with the cell surface, followed by rupture of the

Gordon (ed) Platelets in Biology and Pathology
© *Elsevier/North-Holland Biomedical Press, 1976*

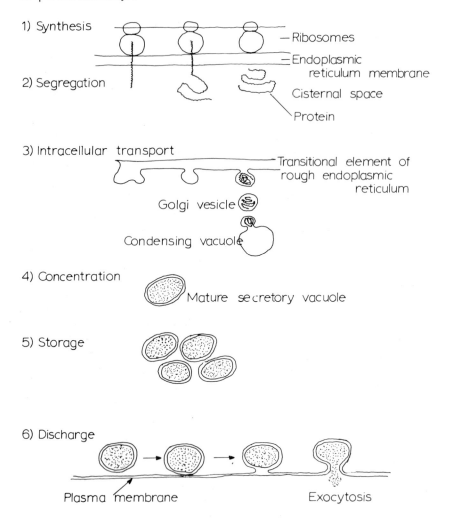

1) Synthesis

Ribosomes

Endoplasmic reticulum membrane

2) Segregation

Cisternal space

Protein

3) Intracellular transport

Transitional element of rough endoplasmic reticulum

Golgi vesicle

Condensing vacuole

4) Concentration

Mature secretory vacuole

5) Storage

6) Discharge

Plasma membrane

Exocytosis

Fig. 1

fused membranes. Palade and coworkers investigated the sequence of events in the selective release of proteins from the pancreatic acinar cell and concluded that there were six steps involved (Palade, 1975; see Fig. 1):

(1) *Synthesis of protein*   Occurs on polysomes attached to membranes of the rough endoplasmic reticulum.

(2) *Segregation*   Newly synthesised polypeptides from the large ribosomal subunit are vectorially transported through the endoplasmic reticulum membrane to the cisternal space.

(3) *Intracellular transport*   The secretory proteins in the cisternal space are transported to the Golgi complex where they can be located in condensing vacuoles.

(4) *Concentration*   Secretory proteins in the condensing vacuoles are concentrated to the level found in mature secretion granules.

(5) *Intracellular storage*   The secretory proteins are temporarily stored in secretion granules, distributed at random in the pre-existing granule population.

(6) *Discharge*   Granule membranes fuse with cell membrane, and granule contents are discharged by exocytosis to the cell exterior.

Palade (1975) suggests that a similar sequence is probably involved in secretion by other cell types, even for granules whose main secretory product is not a protein, since such materials are usually condensed in granules with a specific "packing" protein (Douglas, 1974a).

When investigating the effect of secretory stimulants (secretagogues) on cells, Douglas and Rubin (1961) showed that acetylcholine-induced secretion from chromaffin cells of the adrenal medulla was dependent on the concentration of calcium in the extracellular environment, and that under certain conditions calcium alone could stimulate secretion. They proposed that acetylcholine's action on the plasma membrane of the cell induced inward movement of calcium ions, and compared this to excitation-contraction coupling in muscle. These workers suggested that calcium might be the mediator of 'stimulus-secretion coupling', later defined as 'all the events occurring in the cell exposed to its immediate stimulus that lead finally to the appearance of the characteristic secretory product in the extracellular environment' (Douglas, 1968). Secretion in other cell types was also found to depend on extracellular calcium ions (Mongar and Schild, 1962; Katz, 1962), which suggested that calcium influx might be the universal trigger for releasing biologically active substances from cells.

Exocytosis is now recognised as a secretory mechanism used by cells of widely different form and function (for reviews, see Rubin, 1970; Douglas, 1974b). The aims of the present chapter are to review the platelet release reaction in this context, to consider the suitability of platelets as a cellular model for investigating stimulus-secretion coupling, and to discuss briefly the biological importance of the platelet release reaction. Accordingly, the characteristics of the platelet release reaction will be summarised and compared with the secretory responses of three other cell types – polymorphonuclear leukocytes, mast cells, and the chromaffin cells of the adrenal medulla.

2. The platelet release reaction

Blood platelets can be justifiably regarded as secretory cells, since they selectively release the constituents of their storage granules in response to specific stimuli.

Platelets contain at least two types of storage granule: a group of organelles known as 'alpha granules', and the smaller 'very dense body'. In human platelets, alpha granules are much more numerous than dense bodies. Some of the alpha granules contain lysosomal enzymes (for review, see Gordon, 1975), whereas dense bodies are the amine and nucleotide storage granules, where calcium, ATP, ADP and serotonin are present as high molecular weight aggregates (Pletscher et al., 1971). The existence of a third type of platelet granule has recently been proposed (Bentfield and Bainton, 1975), which is probably a non-lysosomal sub-population of the alpha granules.

Grette (1962) introduced the term 'platelet release reaction' to describe the biochemical reactions occurring when adenine nucleotides, serotonin, proteins and amino acids were rapidly extruded from platelets treated with thrombin, and Kjaerheim and Hovig (1962) showed microscopically that this reaction was not due to platelet lysis. Holmsen and coworkers (1969) showed that the response to thrombin resembled that induced by several other agents, and suggested that there was one basic 'platelet release reaction', characterised by the rapid discharge of the contents of dense bodies and alpha granules from the platelet to the extracellular environment.

The platelet release reaction can be induced in vitro by many stimuli: some are physiologically important while others serve purely as research tools.

The stimuli include:
(1) Adhesion to surfaces, especially to collagen fibrils (see Chapter 2),
(2) Platelet–platelet contact ('aggregation'),
(3) Immune reactions at the platelet membrane (see Chapter 12),
(4) ADP,
(5) Adrenaline,
(6) Thrombin, and certain other proteolytic enzymes,
(7) Divalent cation ionophores.

Day and Holmsen (1971) showed that release of dense body constituents induced by ADP, adrenaline, or by low concentrations of thrombin or collagen, was not accompanied by release of alpha granule constituents, whereas high concentrations of thrombin and collagen caused release of both granule constituents. Holmsen and Day (1970) showed that, in the thrombin-induced release reaction, release of 5HT (a dense body constituent) preceded release of lysosomal enzymes (alpha granule constituents), and suggested that there are two kinetically-distinct phases of release:

Release I – dense body constituents,
Release II – alpha granule constituents.

2.1. Energy requirements

Platelets metabolise glycogen or extracellular glucose by glycolysis, and further via the Krebs cycle and oxidative phosphorylation. Each of these processes contributes about half of the ATP production by resting platelets in vitro. The enzymes of the hexose monophosphate shunt pathway are also present in platelets (Doery et al., 1970; Karpatkin, 1972).

Platelets cannot synthesise adenine nucleotides de novo, but AMP can be synthesised from exogenous adenine (via adenine phosphoribosyl transferase) or from adenosine (via adenosine kinase). AMP can then be converted to ADP and ATP by adenylate kinase. When platelets are incubated with radioactive adenosine or adenine the label is incorporated into adenine nucleotides, but during the platelet release reaction only *non-labelled* adenine nucleotides are released; the labelled adenine nucleotides remain in the platelets (Holmsen et al., 1969). From this we can conclude that there are two main pools of adenine nucleotides in platelets:

(1) A 'metabolic pool'; readily labelled with radioactive adenine or adenosine, not released from platelets during the release reaction, and presumably localised in the mitochondria, cytosol and membranes.

(2) A 'non-metabolic pool', or 'storage pool'; not labelled with radioactive adenine or adenosine, but released during the release reaction. This pool is localised in the dense bodies.

A slow exchange between the metabolic pool and the storage pool can occur (Reimers et al., 1975).

Platelets respond to stimulation by increasing glycolytic and Krebs-cycle activity (Holmsen, 1972). During the release reaction, ATP from the metabolic pool is consumed and metabolised to hypoxanthine (Fig. 2). Holmsen et al. (1969) showed that this ATP – hypoxanthine conversion was associated with release but not with shape-change or aggregation. They suggested that the conversion utilised

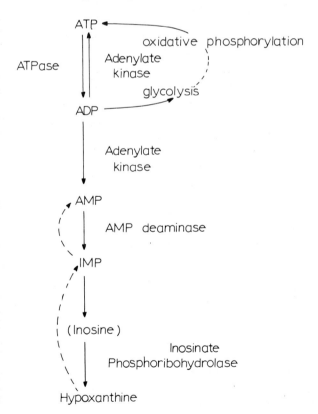

Fig. 2

a specific 'release energy' pool of ATP, and that energy liberated during the conversion was required for the release reaction. Other studies, however, showed that ATP – hypoxanthine conversion occurred, albeit slowly, in resting platelets (Holmsen and Rozenberg, 1968) and in stimulated platelets treated with metabolic inhibitors (Holmsen et al., 1974) – situations where no release reaction occurred. Also, Holmsen (1975) later showed that adenine–hypoxanthine conversion could be inhibited without affecting release, and Ball et al. (1969) showed that a greater conversion of ATP to hypoxanthine occurred during the release reaction when ATP resynthesis was blocked by metabolic inhibitors. It therefore seems that the amount of ATP–hypoxanthine conversion in platelets under various conditions is merely a reflection of the extent to which platelets cannot compensate energy-consuming reactions by rapid ATP resynthesis.

Holmsen and coworkers (1974) and Holmsen (1975) have shown that the platelet shape-change, aggregation, and the release reaction all require a critical level of metabolic ATP, and all are completely inhibited if the steady-state level of ATP falls below this value.

The same group of workers studied the metabolic requirements for release I and release II under different conditions and concluded that the ATP consumed during the release reaction is not utilised in processes directly involved in the release mechanism (Holmsen, 1975); the energy-consuming part of the release reaction apparently occurs in the resting cell, and this energy is stored in the form of a myosin–ADP complex (mechanical energy), being liberated when the cell is activated.

The increased metabolic activity of stimulated platelets is not due to direct stimulation of metabolic pathways by various aggregating agents and release inducers (Holmsen, 1972); rather, the enhanced activity of key enzymes in glycolysis and oxidative phosphorylation is determined by the adenylate energy charge of the system (Atkinson, 1968), where

$$\text{Adenylate energy charge} = \frac{((\text{ATP}) + \frac{1}{2}(\text{ADP}))}{(\text{ATP} + \text{ADP} + \text{AMP})}$$

Any decrease in the adenylate energy charge tends to increase the rates of reactions controlling ATP regeneration – possibly by causing allosteric changes on regulator enzymes (Karpatkin and Langer, 1968). Since the sequence of reactions *shape change → aggregation → release I → release II* is progressively energy-consuming and is associated with a decrease in the adenylate energy charge, there is activation of regulatory enzymes and consequently stimulation of metabolic activity (Weiss, 1975).

2.2. Morphology

The platelet release reaction is associated with loss of platelet granules; these move centripetally and cluster in the centre of the cell, surrounded by a band of microtubules (White, 1971; see Fig. 3). This centralisation has been termed the 'contractile wave', and Hovig (1974) suggested that polymerised cytoplasmic

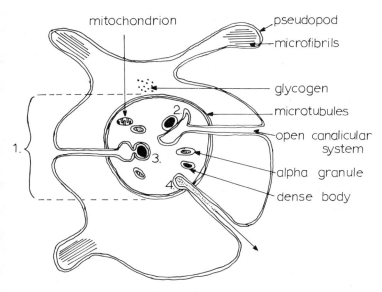

1. Centralisation of platelet organelles.

2. Platelet granule comes into contact with membrane of the open canalicular system

3. Fusion of granule membrane with open canalicular system membrane.

4. Granule contents extruded into the open canalicular system from which they diffuse into the surrounding milieu.

Fig. 3

thrombosthenin (i.e., actomyosin) could be responsible for this (see Chapter 6 for a detailed discussion on the composition and function of platelet contractile proteins). Although the precise means by which the granule contents are extruded remains to be determined, it is generally accepted that the granule membranes fuse with the inner parts of the surface-connected canalicular system, and the contents diffuse out (Fig. 3). The presence of platelet granule contents in the open canalicular system during the release reaction has been demonstrated by White (1972) and by Holme and coworkers (1973).

2.3. Stimulus-secretion coupling

2.3.1. Calcium-dependence

The platelet release reaction can be induced by some stimuli in the presence of high concentrations of EGTA, indicating that it is independent of extracellular calcium, but extracellular calcium is essential for the release reaction which accompanies platelet aggregation (Holmsen and Day, 1968; Robblee et al., 1973). Moreover, no uptake of ^{45}Ca by platelets is detectable during the thrombin-induced release reaction (Murer and Holme, 1970; Robblee et al., 1973). Day and Holmsen (1971) suggested that energy from ATP metabolism along with *intracellular* calcium initiated contraction of platelet thrombosthenin, bringing about centralisation of organelles and approximation of platelet granules to the open canalicular system.

The intracellular calcium storage site in platelets has been variously reported as being membrane-associated (Statland et al., 1969), localised in dense bodies (Martin et al., 1974), and localised in alpha granules (Sato et al., 1975). It is, however, quite conceivable that there are several calcium storage pools in platelets, each of which serves a different function.

2.3.2. Initiating stimuli

Holmsen et al. (1969) proposed that the platelet release reaction be considered as having three stages, namely, *induction, transmission*, and *extrusion*, and suggested that since the mechanisms of intracellular transmission and granular extrusion were apparently similar for all release inducers, differences which were observed must be associated with the induction phase.

Massini and Lüscher (1972) suggested that inducers of the platelet release reaction – with the exception of thrombin and other proteolytic enzymes – have a common requirement for platelet–surface contact to cause the release reaction. The 'surface' in question may be either a separate particulate entity–such as collagen or immune complexes – or, in the case of ADP and adrenaline, it may be the platelets themselves.

That platelet–platelet contact ('propinquity') can induce the platelet release reaction was first observed by O'Brien and Woodhouse (1968) who showed that centrifugation of platelets at 37°C caused release of ADP. Massini and Lüscher (1971) extended these findings and reported that platelets must first be 'conditioned' in some way, before cell contact can induce the release reaction.

In our laboratory we recently investigated the kinetics of the release of platelet 5HT induced by microfibrillar collagen. Two phases of release were evident: the first phase occurred rapidly (<60s) and the second phase accompanied platelet aggregate formation. Reuptake of 5HT between the first and second phase of release was observed. Pre-incubation of platelets with 7.5 mM-EDTA abolished the second phase of release but did not influence the first phase. Since EDTA inhibits platelet aggregation but has no effect on binding of collagen to platelets (MacIntyre and Gordon, 1975), we concluded that the first phase of release was associated with binding of collagen to platelets. Further studies established that the first phase of release was only evident when samples were centrifuged (20°C: 14,800 g) for 60s or longer in the presence of collagen, and we reasoned that centrifugation in the presence of collagen 'conditioned' the platelets to undergo a release reaction upon platelet–platelet contact.

The release of platelet constituents induced by thrombin and other proteolytic enzymes differs from that induced by other stimuli in that platelet-surface contact is not a prerequisite (Massini and Lüscher, 1972) and release can be induced in the absence of extracellular calcium (Murer and Holme, 1970; Robblee et al., 1973). Thrombin is a proteolytic enzyme with specificity for arginyl side chains (Weinstein and Doolittle, 1972), and in order to stimulate the platelet release reaction, thrombin must bind to a specific protein on the platelet membrane (see Chapter 8) and hydrolyse a susceptible peptide (Davey and Lüscher, 1967; Phillips and Agin, 1973). Proteolytic enzymes with similar substrate specificity (e.g., trypsin and papain) also induce the platelet release reaction, but enzymes such as chymotrypsin and plasmin, with little specificity for arginyl residues, have no effect (Martin et al., 1975).

The characteristics of the platelet release reaction induced by immune complexes and complement are reviewed in Chapter 12.

ADP and adrenaline induce release of dense body constituents only (release I), and as they act by stimulating the formation of platelet aggregates, they require extracellular calcium (Smith and Macfarlane, 1974). This type of release reaction is another in which the platelets are 'conditioned' by the stimulus such that subsequent platelet–platelet contact induces release.

Divalent cation ionophores have been reported to induce the platelet release reaction (Feinman and Detwiler, 1974; Massini and Lüscher, 1974; White et al., 1974; Worner and Brossmer, 1975). The release reaction induced by the divalent cation ionophore A23187 occurs in the presence of EGTA, and could therefore be mediated by mobilisation of calcium from an intracellular source (Feinman and Detwiler, 1974). Most studies with A23187 have measured release I only, but Detwiler et al. (1975) suggested that A23187 can mediate all of the platelet responses which can be induced by thrombin.

2.3.3. Intracellular control

The roles of prostaglandin endoperoxides and non-prostanoate derivatives of arachidonic acid in platelet function are fully discussed in Chapter 13. These agents may be the main chemical trigger for the release reaction (Willis, 1974; Hamberg et al., 1975), and their formation is abolished by aspirin, through acetylation of the cyclo-oxygenase enzyme of the prostaglandin synthase complex (Roth et al., 1975).

Aspirin abolishes release I induced by ADP, adrenaline or low concentrations of collagen, but has no effect on release II, or on release I induced by high concentrations of collagen or thrombin (Smith and Willis, 1971; Smith and Macfarlane, 1974; Holmsen et al., 1975). Aspirin also has no effect on the release reaction induced by A23187 (Salzman, 1975).

Agents which elevate cellular cAMP levels inhibit the platelet release reaction (Mills and Smith, 1971; Mills and Macfarlane, Chapter 7). Release induced by ADP, adrenaline, and thrombin can be abolished by PGE_1 which increases cAMP by stimulating adenylate cyclase, but there is some controversy concerning the effect of PGE_1 on release induced by A23187 (White et al., 1974; Friedman and Detwiler, 1975). Release induced by platelet–collagen binding is much less susceptible than aggregation-associated release to inhibition by PGE_1.

In many biological systems the effects of cAMP and cGMP are mutually antagonistic (Goldberg et al., 1973), and Haslam and McClenaghan (1974) showed that release of platelet constituents (release I) induced by collagen is parallelled by an increase in the concentration of platelet cGMP. However, no causal relationship between this increase in platelet cGMP and the platelet release reaction has yet been established (Haslam, 1975).

Platelet structural and contractile proteins are the subject of a detailed review in Chapter 6, but as their role in the platelet release reaction has been the subject of some debate, a few brief comments are appropriate here. The role of microfilaments in cell function has often been investigated using cytochalasin B, which disrupts microfilaments (Wessels et al., 1971), although the actions of this compound are not restricted to microfilaments (Estensen and Plagemann, 1972). Haslam et al. (1975) showed that both release I and release II induced by collagen were potentiated by low concentrations of cytochalasin B, though inhibited by higher concentrations. Similarly, release induced by thrombin and A23187 is potentiated by low concentrations of cytochalasin B (Friedman and Detwiler, 1975). Disruption of microfilaments may facilitate exocytosis, but there is no convincing evidence for this at present. Microtubules are involved in secretory processes in several cells (Allison, 1973), but unusually high concentrations of microtubule binding reagents (e.g., colchicine and Vinca alkaloids) are necessary to inhibit the platelet release reaction induced by collagen, thrombin or A23187 (Friedman and Detwiler, 1975), and consequently it is debatable whether microtubules play a direct role in platelet secretion.

Calcium ions apparently play a vital role in the secretory process (Holmsen, 1972; Haslam, 1975), and one means of controlling platelet secretion would be by regulating the amount of calcium available. Booyse et al. (1973) postulated that this could be achieved by a calcium-binding protein on the platelet membrane which existed in two forms: a phosphorylated form (maintained by a cAMP-dependent protein kinase) which could sequester calcium, and a non-phosphorylated form (maintained by a phosphoprotein phosphatase) which could not. This control system is similar to that proposed by Statland et al. (1969). At equilibrium, the protein would normally be phosphorylated, with little free calcium – insufficient to activate the secretory process. When the equilibrium was disturbed and dephosphorylation occurred, intracellular calcium levels would increase, initiating the release reaction (Fig. 4). Dephosphorylation could be induced in the following ways:

(1) Competing with the binding protein for the cAMP dependent protein kinase – as apparently occurs with ADP, collagen and thrombin (Booyse et al., 1975).

(2) Activation of the phosphoprotein phosphatase – apparently caused by adrenaline in platelets (Booyse et al., 1975) and by cGMP in other tissues (Smith and Ignarro, 1975).

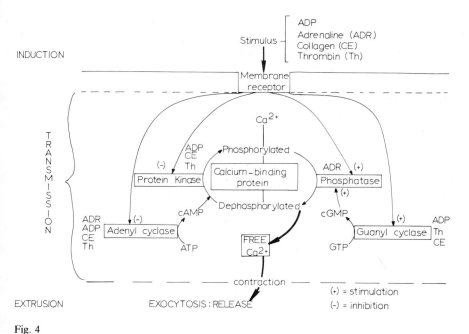

Fig. 4

(3) Reduction in the level of cAMP. It should be noted that if the functional pool of cAMP is only a small proportion of the total, as may be the case in platelets (Haslam, 1975), then a reduction in such a pool would be difficult to detect. Divalent cation ionophores would be expected to mobilise calcium without affecting either the kinase or the phosphatase.

2.3.4. Summary

The mechanisms responsible for the release of platelet constituents are still the subject of considerable research, but current evidence suggest that there could be several routes involved.

Collagen or thrombin can release platelet 5HT and ADP even when platelet prostaglandin biosynthesis is abolished (Smith and Willis, 1971; Willis and Weiss, 1973), indicating that there are prostaglandin synthase-dependent and independent release processes. Release II is not apparently mediated by prostaglandin synthase: Willis et al. (1974) showed that prostaglandin endoperoxides induced release of ADP and 5HT, but not of lysosomal enzymes. Hence, it appears that there are at least two mechanisms that can cause release of ADP and 5HT from platelets, and possibly a separate mechanism involved in the discharge of alpha granule contents. Calcium ions are apparently essential in all these processes, although it should be emphasised that only when release depends on platelet aggregation is extracellular calcium necessary. It is also possible that different release mechanisms may utilise different intracellular calcium pools. Although the precise means by which the intracellular liberation of ionised calcium causes the release reaction remains to be determined, we can conclude that platelet degranulation is an example of calcium-mediated exocytosis.

3. Secretion by polymorphonuclear leukocytes

Neutrophils, the most abundant of the blood leukocytes in man, are about 10 μm or more in diameter and contain 50–200 granules, which vary in size and electron density. Two distinct classes of granule are evident (Bainton et al., 1971; see Fig. 5):

(1) Large (0.5–0.8 μm), electron-dense granules, called primary or azurophilic.
(2) Smaller (0.25–0.4 μm), less-dense granules, called secondary or specific.

Azurophil granules contain acid phosphatase and other acid hydrolases, aryl sulphatase and peroxidase; specific granules contain alkaline phosphatase but not acid hydrolases or peroxidase. Lysozyme is present in both azurophilic and specific granules, though mainly in the latter.

Early in an inflammatory reaction polymorphonuclear leukocytes adhere to venule endothelium in the inflamed area, then migrate through the vessel wall, attracted by chemotaxis to the invading microorganism, which they phagocytose. The bactericidal components of the neutrophil specific granules (lysozyme) are secreted into the phagocytic vacuole and kill the bacterium; its destruction is completed by the lysosomal enzymes of the primary granules.

Polymorphonuclear leukocytes derive over 90% of their energy supply from glycolysis, which allows them to function in anaerobic conditions – for example, in avascular, necrotic tissue. During phagocytosis there is a marked increase in metabolic activity and an increase in oxygen uptake (Hirsch, 1974).

The contents of polymorphonuclear leukocyte granules are discharged intracellularly when the azurophilic and specific granules fuse with the phagocytic vacuoles (Fig. 6), but exocytotic degranulation also occcurs during the phagocytosis of particles (May et al., 1970) or when cells are exposed to immune complexes immobilised on a non-phagocytosable surface (Henson, 1971). The constituents thus released can cause tissue damage (for review see Janoff, 1970).

3.1. Stimulus-secretion coupling

Leukocyte degranulation requires extracellular calcium ions (Smith and Ignarro, 1975; Lichtenstein, 1975; Siraganian and Siraganian, 1975), and Smith and Ignarro (1975) have shown that calcium accumulates in the cells following stimulation.

Leukocyte degranulation can be induced in vitro by a number of stimuli:
(1) Phagocytosis of particulate matter.
(2) Immune complexes.
(3) Divalent cation ionophores.
(4) Lectins.

Henson (1971) showed that when rabbit neutrophil leukocytes were stimulated

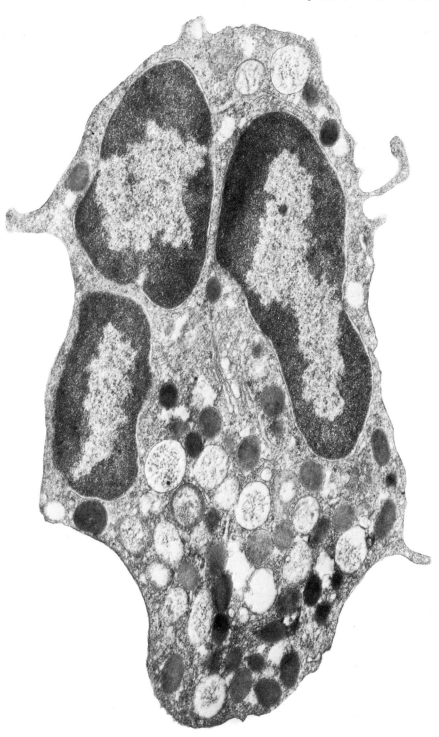

Fig. 5. Rabbit polymorphonuclear leukocyte, obtained by peritoneal lavage following injection of glycogen. Original magnification ×21,000. (Kindly provided by Dr. Kareen Thorne, Strangeways Research Laboratory, Cambridge.)

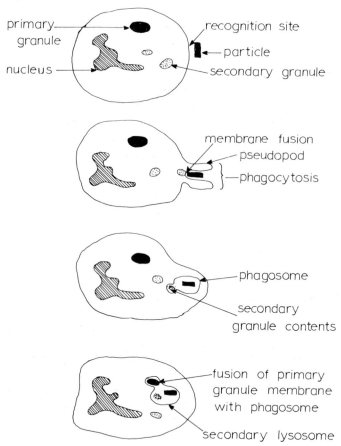

primary granule

recognition site

nucleus

particle

secondary granule

membrane fusion

pseudopod

phagocytosis

phagosome

secondary granule contents

fusion of primary granule membrane with phagosome

secondary lysosome

Fig. 6

by immobilised immune complexes, specific granule constituents (alkaline phosphatase) were released before azurophilic granule constituents (β-glucuronidase).

Smith and Ignarro (1975) compared release of lysosomal enzymes from neutrophil leukocytes induced by immune complexes and A23187, and showed that the secretory process was calcium-dependent, energy-dependent and temperature-dependent. Lichtenstein (1975) obtained similar results when studying histamine release from basophil leukocytes.

Release is accompanied by increased cGMP levels (Smith and Ignarro, 1975), and agents which increase cAMP (e.g., adrenaline, PGE_1, cholera toxin) inhibit release, whereas agents which increase cGMP (e.g., cholinergic reagents, $PGF_{2\alpha}$) enhance release (Gillespie and Lichtenstein, 1973). Colchicine (in micromolar concentrations) inhibits lysosomal enzyme release from neutrophils and histamine release from basophils induced by a variety of stimuli, including immune complexes, phagocytosis, and A23187 (Weissman et al., 1975a; Lichtenstein, 1975). Weissman et al. (1975b) counted microtubules within neutrophils and showed that inhibition of lysosomal enzyme release from neutrophils was associated with transient microtubule disassembly, whereas stimulation of release was associated with polymerisation of cytoplasmic microtubules. D_2O, which stabilises microtubules, enhances secretion from both neutrophils and basophils (Gillespie and Lichtenstein, 1973; Weissman et al., 1975a).

Lichtenstein (1975) observed that agents increasing cAMP levels in basophil leukocytes inhibited release of histamine induced by immune complexes without affecting that induced by A23187; however, colchicine and inhibitors of glycolysis inhibited both processes. He therefore concluded that this release could be separated into two stages:

(1) Antigen-dependent; Ca^{2+}-independent; inhibited by increased cAMP.

(2) Calcium-dependent; antigen-independent; inhibited by disruption of microtubules and by glycolysis inhibitors.

3.2. Summary

The available evidence suggests that increased cellular levels of cGMP and calcium are involved in mediating secretion from leukocytes, whereas increased cAMP levels inhibit this process.

Smith and Ignarro (1975) suggested that influx of Ca^{2+} is a prerequisite for cGMP formation, but the complement component C5a can apparently induce release in the absence of extracellular calcium (Weissman et al., 1975b); this release may, however, involve a different mechanism.

Lichtenstein (1975) and Weissman et al. (1975a,b) suggest that release is associated with transient assembly of microtubules, and that agents causing decreased cAMP or increased cGMP enhance microtubule assembly, whereas agents causing increased cAMP inhibit microtubule assembly. Weissman et al. (1975b) have isolated a cAMP-dependent protein kinase, and suggested that inhibition of release is associated with phosphorylation of an as yet unidentified substrate (cf. Section 2.3.3.).

4. Secretion by mast cells

Mast cells, which are apparently derived from undifferentiated mesenchymal cells, are mainly located in loose connective tissue (Bloom, 1974). There is considerable interspecies variation in mast cell characteristics, but the most commonly studied is the rat peritoneal mast cell: these are around 13 μm in diameter, and contain about 1000 granules, as well as rough endoplasmic reticulum, cytoplasmic microtubules, mitochondria, and Golgi apparatus (see Fig. 7).

Mast cell granules, which originate in the Golgi apparatus (Combs, 1966) contain heparin (Parekh and Glick, 1962) and histamine (Benditt et al., 1956). Other amines are also present in some species–5HT in rat and mouse, and dopamine in sheep and ox. Cytochrome oxidase, acid and alkaline phosphatase,

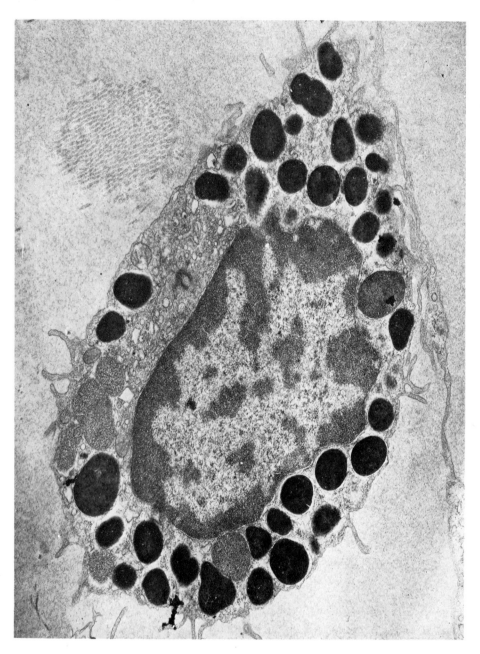

Fig. 7. Mast cell in the mesentery of the rat. Original magnification ×21,000. (Kindly provided by Dr. J.L. Gordon.)

and proteinases have also been found in mast cell granules (Bloom, 1974; Lagunoff and Benditt, 1963).

Although the physiological role of mast cells is unclear, constituents released from mast cells contribute to the inflammatory process: for example, histamine and 5HT can increase capillary permeability and stimulate phagocytosis (Bloom, 1974), and proteolytic enzymes can prolong the vascular component of the inflammatory response by reacting with tissue fluid proteins to generate kinins (Keller, 1966).

4.1. Stimulus-secretion coupling

Discharge of mast cell granules contents can be induced by several agents:
(1) Immune complexes.
(2) Polyamines e.g., compound 48/80.
(3) Dextran.
(4) Proteinases.
(5) Divalent cation ionophores.

Thon and Uvnas (1967) showed that release of histamine from mast cells took place in two stages:

(a) Exposure of granules to the extracellular milieu.

(b) Displacement of amines from granules by exchange between sodium ions and bound histamine (Uvnas, 1974; see Fig. 8). Release of granule constituents is selective–cytoplasmic constituents (e.g., lactic dehydrogenase, potassium and ADP) are retained (Johnson and Moran, 1969), as, indeed, are some of the granule constituents, in the form of an insoluble complex of protein and heparin (Lagunoff, 1972).

Electron microscopy has revealed that secretion of granule contents occurs by exocytosis (Bloom and Chakravarty, 1970; Rohlich et al., 1971), and Douglas (1974b) showed that when mast cells are stimulated by compound 48/80, exocytosis can be either *Simple* (a single granule fusing with the plasma membrane) or *Compound* (several granule membranes fusing together, leading to simultaneous exposure of their contents to the exterior).

Release of histamine from mast cells induced by immune complexes, dextrans, ATP and proteolytic enzymes is calcium-dependent (Foreman and Mongar, 1972; Lagunoff et al., 1975), although Uvnas and Thon (1961) reported that compound 48/80 could induce release in a calcium-free medium. Douglas and Ueda (1973) later showed that 48/80-induced histamine release could be abolished by *prolonged* incubation of the cells with EDTA, implying that 48/80-induced histamine release requires intracellular calcium ions, and Kanno and coworkers (1973) showed that the intracellular injection of Ca^{2+} by means of a micropipette was sufficient to initiate exocytosis. A23187 can also induce exocytosis of histamine from mast cells, provided that extracellular calcium is present and the cells are metabolically active (Foreman et al., 1973; Kagayama and Douglas, 1974). Mast cells derive their metabolic energy both by oxidative phosphorylation and by glycolysis, and the role of energy metabolism in mast cell exocytosis has recently been reviewed by Peterson (1974).

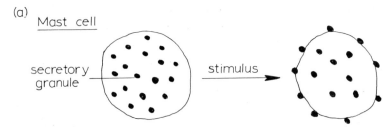

(a)

Mast cell

secretory granule

stimulus

Exposure of granules to extracellular milieu.

(b) Secretory granule

Heparin–protein histamine complex

Displacement of histamine by sodium

Fig. 8

Mast cells contain large amounts of a chymotrypsin-like enzyme, and Lagunoff and Benditt (1963) suggested that this might be involved in exocytosis; Becker and Austen (1966) showed that activation of a chymotrypsin zymogen was necessary for secretory activity. Exogenous α-chymotrypsin can induce release of histamine from mast cells, provided extracellular calcium is present (Lagunoff et al., 1975).

Baxter (1972) showed that adrenergic drugs, theophylline (a phosphodiesterase inhibitor), and dibutyryl cAMP all inhibited dextran-induced histamine release, implying that the intracellular cAMP level was important. This was later confirmed by Johnson et al. (1974) and Kaliner and Austen (1974), although increasing cAMP had no effect on ionophore-induced release (Johnson et al., 1974; Foreman and Gomperts, 1975), which suggests that the cAMP-sensitive stage may be associated with Ca^{2+} influx. Kaliner and coworkers (1972) suggested that increased cGMP levels could enhance release, but adding dibutyryl cGMP apparently had no effect (Renoux et al., 1974).

Phosphatidyl serine enhances secretion induced by antigen and dextran, but not that induced by compound 48/80 (Goth et al., 1971), because phosphatidyl serine's effect occurs only in the presence of calcium (Mongar and Svec, 1972), and compound 48/80 requires minimal extracellular calcium (Douglas and Ueda, 1973). Foreman and Mongar (1973) proposed that histamine release is controlled by 'gates' in the cell membrane which regulate passage of Ca^{2+} into the cell, and Foreman and Gomperts (1975) suggested that phosphatidyl serine acts by delaying the closure of these calcium 'gates'. Since 48/80 apparently utilises cellular calcium stores, and the ionophore A23187 presumably does not need to pass through the calcium 'gate', it is interesting that exocytosis induced by these agents is little affected by an increase in cAMP. This suggests that cellular cAMP levels may control calcium influx (gate opening) (Fig. 9).

The role of microtubules in histamine secretion from mast cells was studied by Tolone et al. (1974), who used colchicine and vinblastine. Both these agents at concentrations around 10^{-5} M inhibited release induced by 48/80, suggesting that microtubules are important in the secretory process. Douglas and Ueda (1973) showed that cytochalasin B had little effect on mast cell secretion under normal aerobic conditions, and although it was inhibitory in cells utilising extracellular glucose, this was apparently due to inhibition of glucose uptake.

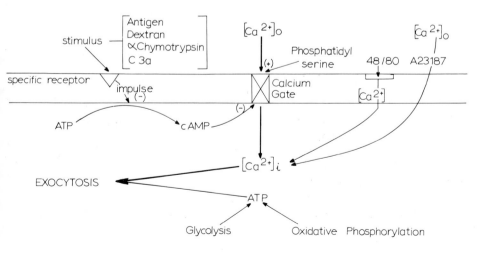

Fig. 9

5. Secretion by adrenal chromaffin cells

There are two types of adrenal medullary chromaffin cells: those with small, electron-dense granules, containing noradrenaline (N-cells); and the more abundant adrenaline-containing cells with larger, less electron-dense granules (A-cells) (Costa, 1973). The granules contain catecholamines, ATP and a 'packing protein', chromogranin (Douglas and Poisner, 1966), as well as a magnesium-dependent ATPase (Trifaro and Poisner, 1967) and dopamine-β-oxidase (Viveros et al., 1968). Lysosomes are also present in chromaffin cells, (Smith and Winkler, 1966) and lysosomal constituents are secreted in parallel with the catecholamines.

5.1. Stimulus-secretion coupling

The physiological stimulus for the secretory response is acetylcholine (liberated from the preganglionic sympathetic fibres which innervate the adrenal medulla) and Rubin (1970) showed that energy metabolism of chromaffin cells was essential for secretion. Several stimuli can cause release of catecholamines from chromaffin cells:

(1) Acetylcholine.
(2) Potassium ions.
(3) Angiotensin.
(4) Histamine.
(5) 5HT.
(6) Proteolytic enzymes (e.g., thrombin and trypsin).
(7) Sympathomimetic amines.
(8) Divalent cation ionophores.

The observation that granule contents were secreted (Douglas, 1968), whereas cytoplasmic constituents were retained implied a selective release process, and Diner (1967) confirmed that exocytosis occurred (for review, see Douglas, 1968).

Douglas and Rubin (1961) showed that extracellular calcium was necessary for acetylcholine to induce release of catecholamines from the adrenal medulla, and Douglas and coworkers (1967) showed that acetylcholine depolarised the chromaffin cell membrane by inducing an influx of sodium and calcium. Sodium influx is not necessary for secretion, however; acetylcholine-induced release is actually enhanced in a sodium-free medium. Methyl xanthines, (caffeine and theophylline), apparently stimulate catecholamine release in the absence of calcium (Poisner, 1973), possibly by liberating calcium from intracellular stores. The microsomes, mitochondria, and chromaffin granules of these cells can all take up calcium, and agents which stimulate catecholamine release in the absence of extracellular calcium all apparently prevent calcium uptake by microsomes (Borowitz, 1969; Poisner and Hava, 1970).

The role of cyclic nucleotides in controlling secretion from the adrenal medullary chromaffin cells is as yet unresolved (Rasmussen, 1970; Williams, 1974), but contractile proteins are undoubtedly important. Douglas and Sorimachi (1972) showed that colchicine inhibited catecholamine release induced by acetylcholine, although it had little effect on that induced by potassium ions. Cytochalasin B was even more effective than colchicine, but again the acetylcholine response was more readily inhibited than the potassium response. Poisner and Cooke (1975) tested several microtubule 'poisons' and showed that catecholamine release was inhibited by concentrations which did not affect other cell functions. They concluded that microtubules were intimately involved in the physiological secretory process in chromaffin cells, and suggested that the lack of effect of microtubule 'poisons' on release induced by potassium was because potassium utilised calcium from a different source than that utilised by acetylcholine. Microtubules are apparently only involved in acetylcholine-induced release (Rahwan et al., 1973).

6. Discussion

This review summarises our present knowledge of the platelet release reaction and compares it with stimulated secretion in other cells, using as examples a mature, circulating cell (the polymorphonuclear leukocyte), an isolated connective-tissue cell (the mast cell), and an innervated cell in an organised tissue (the adrenal medullary chromaffin cell). Each secretory process involves the selective liberation of granule contents in response to specific stimuli.

There are significant differences in the stimuli to which the different cells respond, but the mechanism of intracellular transmission is essentially similar in each case, involving calcium ions, contractile proteins, and (usually) cyclic nucleotides. In addition, the final event in each secretory process is apparently the same – that is, *exocytosis*, or the fusion of the granule membrane with part of the plasma membrane of the cell – although, in the platelet, which has a complex, surface-connected canalicular system, the storage granules move centripetally just before fusion (in contrast to the peripheral migration of granules seen in other cells).

The basic similarity between the platelet release reaction and other examples of stimulated secretion prompts the question 'how can studies with platelets help to elucidate the mechanisms involved in stimulus-secretion coupling'? For answers, we need only turn to other parts of this volume: for example, Crawford discusses in Chapter 6 how studies of platelet microtubules and microfilaments have increased our understanding of the physiological roles of contractile proteins; Mills and Macfarlane (Chapter 7) emphasise the value of platelet studies in investigating the role of cyclic nucleotides in intracellular control mechanisms; and Smith and Silver (Chapter 13) highlight the importance of prostaglandin synthesis in the platelet release reaction, and discuss how recent platelet studies have added a new dimension to prostaglandin research.

Virtually all examples of stimulus-secretion coupling so far investigated are in some respects calcium-dependent, and the variable calcium-dependence of the platelet-release reaction induced by different stimuli makes it possible to address the question of whether there may be different mechanisms of stimulus-secretion

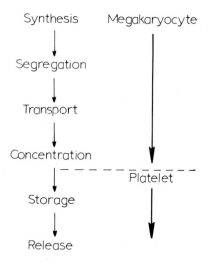

Fig. 10

coupling involving separate calcium sources. Some stimuli cause the platelet release reaction by inducing platelet aggregation, and since aggregation needs extracellular calcium ions, the release reaction induced by such stimuli is inhibited by extracellular chelating agents. Other stimuli apparently liberate calcium ions from intracellular stores, and since platelets contain two easily-distinguished granule populations (whose contents are not always released in parallel), studies with such stimuli could help to establish whether there are different mechanisms of stimulus-secretion coupling (for example, using different calcium stores) for discharging the contents of separate granule populations.

One advantage of using platelets in studies of stimulus-secretion coupling is that they are readily obtained as a homogeneous population of intact cells, without any tissue disruption being necessary. Unlike the other cells discussed in this review, platelets are unsuitable for studying the early stages of the secretion process because, being anucleate, they are incapable of protein synthesis, segregation, and concentration (Palade, 1975); these processes take place in the precursor megakaryocyte (Fig. 10). However, platelets admirably perform the functions of storage and release and can justifiably be regarded as excellent cellular models for investigating the steps involved in these processes; from the identification and function of membrane receptors for specific stimuli, through the mechanisms of intracellular transmission, to the final discharge of granule contents.

References

Allison, A.C. (1973) in Locomotion of tissue cells, Ciba Foundation Symposium 14, 109.
Atkinson, D.E. (1968) Biochemistry, 7, 4030.

Bainton, D.F., Ullyot, J.L. and Farquhar, M.G. (1971) J. Exp. Med., *134*, 907.
Ball, G., Fulwood, M., Ireland, D.M. and Yates, P. (1969) Biochem. J., *114*, 669.
Baxter, J.H. (1972) Proc. Soc. Exp. Biol. Med., *141*, 576.
Becker, E.L. and Austen, K.F. (1966) J. Exp. Med., *124*, 379.
Benditt, E.P., Arase, M. and Roeper, E. (1956) J. Histochem. Cytochem., *4*, 419.
Bennett, H.S. (1956) J. Biophys. Biochem. Cytol., Suppl. *2*, 99.
Bentfield, M.E. and Bainton, D.F. (1975) J. Clin. Invest., *56*, 1635.
Bito, L.Z. (1975) Prostaglandins, *9*, 851.
Bloom, G.D. (1974) in The Inflammatory Process (Zweifach, B.W., Grant, L. and McCluskey, R.T., eds), p. 545, Academic Press, New York.
Bloom, G.D. and Chakravarty, N. (1970) Acta Physiol. Scand., *78*, 410.
Booyse, F.M., Guilani, D., Marr, J.J. and Rafelson, M.E. (1973) Ser. Haemat., *6*, 351.
Booyse, F.M., Marr, J.J., Tomlinson, D., Yang, D.C. and Rafelson, M.E. (1975) Thromb. Diath. Haemorrh., *34*, 558.
Borowitz, J.L. (1969) Biochem. Pharmacol., *18*, 75.
Combs, J.W. (1966) J. Cell. Biol., *31*, 563.
Costa, J.L. (1973) Comp. Gen. Endocrinol., *20*, 498.
Davey, M.G. and Lüscher, E.F. (1967) Nature, *216*, 857.
Day, H.J. and Holmsen, H. (1971) Semin. Haematol., *4*, 3.
De Duve, C. (1963) in Endocytosis in Lysosomes, Ciba Foundation Symposium, p. 126.
Detwiler, T.C., Martin, B.M. and Feinman, R.D. (1975) in Biochemistry and Pharmacology of platelets, Ciba Foundation Symposium, *35*, p. 77.
Diner, O. (1967) C.R.S. Acad. Sci., *265*, 616.
Doery, J.C.G., Hirsh, J. and De Gruchy, G.C. (1970) Haematologica, *4*, 405.
Douglas, W.W. (1968) Brit. J. Pharmacol., *34*, 451.
Douglas, W.W. (1974a). Biochem. Soc. Symp. *39*, 1.
Douglas, W.W. (1974b) in Secretory Mechanisms of Exocrine Glands (Thorn, N.A. and Peterson, D.H., eds), p. 116, Munksgaard, Copenhagen.
Douglas, W.W., Kanno, T. and Sampson, S.R. (1967) J. Physiol., *188*, 107.
Douglas, W.W. and Poisner, A.M. (1966) J. Physiol., *183*, 236.
Douglas, W.W. and Rubin, R.P. (1961) J. Physiol. *159*, 40.
Douglas, W.W. and Sorimachi, M. (1972) Brit. J. Pharmacol., *45*, 129.
Douglas, W.W. and Ueda, Y. (1973) J. Physiol., *234*, 97P.
Estensen, R.D. and Plagemann, P.G.W. (1972) Proc. Natl. Acad. Sci. U.S.A. *69*, 1430.
Feinman, R.D. and Detwiler, T.C. (1974) Nature, *249*, 172.
Foreman, J.C. and Gomperts, B.D. (1975) Int. Arch. Allergy, *49*, 179.
Foreman, J.C. and Mongar, J.L. (1972) J. Physiol., *224*, 753.
Foreman, J.C., Mongar, J.L. and Gomperts, B.D. (1973) Nature, *245*, 249.
Friedman, F. and Detwiler, T.C. (1975) Biochemistry, *14*, 1315.
Gillespie, E. and Lichtenstein, L.M. (1973) Int. Arch. Allergy, *45*, 95.
Goldberg, N.D., O'Dea, R.F. and Haddok, M.K. (1973) Adv. Cyclic Nucleotide Res., *3*, 155.
Gordon, J.L. (1975) in Lysosomes (Dingle, J.T. and Dean, R.T., eds), Vol. 4, p. 3, North-Holland, Amsterdam.
Goth, A., Adams, H.R. and Knoohuizen, M. (1971) Science, *173*, 1034.
Grette, K. (1962) Acta Physiol. Scand. Suppl., *56*, 195.
Hamberg, M., Svensson, J. and Samuelsson, B. (1975) Proc. Natl. Acad. Sci. U.S.A., *72*, 2994.
Haslam, R.J. (1975) in Biochemistry and Pharmacology of platelets. Ciba Foundation Symposium, *35*, p. 121.
Haslam, R.J., Davidson, M.M.L. and McClenachan, M.D. (1975) Nature, *253*, 455.
Haslam, R.J. and McClenachan, M.D. (1974) Biochem. J., *138*, 317.
Henson, P.M. (1971) J. Immunol., *107*, 1535.
Hirsch, J.G. (1974) in The Inflammatory Process (Zweifach, B.W., Grant, L. and McCluskey, R.T., eds), p. 411, Academic Press, New York.
Holme, R., Sixma, J.J., Murer, E.H. and Hovig, T. (1973) Thromb. Res., *3*, 347.
Holmsen, H. (1972) Clin. Haematol., *1*, 235.
Holmsen, H. (1975) in Biochemistry and Pharmacology of platelets. Ciba Foundation Symposium 35, p. 175.
Holmsen, H. and Day, H.J. (1968) Nature, *219*, 760.
Holmsen, H. and Day, H.J. (1970) J. Lab. Clin. Med., *75*, 840.
Holmsen, H., Day, H.J. and Stormorken, H. (1969) Scand. J. Haematol. Suppl., *8*, 3.

Holmsen, H. and Rozenberg, M.C. (1968) Biochim. Biophys. Acta, *157*, 266.
Holmsen, H., Setkowsky, C.A. and Day, H.J. (1974) Biochem. J., *144*, 385.
Holmsen, H., Setkowsky, C.A., Lages, B., Day, H.J., Weiss, H.J. and Scrutton, M.C. (1975) Blood, *46*, 131.
Hovig, T. (1974) in Platelets: production, function, transfusion and storage (Baldini, M.G. and Ebbe, S., eds), p. 221, Grune and Stratton, New York.
Janoff, A. (1970) Ser. Haematol., *3*, 96.
Johnson, A.R. and Moran, N.C. (1969) Fed. Proc., *28*, 1716.
Johnson, A.R., Moran, N.C. and Meyer, S.E. (1974) J. Immunol., *112*, 511.
Katz, B. (1962) Proc. Roy. Soc. B., *155*, 455.
Kagayama, M. and Douglas, W.W. (1974) J. Cell Biol., *62*, 519.
Kaliner, M. and Austen, K.F. (1974) J. Immunol., *112*, 664.
Kaliner, M., Orange, R.P. and Austen, K.F. (1972) J. Exp. Med., *136*, 556.
Kanno, T., Cochrane, D.E. and Douglas, W.W. (1973) Canad. J. Physiol. Pharmacol., *51*, 1001.
Karpatkin, S. (1972) in Hematology (Williams, W.J., Beutler, E. and Erslev, A.J., eds), p. 1006, McGraw-Hill, New York.
Keller, R. (Ed.) (1966) Tissue mast cells in immune reactions. Karger, Basel.
Kjaerheim, A. and Hovig, T. (1962) Thromb. Diath. Haemorrh., *7*, 1.
Lagunoff, D. (1972) Biochem. Pharmacol., *21*, 1889.
Lagunoff, D. and Benditt, E.P. (1963) Ann. N.Y. Acad. Sci., *103*, 185.
Lagunoff, D., Chi, E.Y. and Wan, H. (1975) Biochem. Pharmacol., *24*, 1573.
Lichtenstein, L.M. (1975) Int. Arch. Allergy, *49*, 143.
MacIntyre, D.E. and Gordon, J.L. (1975) Thromb. Diath. Haemorrh., *34*, 332.
Martin, J.H., Carson, F.L. and Race, G.J. (1974) J. Cell Biol., *60*, 775.
Martin, B.M., Feinman, R.D. and Detwiler, T.C. (1975) Biochemistry, *14*, 1308.
Massini, P. and Lüscher, E.F. (1971) Thromb. Diath. Haemorrh., *25*, 13.
Massini, P. and Lüscher, E.F. (1972) Thromb. Diath. Haemorrh., *27*, 121.
Massini, P. and Lüscher, E.F. (1974) Biochim. Biophys. Acta., *372*, 109.
May, C., Levine, B.B. and Weissman, G. (1970) Proc. Soc. Exp. Biol. Med., *133*, 758.
Mills, D.C.B. and Smith, J.B. (1971) Biochem. J., *121*, 185.
Mongar, J.L. and Svec, P. (1972) Brit. J. Pharmacol., *46*, 741.
Mongar, J.L. and Schild, H.O. (1962) Physiol. Rev., *42*, 226.
Murer, E.H. and Holme, R. (1970) Biochim. Biophys. Acta., *222*, 197.
O'Brien, J.R. and Woodhouse, M.A. (1968) Exp. Biol. Med., *3*, 90.
Palade, G. (1958) in Subcellular Particles (Hayashi, T., ed), p. 64, Ronald Press, New York.
Palade, G. (1975) Science, *189*, 347.
Parekh, A.C. and Glick, D. (1962) J. Biol. Chem., *237*, 280.
Peterson, C. (1974) Acta. Physiol. Scand. Suppl., *413*.
Phillips, D.R. and Agin, P.P. (1973) Ser. Haematol., *3*, 292.
Pletscher, A., Da Prada, M., Berneis, K.H., Steffen, H., Lutold, B. and Weder, H.G. (1974) Adv. Cytopharmacol., *2*, 257.
Poisner, A.M. (1973) Proc. Soc. Exp. Biol. Med., *142*, 103.
Poisner, A.M. and Cooke, P. (1975) Ann. N.Y. Acad. Sci., *253*, 653.
Poisner, A.M. and Hava, M. (1970) Mol. Pharmacol., *6*, 407.
Rahwan, R.G., Borowitz, J.L. and Miya, T.S. (1973) J. Pharmac. Exp. Ther., *184*, 106.
Rasmussen, H. (1970) Science, *170*, 404.
Reimers, H.J., Mustard, J.F. and Packham, M.A. (1975) J. Cell. Biol., *67*, 61.
Renoux, M.L., De Montis, G. and Margelli, D. (1974) Biomedicine, *21*, 410.
Robblee, L.S., Shepro, D., Belamarich, F.A. and Towle, C. (1973) Ser. Haemat., *6*, 311.
Rohlich, P., Anderson, P. and Uvnas, B. (1971) J. Cell Biol., *51*, 465.
Roth, G.J., Stanford, N. and Majerus, P.W. (1975) Proc. Natl. Acad. Sci. U.S.A., *72*, 3073.
Rubin, R.P. (1970) Pharmacol. Rev., *22*, 389.
Salzman, E.W. (1975) in Proceedings of the international conference on prostaglandins (Samuelsson, B. and Paoletti, R., eds), Raven Press, New York.
Sato, T., Herman, L., Chandler, J., Stracher, A. and Detwiler, T.C. (1975) J. Histochem. Cytochem., *23*, 103.
Siraganian, R.P. and Siraganian, P.A. (1975) J. Immunol., *114*, 886.
Smith, A.D. and Winkler, H. (1966) J. Physiol., *183*, 179.
Smith, J.B. and Macfarlane, D.E. (1974) in The Prostaglandins (Ramwell, P.W., ed), Plenum Press, New York.

Smith, J.B. and Willis, A.L. (1971) Nature New Biol., *231*, 235.
Smith, R.J. and Ignarro, L.J. (1975) Proc. Natl. Acad. Sci. U.S.A., *72*, 108.
Statland, B.E., Heagen, B.M. and White, J.G. (1969) Nature, *223*, 521.
Stormorken, H. (1969) Scand. J. Haematol. Suppl., *9*, 3.
Thon, I.L. and Uvnas, B. (1967) Acta. Physiol. Scand., *71*, 303.
Tolone, G., Bondsera, L. and Parrinello, N. (1974) Experientia, *30*, 426.
Trifaro, J.M. and Poisner, A.M. (1967) Mol. Pharmacol., *3*, 572.
Uvnas, B. (1974) Life Sci., *14*, 2355.
Uvnas, B. and Thon, I.L. (1961) Exp. Cell. Res., *23*, 45.
Viveros, O.H., Arqueros, L. and Kirshner, N. (1968) Life Sci., *7*, 609.
Weinstein, M.J. and Doolittle, R.F. (1972) Biochim. Biophys. Acta., *258*, 577.
Weiss, H.J. (1975) New Engl. J. Med., *293*, 531.
Weissman, G., Goldstein, I., Hoffstein, S. and Tsung, P.K. (1975a) Ann. N.Y. Acad. Sci., *253*, 750.
Weissman, G., Goldstein, I., Hoffstein, S., Chauvet, G. and Robineaux, (1975b) Ann. N.Y. Acad. Sci., *256*, 222.
Wessels, N.K., Spooner, B.S., Ash, J.F., Bradley, M.P., Luduena, M.A., Taylor, E.L., Wren, J.R. and Yamada, K.M. (1971) Science, *171*, 135.
White, J.G. (1971) in The Circulating Platelet (Johnson, S.A., ed), p. 45, Academic Press, New York.
White, J.G. (1972) Am. J. Pathol., *69*, 41.
White, J.G., Rao, G.H.R. and Gerrard, J.M. (1974) Am. J. Path., *77*, 135.
Williams, J.A. (1974) in Secretory Mechanisms of Exocrine Glands (Thorn, N.A. and Peterson, O.H., eds), p. 389, Munksgaard, Copenhagen.
Willis, A.L. (1974) Prostaglandins, *5*, 1.
Willis, A.L., Vane, F.M., Kuhn, D.C., Scott, C.G. and Petrin, M. (1974) Prostaglandins, 8, 453.
Willis, A.L. and Weiss, H.J. (1973) Prostaglandins, *4*, 783.
Worner, P. and Brossmer, R. (1975) Thromb. Res., *6*, 297.

PART II

Platelet constituents, cellular control mechanisms and biological significance

CHAPTER 4

Characterisation of plasma membranes from platelets*

G.A. JAMIESON and D.F. SMITH

American National Red Cross, Blood Research Laboratory, 9321 Old Georgetown Road, Bethesda, Maryland 20014, U.S.A.

1. Introduction

Knowledge of the structure and function of the platelet plasma membrane has been developed from studies on intact platelets and, more recently, by the characterization of plasma membranes isolated following various techniques of platelet homogenization. In this chapter we have endeavored to describe the general features of the surface membrane in the intact platelet, the methods for its isolation and analytical characterization, and certain specialized aspects of individual components of the surface membrane and their possible role in platelet function although these may overlap with chapters giving more detailed accounts of individual aspects of platelet function.

The platelet is apparently unique among cells in being formed by the fragmentation of its precursor rather than by the maturation of a more primitive cell; the megakaryocyte divides within the bone marrow, each megakaryocyte producing a total of about 2000 platelets (Harker, 1971). During the maturation of the megakaryocyte, demarcation membranes are formed by invagination of its plasma membrane (Behnke, 1968b) although an origin from internal structures has been suggested (Schulz, 1966). These demarcation membranes are rich in carbohydrate and define the outer membrane of the developing platelet.

The trilaminar structure of the platelet plasma membrane is morphologically indistinguishable from that of other cells and is 7–9 nm in thickness. However, the surface membrane of the platelet is characterized by deep invaginations into the interior of the platelet leading to a complex network known as the surface-connected system or canalicular system. One may ask whether these invaginations represent uncompleted demarcation membranes remaining from the megakaryocyte. The canalicular system gives the platelet a 'sponge-like' quality which may assist in the transport within the circulation of clotting factors, such as fibrinogen, and other plasma proteins. It certainly gives to the platelet a high

---

* Contribution No. 326 from The American National Red Cross.

Gordon (ed) Platelets in Biology and Pathology
© *Elsevier/North-Holland Biomedical Press, 1976*

surface to volume ratio and brings the interior of the platelet and the exterior milieu into close proximity.

Outside the trilaminar membrane, both on the platelet surface and in the channels of the surface connected system, is an extensive exterior coat or glycocalyx which is 20–50 nm in depth and is thus about 3–8 times the thickness of the membrane. This surface is thought to be rich in carbohydrate on the basis of staining with specific cytochemical reagents (Behnke, 1967; Rambourg and Leblond, 1967; Hovig, 1968). Emerging evidence, to be discussed later, suggests that components of this exterior coat may be important in platelet function. It can be removed by careful proteolysis without extensive changes in the ultrastructure of the membrane (Hovig, 1968). At the present time it is not clear whether the glycocalyx should be regarded as an integral component of the platelet membrane or as being more-or-less loosely associated with it.

In its normal environment the platelet, together with its exterior coat, is surrounded by an ill-defined nimbus of plasma proteins which has been called the plasmatic atmosphere; differences between the reactions of platelets in plasma and washed platelets may arise from the loss of components in this compartment (Ardlie and Han, 1974).

Recent studies using freeze-fracture and freeze-etching techniques (Hoak, 1972, Reddick and Mason, 1973; Feagler et al., 1974) have been particularly valuable in allowing the visualization of surface details of the plasma membrane and its relationship to the canalicular or surface-connected system (Fig. 1). Although little is known about their role or structure, surface-associated knobs or particles have been found embedded in the outer surface of the membrane and extending into the canalicular system while the inner surface contained numerous fibrillar structures. These particles are absent from the surface of platelets which do not aggregate, either because they have been obtained from thrombasthenic patients or are normal platelets which have been treated with an anti-aggregating drug.

Thus, the platelet surface may be regarded as comprising three different zones; the plasmatic atmosphere which is retained by platelets only under special conditions of isolation and is required for ADP-induced aggregation, the glycocalyx which remains with the platelet during most isolation procedures and may be the site of thrombin action and lectin-induced agglutination, and the platelet membrane itself which contains the structural elements associated with transport, release and the exchange of information between the interior and exterior of the platelet.

In addition to the plasma membrane, platelets contain membranes associated with their Golgi apparatus, their granules and dense bodies and with their dense tubular system; however, virtually nothing is known about the membranes of these last three compartments.

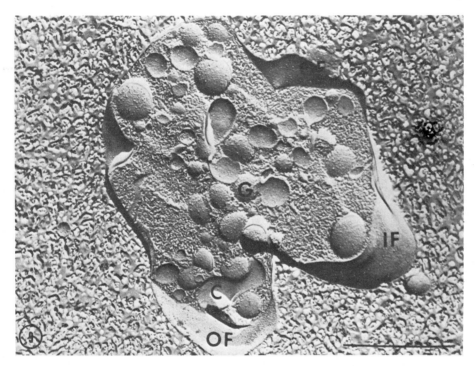

Fig. 1. Replica of a freeze-etched normal platelet suspended in 25% glycerol. Inner faces (IF) and outer faces (OF) of the fractured platelet surface membrane contain scattered intramembranous particles. Fractured membranes of granules (G) and the canalicular system (C) also contain scattered intramembranous particles. Scale bar, 1.0 μm; ×34,000. Reprinted, with permission, from J. Cell Biol., 60, 541, 1974 (Feagler, J.R., Tillack, T.W., Champlin, D.D. and Majerus, P.W.).

2. Platelet charge

It is only when charged groups are present in the outer nanometer or so of a cell surface that they contribute effectively to the electrophoretic charge, or zeta potential. Thus any change in the arrangement of charged groups at the cell surface, such as might arise following adhesion or aggregation, might lead to changes in electrophoretic mobility.

The platelet surface contains a range of ionic organic groups (Mehrishi, 1971) and platelets have a high net negative charge with an isoelectric point at pH 3.6 and an electrophoretic mobility of 0.85 μm/sec/V/cm at pH 7 (Seaman and Vassar, 1966). This charge is at least partially due to sialic acid residues since treatment with neuraminidase removes about 10^5 molecules of sialic acid per μm^2 and results in 50% reduction in electrophoretic mobility with a concomitant increase in the isoelectric point to pH 4.2. Calculations show that total surface sialic acid is about 1.9×10^6 molecules of sialic acid per μm^2, which is approximately 10-fold the surface density on red cells. Although these values were obtained with intact platelets similar values have been found for the isoelectric points of isolated platelet membranes by the techniques of isoelectric focusing, both before and after treatment with neuraminidase (Jamieson and Groh, 1971) suggesting that the charge distribution in the glycocalyx remains intact during the isolation of the membrane.

The electrophoretic mobility of platelets is affected by aggregating agents (Hampton and Mitchell, 1966; Seaman and Vassar, 1966), by aging in vitro (Mason and Shermer, 1971) and in certain pathological conditions. For example, the giant platelets of congenital macrothrombocytic thrombopenia (Bernard-Soulier syndrome) have a reduced electrophoretic mobility which may reflect a decreased density of sialic acid on the platelet surface since the total sialic acid content is the same as that of normal platelets (Gröttum and Solum, 1969). On the other hand, the electrophoretic mobility of platelets from patients suffering from Glanzmann's thrombasthenia is identical with that of normal platelets, and they have been reported to have the same content of sialic acid (Zucker and Levine, 1963), although more recent studies indicate that these patients lack a major glycoprotein on the platelet membrane (Nurden and Caen, 1974).

This bound sialic acid probably constitutes the viral receptor site of the platelet (Terada et al., 1966) and is the source of its hemagglutination inhibition activity (Uhlenbruck, 1961); an active receptor fraction has been isolated from a crude preparation of platelet membranes by solubilization with aqueous pyridine (Pepper and Jamieson, 1968). Thrombocytopenia is a frequent concomitant of viral infections (Broun and Broun, 1962) and this condition is also induced in mice by injections of neuraminidase. A concomitant decrease in the incidence of metastases is observed (Gasic and Gasic, 1962) which may reflect a role for platelets in the spread of malignant disease (Gasic et al., 1973). High concentrations of Maloney mouse leukemia virus have been found in association with the demarcation membranes of mouse megakaryocyte (Schulz, 1968) reflecting, perhaps, the concentration of carbohydrate in this region.

3. Preparation of platelet plasma membranes

The ability of platelets to undergo morphological changes in response to a wide variety of stimuli makes the initial preparation of homogenous platelet suspensions a critical step in their subcellular fractionation. In order to reduce the production of artifacts, which might arise due to stimulation of the release reaction or aggregation prior to homogenization, platelets are removed from contaminating cells by differential centrifugation and washed repeatedly in isotonic solutions containing low concentrations of EDTA (0.2–3 mM). While EDTA presumably inhibits the release reaction, the use of buffers at low pH (6.5–6.8) has been shown to facilitate resuspension of platelet pellets and inhibit aggregation (Kaulen and Gross, 1973).

The major difficulty in the subcellular fractionation of blood platelets is their remarkable resistance to homogenization thought to be due to their small size (Barber et al., 1971) and the presence of contractile elements within the cells (Salganicoff and Fukami, 1972). The procedures which have been employed to produce preparations of lysed platelets include freezing and thawing cycles (Schultz and Heipler, 1959; French et al., 1970), homogenization in a Potter-type homogenizer fitted with a 'non-clearance' Teflon pestle (Marcus et al., 1966), blendor homogenization (Harris and Crawford, 1973; Siegal et al., 1971; Minter and Crawford, 1971; Day et al., 1969), sonication (Buckingham and Maynert, 1964; Solatunturi and Paasonen, 1966; DaPrada and Pletscher, 1968), homogenization with a French pressure cell (Salganicoff and Fukami, 1972; Salganicoff et al., 1975; Fukami and Salganicoff, 1973), nitrogen cavitation (Broekman et al., 1974) and hypotonic lysis of glycerol-loaded platelets (Barber and Jamieson, 1970).

Only a few studies have been performed which make direct comparison of certain of these methods for platelet lysis. Day et al., (1969) compared the 'non-clearance', pestle homogenization with blendor homogenization. The distribution of 'marker enzymes' in subcellular fractions obtained following discontinuous and continuous sucrose gradient centrifugation and ultrastructural studies of the resulting particulate fractions were studied. These investigators concluded that the pestle homogenization (Marcus et al., 1969) provided the best conditions for lysis when the entire platelet contents were to be submitted to subcellular fractionation. This method was found superior to blendor homogenization as it produced higher yields of plasma membrane fraction and particulate-bound enzymes, provided the best organelle preservation and best separation of α-granules.

Barber et al. (1971) in another comparative study investigated sonication, nitrogen cavitation in a high pressure bomb, the 'non-clearance' pestle homogenizer, simple osmotic lysis and hypotonic lysis of glycerol loaded platelets as methods for the preparation of platelet homogenates for isolation of platelet plasma membrane fractions. The platelet homogenates obtained by these different methods were submitted to centrifugation on continuous or discontinuous sucrose density gradients and the resulting plasma membrane fractions were compared by ultrastructural analysis, enzymatic activity, chemical analysis and viral hemagglutination inhibition. These authors described simple osmotic lysis in distilled water as an inefficient method of platelet lysis and nitrogen cavitation as a non-reproducible method when applied to platelets with respect to degree of lysis and yield of plasma membrane fraction. Based on the number of intact platelets present after each homogenization method, the glycerol-lysis technique proved the most effective at 85% lysis compared to sonication and pestle homogenization at 79% and 75% respectively. These three methods, which were studied in detail, all produced multiple plasma membrane bands on sucrose gradients with densities between 1.090 and 1.020, suggesting that fragmentation of the plasma membrane may have occurred during homogenization.

In order to decrease possible fragmentation of surface membrane during homogenization, the platelets were treated with surface stabilizing agents (Warren et al., 1966) such as $ZnCl_2$ and fluorescein mercuric acetate (FMA). Treatment of platelets with these agents apparently decreased the multiplicity of membrane bands on sucrose gradients when homogenates were prepared by sonication or pestle homogenization. However, the two characteristic membrane fractions at densities of 1.090 and 1.120 were observed with the glycerol-lysis method using treated or untreated platelets.

These data suggested that the multiple membrane bands observed on sucrose density gradients are probably not the result of fragmentation. The major disadvantage in using surface stabilizing agents proved to be the decreased yield of plasma membranes possibly due to the reduced lysis observed when treated platelets were disrupted by glycerol-lysis, sonication, or nitrogen decompression. Furthermore, this procedure resulted in either inhibition or complete destruction of enzyme activity.

These authors concluded that while none of the methods evaluated for platelet disruption nor the use of surface stabilizing agents yielded a single membrane population, the glycerol-lysis technique was found most effective with respect to efficiency of cell lysis, yield of plasma membrane fraction with production of the largest membrane fragments, and ease of operation and reproducibility.

More recently Kaulen and Gross (1973) compared freezing-and-thawing cycles, sonication, 'non-clearance' pestle homogenization and hypotonic lysis of glycerol-loaded platelets as methods for platelet disruption. In agreement with Barber et al. (1971), these investigators concluded that the glycerol-lysis method was the most efficient in platelet disruption while producing only minor destruction of intracellular organelles.

The use of the French pressure cell (Salganicoff et al., 1975) and nitrogen cavitation (Broekman et al., 1974) have recently been shown to be effective methods of platelet lysis for the isolation of intracellular organelles associated with the platelet granular fraction. Broekman et al. (1974), using nitrogen cavitation, fractionated the entire homogenate on a linear sucrose gradient (30–60%) and obtained a morphologically homogenous preparation of α-granules and a highly enriched fraction of mitochondria. Salganicoff et al. (1975) disrupted pig platelets with a French pressure cell and obtained a granular fraction by differential centrifugation which yielded coupled mitochondria, α-granules and dense bodies while retaining 80% of the granule components in a particulate form. Resolution of the granular fractions on sucrose discontinuous gradients, while not successful in isolating a morphologically homogeneous preparation of any of the subcellular organelles, did provide separation of a mitochondria-enriched fraction and a dense-body enriched-fraction. While these homogenization methods may be useful for isolation of intracellular organelles, they have not been extensively studied for the preparation of plasma membrane fractions. In particular, the method described by Salganicoff et al. (1975), which was developed primarily for the isolation of platelet mitochondria (Salganicoff and Fukami, 1972), utilized treatment of platelets with the proteolytic enzyme, Nagarse, prior to homogenization to weaken the plasma membrane. While this procedure presumably maintained the integrity of the subcellular particles, it must certainly produce partially degraded plasma membrane preparations.

Probably the most widely utilized methods for platelet disruption and plasma membrane preparation are the 'non-clearance' homogenizer method (Marcus et al., 1966) and the glycerol-lysis method (Barber and Jamieson, 1970). The 'non-clearance' homogenization is obtained by using a Teflon pestle which fits the homogenization vessel only at low temperature and then expands during the homogenization procedure. This process depends upon uniform contraction and expansion of the teflon pestle to maintain a constant side-to-wall clearance. Homogenization was performed for 5 min at 1700 rev/min and the resulting homogenate was centrifuged to remove non-disrupted platelets and debris. The supernatant was then fractionated on a linear sucrose gradient (30–60%) to obtain the plasma membrane fraction at buoyant density of 1.13–1.12 and a granular fraction at 1.21–1.17 which were washed in appropriate buffers and collected by centrifugation.

The glycerol-lysis technique involves the slow intracellular accumulation of glycerol into platelets by centrifugation through a continuous glycerol gradient (0–40%) followed by lysis by an isotonic sucrose solution. Platelet membranes have a very slow transit time for glycerol, of the order of minutes, whereas the transit time for water is in microseconds. Hence, the net effect of the above treatment is for a rapid influx of water, and a slow efflux of glycerol, resulting in an 'explosive' lysis from the interior of the platelet. The plasma membrane, cellular cytoplasm and cellular debris are then separated by density step (27% sucrose; d, 1.106) centrifugation.

The membrane fraction from the density step procedure could be further separated into two equal subfractions of d, 1.090 and 1.120 on a continuous sucrose gradient (15–40%; d, 1.06–1.15). Both these subfractions appeared to be derived from the platelet surface membrane. Although these subfractions were identical by chemical and enzymatic analyses, isolectric points and in protein distribution as determined by gel electrophoresis, they differed in their protein:lipid ratios which were thought to be responsible for their observed differences in density on sucrose gradients. They did not appear to be 'inside-out, outside-out' vesicles on the basis of their equal accessibility to neuraminidase and trypsin and to iodination catalyzed by lactoperoxidase (Barber and Jamieson, 1971a). However, they did differ in ultrastructure, the lighter (d, 1.090) having an average diameter of 1.7 μm, close to that of the intact platelet, and with concentric double membrane structures, while the heavier (d, 1.120) consisted of single membrane structures of average diameter 0.7 μm (Fig. 2).

The two membrane subfractions had identical procoagulant activities but differences were shown in the lipids extracted from each, the lipids from the low density fraction having a higher procoagulant activity than those from the high density fraction (Barber et al., 1972). The origin of the two subclasses is unknown, but they may reflect regions of anatomical specialization which has been proposed for platelet cell-surfaces (Nakao and Angrist, 1960) or heterogeneity of platelet populations thought to arise from megakaryocytopoiesis (Paulus and Kinet-DeNoel, 1973; Boneu et al., 1973) or from platelet senescence (for review see Karpatkin, 1972). However, the cell surface origin of the two subclasses is supported by the ability of both fractions to be labeled with FMA and ^{125}I when platelets were treated with the surface stabilizing agent (Barber et al., 1971) or labeled by lacto peroxidase catalyzed iodination (Barber and Jamieson, 1971a).

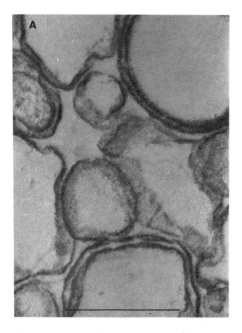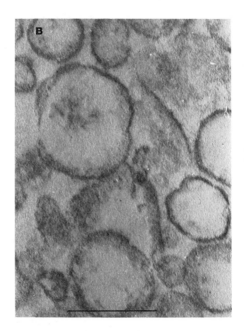

Fig. 2. Electron photographs of platelet membranes isolated by the glycerol lysis technique and continuous density centrifugation. Contaminating subcellular structures are absent; ×18,000. (A) Membrane band, d, 1.090. Note the appearance of double membrane structures. Scale bar, 2 μm. (B) Membrane band, d, 1.120. Note absence of double membrane structures. Scale bar, 1 μm. Reprinted, with permission, from J. Biol. Chem., 245, 6357, 1970 (Barber, A.J. and Jamieson, G.A.).

More recently, pig platelet membranes prepared by the blendor technique (Harris and Crawford, 1973) were subfractionated by zonal centrifugation (Taylor and Crawford, 1974) into two components. These subfractions demonstrated significant differences in the relative distribution of two phosphodiesterase activities and specific radioactivity when isolated from platelets which had been labeled with ^{125}I. These authors suggested that one component may be of intracellular origin.

4. Enzymes of the platelet plasma membrane

While most of the membrane preparations described have depended largely upon ultrastructural analysis and chemical composition for identification of platelet plasma membrane and granular fractions, considerable attention has been given to the distribution of 'marker-enzymes' during fractionations of platelet homogenates. These investigations have been frustrated by the observation that certain enzymatic activities which are well localized and appear to be entirely associated with subcellular organelles in other cell types demonstrate soluble activity when blood platelets are fractionated. This property has been observed for several enzymes known to be localized in lysosomal fractions of other tissues (Marcus, 1966; Siegel and Lüscher, 1967).

The absence of a well defined 'marker-enzyme' is particularly evident in the case of the plasma membrane. 5'-Nucleotidase is known to be associated with the plasma membrane of liver (Emmelot and Bos, 1966; Goldfischer et al., 1964) but several investigators have reported low levels of this enzyme in platelets, primarily in the soluble fraction (Day et al., 1969; Harris and Crawford, 1973).

The enzymes of the plasma membrane have been most extensively studied in membranes isolated by the glycerol-lysis method (Barber and Jamieson, 1970; Kaulen and Gross, 1973). These investigations indicated an enrichment of phosphodiesterase (8-fold), acid phosphatase (4-fold), Na^+, K^+-ATPase (2-fold) and Mg^{2+}-ATPase (4-fold) in the plasma membrane fraction but represented only 12%, 34%, 20% and 12% of the total activity of the lysate, respectively. The relatively low recoveries of enzymatic activity may be a function of the yield of plasma membranes in these fractions since Kaulen and Gross (1973) reported 90% of the Mg^{2+}-ATPase and 80% of the acid phosphatase were associated with the platelet particulate fraction. More recently Taylor and Crawford (1974) have provided more evidence for the plasma membrane localization of phosphodiesterase in pig platelets by demonstrating not only an increase in specific activity of this enzyme in plasma membrane fraction but a distribution of activity on zonal centrifugation that followed closely the distribution of the specific activity of ^{125}I where the intact platelets were labeled by lactoperoxidase catalyzed iodination prior to fractionation. The latter investigation, however, did not provide recovery data for this activity either in the soluble or particulate fraction.

These observations suggest that platelet enzymes may have distributions significantly different from those observed in other tissues and indicate the necessity for more detailed investigations of the subcellular location of platelet enzymes. While very few histochemical studies on platelet enzymes have been made, this approach, combined with biochemical analysis of morphologically defined subcellular fractions, may be valuable in defining the subcellular compartmentation of platelet enzymes.

Compositional analysis of the isolated platelet plasma membrane indicated that this organelle is a glycolipoprotein containing 52% lipid, 36% protein and 7% carbohydrate (Barber and Jamieson, 1970). A comparison of the chemical composition of the two plasma membrane fractions, isolated by the glycerol lysis technique, with the lysate and the debris and soluble fractions is shown in Table 1.

5. Glycoproteins of the platelet surface

As mentioned above, indirect evidence for the presence of glycoproteins on the platelet surface arose from the use of specific cytochemical stains combined with electron microscopy and from studies on platelet electrophoresis and viral-induced agglutination.

Further indirect evidence for surface carbohydrate on the platelet has been

TABLE 1
Yields of components of fractions obtained during the purification of membranes from human blood platelets

Component	Lysate	Soluble		Debris (mg)		Upper band (d, 1.090)	Lower band (d, 1.120)	Recovery (%)
Dry weight	3594	1057	(29.4)	2085	(58.0)	92.56 (2.6)	90.56 (2.5)	92.5
Protein	2571	967	(37.6)	1390	(54.1)	29.53 (1.2)	36.31 (1.4)	94.2
Phospholipid	730	21	(2.8)	394	(54.0)	41.53 (5.7)	35.62 (4.9)	67.4
Cholesterol	133	0.3	(0.3)	77.4	(58.2)	10.23 (7.7)	8.04 (6.1)	72.2
RNA	5.62	0.63 (11.3)		3.26 (58.1)		0.31(5.5)	0.35 (6.2)	81.1
DNA	3.29			2.21 (67.3)				67.3
Neutral sugars	108.8	13.0 (12.0)		75.9 (69.7)		4.75 (4.4)	4.38 (4.0)	90.1
Hexosamine	39.78	10.23 (25.7)		23.08 (58.1)		1.75 (4.4)	1.63 (4.1)	92.2
Sialic acid	10.92	3.02 (27.7)		6.40 (58.6)		0.51 (4.6)	0.47 (4.3)	95.1

[a]Figures in parentheses are percentages of component in each fraction
Determinations were carried out on platelets derived from 30 platelet units ($\sim$ 15 liters of blood)
Reprinted, with permission, from J. Biol. Chem., 245, 6357, 1970.

provided by studies on the reaction of platelets with lectins having different carbohydrate specificities (Greenberg and Jamieson, 1974). These studies have shown that platelets are strongly agglutinated by wheat germ agglutinin, which has N-acetylglucosamine or sialic acid as its haptenic determinants, by *Ricinus communis*, which has galactose as its haptenic determinant, and by the lectin of *Phaseolus coccineus*; this last lectin has no known monosaccharide determinant but is inhibited by an extended glycopeptide of the red cell surface (Kubanek et al., 1973). Lectins with specificities towards glucose and mannose (concanavalin A, *Lathyrus sativus*, *Lens culinaris* and *Pisum sativum*) did not cause platelet agglutination nor the release of ADP, but did cause the release of serotonin at high concentrations suggesting that different receptor sites may exist on the platelet surface for the release of the two metabolites; another galactose-specific lectin (*Agaricus bisporus*) also fell into this class. Interestingly, although concanavalin A did not cause the agglutination of intact platelets it did cause the agglutination of isolated membranes. This is consistent with the suggestion that this lectin may be a marker for galactosyltransferase in certain cells (Lamont et al., 1974) since the galactosyltransferase of the platelet is only manifest in isolated membranes but not in intact platelets (Barber and Jamieson, 1971c) which suggests that the enzyme is located on the inner aspect of the membrane or is buried within the intact membrane in a form which is revealed following the trauma of isolation. Soybean lectin, with an N-acetylgalactosamine determinant, was virtually without effect on platelet agglutination or release.

Quantitative ultrastructural studies have also been carried out on the binding of lectins to platelets. The erythroagglutinating lectin (E-PHA) of *Phaseolus vulgaris* and the leukoagglutinating lectin (L-PHA) bind to intact platelets causing platelet aggregation and the inhibition of adenyl cyclase, changes which also occur during aggregation induced by thrombin (Majerus and Brodie, 1972). About

600,000 molecules of E-PHA per platelet bind to the surface with an apparent dissociation constant of 0.5×10^{-7} M while about 300,000 molecules of L-PHA bind with an apparent dissociation constant of 4×10^{-7} M. Although the lectin of *Lens culinaris* does not cause aggregation it does bind tightly (400,000 molecules per platelet, $K_{diss} = 1.4 \times 10^{-7}$ M) and there is an approximate doubling of receptor sites for this lectin on prior treatment of the platelet with thrombin or L-PHA. Subsequent studies showed differences in the rate and extent of serotonin release induced by thrombin and PHA and in resulting platelet morphology (Tollefsen et al., 1974). The use of ferritin-conjugated PHA and the freeze fracture technique demonstrated that the morphological changes induced by thrombin involved a decrease in the number of lectin receptor sites on the platelet surface and a marked increase in their number in the canalicular system (Feagler et al., 1974). It was suggested that this may arise from the fusion of granule membranes with the plasma membranes of the canalicular system.

Direct evidence for the presence of surface glycoproteins on the platelet was obtained by the isolation of glycopeptides following treatment with trypsin, pronase and papain (Pepper and Jamieson, 1970), plasmin and thrombin (Jamieson et al., 1971) and chymotrypsin (Barber and Jamieson, 1971a). In each case the glycopeptides obtained were generally similar to those obtained with trypsin, the most extensively studied system (Pepper and Jamieson, 1970). Three size classes of glycopeptides were obtained with molecular weights of 120,000 (glycopeptide I), 22,500 (glycopeptide II) and 5000 (glycopeptide III); the highest molecular weight glycopeptide (glycopeptide I) has been termed a macroglycopeptide since its molecular weight appears to be an order of magnitude higher than those of glycopeptides from plasma proteins or red cell stroma. The platelet glycopeptides showed several analytical differences between each class; the macroglycopeptide (glycopeptide I) contained about 70% carbohydrate with galactose as essentially its sole neutral sugar with equimolar amounts of galactosamine and glucosamine, presumably as their *N*-acetyl derivatives, and with heterosaccharide residues joined to the polypeptide backbone in *O*- and *N*-glycosidic linkages. On the other hand, the glycopeptide of lowest molecular weight (glycopeptide-III) contained equimolar amounts of galactose and mannose, had asparagine as its principal amino acid and appeared to contain only *N*-glycosidic linkages; the glycopeptide of intermediate molecular weight (glycopeptide-II) was also intermediate in properties but was not studied extensively because it was present in relatively small amounts.

The presence of mucopolysaccharides on the outer surface of the platelet has frequently been suggested on the basis of ultrastructural studies with specific cytochemical reagents. In the proteolytic studies summarized above, it was found that treatment with enzymes which caused the release reaction (trypsin, pronase, papain, plasmin) resulted in the solubilization of a carbohydrate component (glycopeptide-*O*) which was eluted from Sephadex G200 at the void volume and had properties consistent with being the chondromucopeptide derived from chondroitin sulfate (Jamieson et al., 1971). On the other hand, this component was not obtained with chymotrypsin, which does not cause the release reaction, or among the tryptic products of isolated membranes. These results suggest that mucopolysaccharides are not components of the platelet surface but are probably released from the granules under appropriate circumstances.

Differences between the glycopeptides I, II and III were also shown in their effect on the agglutination of platelets induced by plant lectins (Greenberg and Jamieson, 1974). Platelet agglutination induced by wheat germ agglutinin was inhibited by the macroglycopeptide but not by glycopeptide II, while the agglutination induced by *Phaseolus coccineus* was inhibited by glycopeptide II but not by the macroglycopeptide; glycopeptide III was without effect in either case.

The arrangement of the parent glycoproteins, and other proteins, at the platelet surface has been the object of several studies involving the lactoperoxidase-catalyzed iodination of intact platelets and their isolated membranes. Although considerable information has been obtained, the method has several pitfalls which require caution in the interpretation of the data. For example, the degree of iodination is determined more by the content of aromatic groups in the surface component than by its 'accessibility', as such, and the possibility should not be ignored that congruent peaks of radioactivity and PAS staining may nevertheless be on different molecules.

Lactoperoxidase-catalyzed iodination of intact platelets and subsequent gel electrophoresis in SDS leads to the labeling of a heterogenous group of polypeptides and of three glycoprotein bands with molecular weights approximately 150,000, 120,000 and 95,000 (Nachman and Ferris, 1972; Phillips, 1972; Nachman et al., 1973) all of which are accessible to trypsin (Phillips, 1972). The glycoprotein fraction of lowest molecular weight (95,000) was much more highly iodinated than the other two glycoproteins (Phillips, 1972) although it is present in the lowest amount, as judged from SDS staining; on this basis the term 'major' surface glycoprotein for this component (Nachman et al., 1973) is erroneous. This glycoprotein was partially purified following extraction of the membranes with lithium iodosalicylate and was used to raise antibodies which could themselves induce platelet agglutination (Nachman et al., 1973).

The glycoprotein component of highest molecular weight (approx. 150,000) is the one which stains most strongly with the PAS reagent. It has been found to occur in both membrane-bound and soluble forms in platelet homogenates and has been purified from the soluble fraction (Lombart et al., 1974). The soluble form is thought to be present on the platelet surface based on its labelling with [^{14}C]glycine ethyl ester by transglutaminase and on its accessibility to neuraminidase and to carboxypeptidase, which does not cause the release of intracellular components (Okumura and Jamieson, 1975). The term *glycocalicin* has been suggested for this component on the basis of its origin as a component of the platelet glycocalyx.

Glycocalicin is cleaved by trypsin to yield a macroglycopeptide containing 70% carbohydrate, apparently identical with that obtained from intact platelets, and a large peptide of molecular weight 48,000 which contains a small amount of carbohydrate (approx. 9%). Overall this tryptic peptide lacks the preponderance of hydrophobic amino acids present in the tryptic peptide from the red cell glycoprotein (Winzler, 1969; Marchesi et al., 1972) but may contain more limited hydrophobic domains which are responsible for membrane binding.

Glycocalicin probably constitutes the thrombocyte-specific antigen previously reported as a soluble component of platelet homogenates (Milgrom et al., 1968; Hanna and Nelken, 1971). Antiglycocalicin antibodies raised in chickens recognize two determinants in the glycoprotein, one against the macroglycopeptide portion and the other against the peptide portion (Okumura and Jamieson, 1975). These antibodies agglutinate intact platelets and isolated membranes, which suggests the immunological cross-reactivity of the soluble and membrane-bound forms of the glycoprotein. Glycocalicin also gives precipitin reactions with wheat germ agglutinin and *Agaricus bisporus* and is presumably a receptor site of these lectins (Greenberg and Jamieson, 1974).

6. *Lipids of the platelet plasma membrane*

In addition to their role in primary hemostasis, blood platelets provide an active lipoprotein surface component which interacts with plasma coagulation factors to activate the prothrombin by the intrinsic and, perhaps, the extrinsic pathways. This activity has been termed *platelet factor 3* and resides in the platelet plasma membrane (Marcus et al., 1966; Barber et al., 1972) but Marcus et al., (1971) have properly emphasized that this 'factor' is not a biochemically distinct entity and that platelet procoagulant activity is a more exact nomenclature. Since the mechanism of its conversion from an inactive to an active form during platelet aggregation is not known, the isolation of well-characterized platelet plasma membranes and the investigation of their lipid components has received much attention in recent years.

Marcus et al. (1969) have identified the individual fatty acids as well as the principal lipid classes in isolated platelet plasma membranes. The ratio of lipid to protein was 0.58 with phospholipids comprising 78% of the total lipid and cholesterol accounting for 90% of the neutral lipid. The molar ratio of cholesterol to phospholipid in these membranes was 0.53 which is in agreement with the value obtained by Barber and Jamieson (1970) and Kaulen and Gross (1973) and in the range previously reported for the plasma membrane of several other cell types (Ashworth and Green, 1966; Pfleger et al., 1968).

Phospholipids on the platelet surface may play a role in platelet function since treatment of platelets with phospholipase C resulted in the release of ADP and serotonin together with morphological indications of degranulation (Shick and Yu, 1974). The pattern of phospholipids isolated from platelet plasma membranes is summarized in Table 2 (Marcus, 1969) and is essentially the same as the pattern reported by Kaulen and Gross (1973), who prepared membranes by the glycerol lysis method. The pattern indicates a high sphingomyelin content which is characteristic of plasma membrane from other sources (Pfleger et al., 1968; Chertham et al., 1969; Henning et al., 1970). Since the phospholipid composition

TABLE 2
Distribution of phospholipids in isolated platelet plasma membranes

Phospholipid	% of lipid phosphorous
Phosphatidylethanolamine	26.8
Phosphatidyl serine	9.0
Phosphotidyl inositol	5.2
Lecithin	40.0
Sphingomyelin	17.1
Lysolecithim	0.4
Cardiolipin	0.3

After Marcus et al., 1969.

of the isolated membranes is similar to the whole platelet (Marcus et al., 1969; Kaulen and Gross, 1973), the latter authors have suggested that membranes with low sphingomyelin contents; i.e., mitochondria and endoplasmic reticulum (Johnson and Cornatzer, 1969), are not present in platelets. This is supported by ultrastructural analysis of platelets (Hovig, 1968). Based on the high sphingomyelin content of the platelet membrane and the storage and secretion function of the platelet, Kaulen and Gross (1973) have also concluded that the platelet represents an extremely specialized cell with an abundance of membranes belonging to the 'exoplasmic' type (deDuve, 1969) which are represented by plasma, lysosomal and Golgi apparatus membranes.

Gangliosides, glycosphingolipids which contain sialic acid, have been suggested as being serotonin receptors in neuronal tissue (Woolley and Gommi, 1964) although this has been questioned (Fiszer and DeRobertis, 1969). In view of the importance of serotonin in platelet function, several analytical studies have been carried out on neutral and acid glycosphingolipids in intact platelets because of the difficulty of obtaining adequate amounts of membrane-derived material for analysis (Marcus et al., 1972; Snyder et al., 1972; Tao et al., 1973), although it is generally agreed that glycosphingolipids are components of the plasma membrane of cells (Stoffel, 1971). Of the neutral glycosphingolipids, lactosylceramide and globoside were the most abundant with lesser amounts of glucosyl ceramide and trihexosyl ceramide. Gangliosides comprised 0.5% of the total platelet lipids and about 6% of the total sialic acid content with hematoside comprising 92% of the ganglioside fraction. Equilibrium dialysis studies showed that hematoside and disialolactosyl ceramide isolated from the platelet bind only weakly to serotonin and much less than similar fractions from beef kidney (Marcus et al., 1972). The content of hematoside in platelets is increased by treatment with trypsin (2-fold) chymotrypsin (3-fold) and thrombin (5-fold) (Tao et al., 1973). Time studies showed that the increase in hematoside was complete in ten minutes and was accompanied by a concomitant decrease in ceramide and lactosyl ceramide (Chatterjee and Sweeley, 1973).

Recent studies have suggested that carbohydrate derivatives of dolichol and retinol may function as intermediates; i.e., glycosyl donors, in the biosynthesis of glycolipid (Yogeeswaran et al., 1974) and glycoprotein (Baynes et al., 1973;

Behrens et al., 1973; Warchter et al., 1973; Hsu et al., 1974; Wolf et al., 1974; Lucas et al., 1975; Spiro, 1975). It has recently been shown that intact platelets and isolated platelet plasma membranes are capable of synthesizing dolicholphosphoglucose and retinol phosphomannose when incubated with UDP-glucose and GDP-mannose, respectively (DeLuca et al., 1975). Although glycoproteins were apparently synthesized from mannose in intact platelets, the transfer of mannose from the isolated mannolipid to endogenous acceptors has not yet been demonstrated. Using isolated plasma membranes and UDPG it was found that dicholphosphoglucose was synthesized; however, glucosyltransfer from this intermediate was also not observed with either endogenous or exogenous acceptors.

While surface glycoproteins and glycolipids appear to play an important role in certain aspects of platelet function, the metabolism of carbohydrate portions of these molecules has not been investigated in detail. However, the stimulation of glycolipid synthesis by proteases which induced platelet aggregation (Chatterjee and Sweeley, 1973) support the suggestion that glycosyltransferase (Jamieson et al., 1971; Bosmann, 1971; 1972) may play an important role in platelet function. The possible involvement of glycophospholipid intermediates in these processes should also be investigated further.

7. Possible role of glycosyltransferases in platelet function

In the chronology of the events of hemostasis, the first event affecting the platelet membrane is probably the adhesion of platelets to collagen or other subendothelial structures of the vessel wall leading, subsequently, to the aggregation of platelets to those already adhering. A major limitation in the elucidation of these mechanisms has been the absence of adequate methods for their differential assay. Aggregation has been almost universally assayed by the decrease in the optical density of platelet-rich plasma following the addition of aggregating agents such as ADP or collagen (Born, 1962). This system has been modified by the addition of EDTA so as to measure adhesion to collagen (Spaet and Lejnieks, 1969) which has also been measured by optical (Lyman et al., 1971) or radioactive (Cazenave et al., 1973) counting of platelets adhering to surfaces coated with collagen. However, the role of divalent cations in this phenomenon is not yet clear. Direct measurement of the binding of radiolabeled collagen to platelets has also been made (Gordon and Dingle, 1974).

Probably the best assay is the ex vivo system of Baumgartner (1973) which involves the morphometric analysis of electron photomicrographs of platelet adhesion or microaggregation on an everted segment of rabbit blood vessel from which endothelial cells have been removed. While this system gives an excellent representation of events in vivo, it is tedious and difficult in application since it requires extensive use of the electron microscope.

Blood platelets adhere both to the collagen of the basement membrane and to fibrillar collagen (Hugues and Mahieu, 1970), the latter causing a more extensive formation of platelet microaggregates while the former causes the adhesion of individual platelets (Baumgartner and Haudenschild, 1972; Huang et al., 1974).

The characteristic disaccharide of collagen and basement membrane is glucosylgalactosylhydroxylysine. Studies on the biosynthesis of glomerular basement membrane (Spiro and Spiro, 1971) have suggested that the glycosylation of collagen involves the transfer of galactose or glucose from the appropriate sugar nucleotide to hydroxylsine, or galactosylhydroxylysine, acceptors in collagen. The two enzymes involved in these transfer reactions, collagen:glucosyltransferase and collagen:galactosyltransferase, have been found in platelet membranes isolated by the glycerol lysis technique (Barber and Jamieson, 1971a; 1971b; 1971c; Bosmann, 1971). Since it is not detectable on intact platelets, it is probable that the collagen:galactosyltransferase is buried within the membrane or is present on its inner aspect and the role of this enzyme in platelet function is not known (Barber and Jamieson, 1971c).

A theory has been proposed that platelet:collagen adhesion is mediated by a lectin-like interaction between the collagen:glucosyltransferase of the platelet and incomplete heterosaccharide chains (galactosyl residues) present in collagen (Jamieson et al., 1971). This theory is based on the parallel requirements in adhesion and transferase activity for both free sulphydryl groups and free epsilon amino groups, and on the inhibition of adhesion by collagen glycopeptides. This theory is an extension of the original ideas of Roseman (1970) on the role of transferases in intercellular adhesion and of Ashwell (for review, see Ashwell and Morell, 1974) on the role of galactosyl residues in recognition processes.

Several studies have been directed towards determining the validity of this hypothesis although they have, without exception, addressed themselves to the study of collagen-induced aggregation rather than the adhesion of platelets to collagen, as originally proposed.

The ability of collagen to induce platelet aggregation is destroyed by oxidation of the terminal galactose residues to 6-aldehydo galactose with galactose oxidase, but is re-established by their reduction back to galactose. This has been interpreted as indicating a role for the galactosyl residues of collagen in platelet aggregation (Chesney et al., 1972) but more recent data (Muggli and Baumgartner, 1973) suggest that the oxidation interferes with the formation of collagen fibrils and that the fibrillar structure is required for aggregation.

Galactosylhydroxylsine, the proposed receptor on collagen, binds to the platelet surface while the completed glycopeptide, glucosylgalactosyl hydroxylysine, does not; on the other hand, collagen from which the carbohydrate has been removed by periodate oxidation is still able to support aggregation. These observations have led to the suggestion that the carbohydrate may function as a recognition site rather than an attachment site (Puett et al., 1973). Finally, the purified α1-chain of chick skin collagen has been reported to aggregate platelets and, of the peptides derived from it by cyanogen bromide treatment, only the glycopeptide α1-CB5 was reported to be active (Katzman et al., 1973; Kang et al., 1974).

Thus the question of a role for the carbohydrate of collagen or basement membrane in platelet adhesion and aggregation remains open. An essential requirement of the glycosyltransferase theory is that the first step is the interaction of the enzyme on the platelet surface with the acceptor, galactosylhydroxylysine; the other substrates of the transferase reaction, namely UDPG and Mn^{2+}, would then react subsequently but would not be required for the formation of an enzyme-acceptor complex. A soluble form of the enzyme has been purified approximately 100-fold; preliminary studies (Smith et al., 1975) show that the reaction mechanism is either ordered BiBi or a rapid equilibrium random BiBi with a dead-end EBQ complex. Thus, while UDP and, possibly, ADP inhibit the overall transferase reaction, these reagents may increase the affinity of the cell surface enzyme for its acceptor on collagen by either mechanism. In view of these two possibilities it is of interest that ADP has been found to potentiate collagen induced aggregation (Packham et al., 1973).

The possibility that other glycosyltransferases of the platelet surface may be involved in platelet–platelet aggregation has been suggested based on the presence of a sialytransferase which transfers sialic acid to exogenous glycopeptides from fetuin or prothrombin (Bosmann, 1972) although this was not tested with endogenous glycopeptides of the platelet surface. However, some support for this hypothesis has been provided by the finding that bovine Factor VIII, but not human Factor VIII, can aggregate human platelets (Donati et al., 1973; Forbes and Prentice, 1973). On the other hand, removal of terminal sialic acid from human Factor VIII results in strong aggregating activity while treatment of this product, or bovine Factor VIII, with galactose oxidase destroys the aggregating activity (Vermylen et al., 1973). These results may be interpreted as indicating a role for a sialyltransferase of the platelet surface in this type of aggregation.

Other studies have been directed towards elucidating the mechanism of binding of ADP and of thrombin, both of which play a major role in platelet aggregation. The binding of ADP to isolated platelet membranes was maximal at 37°C over 60 min with a binding constant of $6.5 \times 10^6 M^{-1}$ and approximately 100,000 binding sites per platelet (Nachman and Ferris, 1974). Binding to the membrane was reduced by over 50% by modification of sulfhydryl groups. Inhibitors of platelet aggregation, such as AMP, ATP and chloroadenosine at 10^{-4} M reduced ADP-binding by 50% or more whereas cyclic AMP, α,β-methylene ADP, adenosine and PGE_1 were without effect suggesting that they do not compete at the same site on the membrane. However, another report (Horak and Barton, 1974) suggests that α,β-methylene ADP does compete with ADP in the intact platelet. This discrepancy remains to be resolved.

8. Immunochemistry of the platelet surface

Plasma proteins present in the plasmatic atmosphere, particularly fibrinogen, produce antibodies when intact washed platelets are used as an antigen. In addition, the platelet surface contains HL-A antigens identical with those found in lymphocytes and other tissues (Svejgaard, 1969) and these are of major importance in determining the therapeutic effectiveness of repeated platelet transfusions (Yankee, 1974).

At least three immunogenetic systems unique to platelets have been recognized. These are the PL^A, PL^E and Ko systems and appear to be products of genes located on three different chromosomes. The antigens PL^{A1}, PL^{E1} and Ko^b occur with a frequency of 97–99% in the population whereas their alleles have much lower frequencies, PL^{A2} (26%), PL^{E2} (5%) and Ko^a (14%) and may be involved in neonatal thrombocytopenic purpura due to transplacental sensitization (Shulman et al., 1964).

Although nothing is known of the nature of the determinants of these three immunogenetic systems, some progress has been made regarding the structure of the so-called thrombocyte-specific antigen. An antibody specific for platelets is obtained if human platelets are injected into another species, preferably one phylogenetically distant such as the chicken, and the resulting antiserum is carried through multiple adsorptions with plasma and various cells and tissues to remove nonspecific antibodies (Hanna and Nelken, 1971). Two antigens were recognized, a protein of molecular weight about 30,000 and a glycoprotein with a molecular weight about 117,000. In view of its origin in the cell sap, this antigen is probably identical to the glycoprotein of molecular weight 148,000 which has been isolated from the same source of the glycocalyx (Lombart et al., 1974). Antibodies to the purified glycoprotein contain determinants directed against both the protein and carbohydrate portions of the antigen (Okumura and Jamieson, 1975) and the glycopeptide inhibits the chicken antithrombocyte antisera prepared by Hanna and Nelken (Pepper and Jamieson, 1970). This antigen appears to occur in membrane-bound and soluble forms at the platelet surface.

Although it is not possible to compare the two antisera, a specific antibody to human platelets has also been prepared from intact washed platelets as the antigen and using immunosuppression to avoid the formation of non-specific antibodies (Dzoga et al., 1972). This antiserum also gave two distinct precipitin lines and was used following conjugation with fluorescein or with ferritin to localize the antigen on the platelet surface and in the canalicular system (Stoltzner et al., 1972).

A rabbit antibody to components of the cell sap of human platelets has been used to activate complement leading to complement-induced deletions in the pattern of polypeptide banding of the particulate (membrane) fraction in SDS gels (Zimmerman and Müller-Eberhard, 1973) which are reminiscent of, but distinct from, those found with thrombin but, like them, are obtained only when the platelets are intact and not when a platelet homogenate is exposed to complement. Platelets from patients with paroxysmal nocturnal hemoglobinuria are much more sensitive to complement than are normal platelets and a similar degree of sensitivity occurs following treatment of normal platelets with papain (Aster and Enright, 1969). Immunologic mechanisms of platelet damage and the principles of immune adherence of platelets, which are beyond the scope of this chapter, were discussed by Osler and Siraganian (1972) and by Mylylla (1973); the subject has now been brought up to date in a comprehensive review by D.L. Brown (see Chapter 12 of this volume).

References

Ardlie, N.G. and Han, P. (1974) Brit. J. Haemat., *26*, 357.
Ashwell, G. and Morell, A.G. (1974) Adv. Enzyme., *41*, 99.
Ashworth, L.A.E. and Green, C. (1966) Science, *151*, 210.
Aster, R.H. and Enright, S.E. (1969) J. Clin. Invest., *48*, 1199.
Barber, A.J. and Jamieson, G.A. (1970) J. Biol. Chem., *245*, 6357.
Barber, A.J. and Jamieson, G.A. (1971a) Biochemistry, *10*, 4711.
Barber, A.J. and Jamieson, G.A. (1971b) Biochim. Biophys. Acta, *252*, 533.
Barber, A.J. and Jamieson, G.A. (1971c) Biochim. Biophys. Acta, *252*, 546.
Barber, A.J., Käser-Glanzmann, Jakabova, M. and Lüscher, E.F. (1972) Biochim. Biophys. Acta, *286*, 312.
Barber, A.J., Pepper, D.S. and Jamieson, G.A. (1971) Thromb. Diath. Haemorrh., *26*, 38.
Baumgartner, H.R. (1973) Microvascular Res., *5*, 167.
Baumgartner, H.R. and Haudenschild, C. (1972) Ann. N.Y. Acad. Sci., *201*, 22.
Baynes, J.W., Hsu, A-F. and Heath, E.C. (1973) J. Biol. Chem., *248*, 5693.
Behnke, O. (1967) Anat. Rec., *158*, 121.
Behnke, O. (1968) J. Ultrastruct. Res., *24*, 412.
Behrens, N.H., Carminatti, H., Staneloni, R.J., Leloir, L.F. and Cantarella, A.I. (1973) Proc. Natl. Acad. Sci. U.S.A., *70*, 3390.
Boneu, B., Boneu, A., Raisson, Cl., Guiraud, R. and Bierme, R. (1973) Thromb. Res., *3*, 605.
Born, G.V.R. (1962) Nature, *194*, 927.
Bosmann, H.B. (1971) Biochem. Biophys. Res. Commun., *43*, 1118.
Bosmann, H.B. (1972) Biochim. Biophys. Acta, *279*, 456.
Broekman, M.J., Westmoreland, N.P. and Cohen, P. (1974) J. Cell Biol., *60*, 507.
Broun, G.D. and Broun, G.O. (1962) Proc. 8th Int. Congr. Hematol., 1960, p. 1756.
Buckingham, S. and Maynert, E.W. (1964) J. Pharmacol. Exp. Ther., *143*, 332.
Cazenave, J-P., Packham, M.A. and Mustard, J.F. (1973) J. Lab. Clin. Med., *82*, 978.
Chatterjee, S. and Sweeley, C.C. (1973) Biochem. Biophys. Res. Commun., *53*, 1310.
Cheetham, R.D., Keenan, T.W., Nyquist, S. and Morre, D.J. (1969) J. Cell Biol., *43*, 21a.
Chesney, C. McI., Harper, E. and Colman, R.W. (1972) J. Clin. Invest., *51*, 2693.
DaPrada, M. and Pletscher, A. (1968) J. Pharmac., *34*, 591.
Day, H.J., Holmsen, H. and Hovig, T. (1969) Scand. J. Haemat. Suppl., *7*, 1.
deDuve, C. (1969) in Lysosomes in Biology and Pathology (Dingle, J.T. and Fell, H.B., eds), p. 3, North-Holland, Amsterdam.
DeLuca, S., DeLuca, L. and Jamieson, G.A. (1976) Biochim. Biophys. Acta, in press.
Donati, M.B., de Gaetano, G. and Vermylen, J. (1973) Thromb. Res., *2*, 97.
Dzoga, K., Stoltzner, G. and Wissler, R.W. (1972) Lab. Invest., *27*, 351.
Emmelot, P. and Bos, C.J. (1966) Biochem. Biophys. Acta, *120*, 369.
Feagler, J.R., Tillack, T.W., Chaplin, D.D. and Majerus, P.W. (1974) J. Cell Biol., *60*, 541.
Fiszer, S. and DeRobertis, E. (1969) J. Neurochem., *16*, 1201.
Forbes, C.D. and Prentice, C.R.M. (1973) Nature, New Biol., *241*, 149.
French, P.E., Holmsen, H. and Stormorken, H. (1970) Biochim. Biophys. Acta, *206*, 438.
Fukami, M.H. and Salganicoff, L. (1973) Blood, *42*, 913.
Gasic, G.J. and Gasic, T.B. (1962) Proc. Natl. Acad. Sci. U.S.A., *48*, 1172.
Gasic, G.J., Gasic, T.B., Galanti, N., Johnson, T. and Murphy, S. (1973) Int. J. Cancer, *11*, 704.
Goldfisher, S., Essner, E. and Novikoff, A.B. (1964) J. Histochem. Cytochem., *12*, 72.
Gordon, J.L. and Dingle, J.T. (1974) J. Cell Sci., *16*, 157.
Greenberg, J.H. and Jamieson, G.A. (1974) Biochim. Biophys. Acta, *345*, 231.
Gröttum, K.A. and Solum, N.O. (1969) Brit. J. Haematol., *16*, 277.
Hampton, J.R. and Mitchell, J.R. (1966) Brit. Med. J., *1*, 1074.
Hanna, N. and Nelken, D. (1971) Immunology, *20*, 533.
Harker, L.A. (1971) in The Platelet (Brinkhous, K.M., Shermer, R.W. and Mostofi, F.K., eds), p. 13, Williams and Wilkins, Baltimore.
Harris, G.L.A. and Crawford, N. (1973) Biochim. Biophys. Acta, *291*, 701.
Henning, R., Kaulen, H.D. and Stoffel, W. (1970) Hoppe-Seyler's, Z. Physiol. Chem., *351*, 1191.
Hoak, J.C. (1972) Blood, *40*, 514.
Horak, H. and Barton, P.G. (1974) Biochim. Biophys. Acta, *373*, 471.
Hovig, T. (1968) Ser. Haemat., *1*, 3.

Hsu, A-F., Baynes, J.W. and Heath, E.C. (1974) Proc. Natl. Acad. Sci. U.S.A., *71*, 2391.
Huang, T.W., Lagunoff, D. and Benditt, E.P. (1974) Lab. Invest., *31*, 156.
Hugues, J. and Mahieu, P. (1970) Thromb. Diath. Haemorrh., *24*, 395.
Jamieson, G.A., Fuller, N.A., Barber, A.J. and Lombart, C. (1971) Ser. Haemat., *4*, 125.
Jamieson, G.A. and Groh, N. (1971) Anal. Biochem., *43*, 259.
Jamieson, G.A. and Okumura, T. (1975) J. Biol. Chem., in press.
Jamieson, G.A., Urban, C.L. and Barber, A.J. (1971) Nature New Biol., *234*, 5.
Johnson, J.D. and Cornatzer, W.E. (1969) Proc. Soc. Exptl. Biol. Med., *131*, 474.
Kang, A.H., Beachey, E.H. and Katzman, R.L. (1974) J. Biol. Chem., *249*, 1054.
Karpatkin, S. (1972) Ann. Rev. Med., *23*, 101.
Katzman, R.L., Kang, A.H. and Beachey, E.H. (1973) Science, *181*, 670.
Kaulen, H.D. and Gross, R. (1973) Thromb. Diath. Haemorrh., *30*, 199.
Kubanek, J., Entlicher, G. and Kocourek, J. (1973) Biochim. Biophys. Acta, *304*, 93.
Lamont, J.T., Perrotto, J.L., Weiser, M.M. and Isselbacher, K.J. (1974) Proc. Natl. Acad. Sci. U.S.A., *71*, 3726.
Lombart, C., Okumura, T. and Jamieson, G.A. (1974) FEBS Lett., *41*, 31.
Lucas, J.J., Waechter, C.J. and Lennarz, W.J. (1975) J. Biol. Chem., *250*, 3173.
Lyman, B., Rosenberg, L. and Karpatkin, S. (1971) J. Clin. Invest. 50, 1854.
Majerus, P.W. and Brodie, G.N. (1972) J. Biol. Chem., *247*, 4253.
Marchesi, V.T., Tillack, T.W., Jackson, R.L., Segrest, J.P. and Scott, R.E. (1972) Proc. Natl. Acad. Sci. U.S.A., *69*, 1445.
Marcus, A.J., Safier, L.B. and Ullman, H.L. (1971) in The Circulating Platelet (Johnson, S.A., ed), p. 241, Academic Press, New York.
Marcus, A.J., Ullman, H.L. and Safier, L.B. (1969) J. Lipid Res., *10*, 108.
Marcus, A.J., Ullman, H.L. and Safier, L.B. (1972) J. Clin. Invest. *51*, 2602.
Marcus, A.J., Zucker-Franklin, D., Ullman, H.L. and Safier, L.B. (1966) J. Clin. Invest., *45*, 15.
Mason, R.G. and Shermer, R.W. (1971) in The Platelet (Brinkhous, K.M, Shermer, R.W. and Mostofi, F.K., eds), p. 123, Williams and Wilkins, Baltimore.
Mehrishi, J.N. (1971) Thromb. Diath, Haemorrh., *26*, 370.
Milgrom, F., Campbell, W.A. and Witebsky, E. (1968) Vox Sang., *15*, 418.
Minter, B.F. and Crawford, N. (1971) Biochem. Pharmacol., *20*, 783.
Muggli, R. and Baumgartner, H.R. (1973) Thromb. Res., *3*, 715.
Myllyla, G. (1973) Scand. J. Haemat. Suppl., *19*, 7.
Nachman, R.L. and Ferris, B. (1972) J. Biol. Chem., *247*, 4468.
Nachman, R.L. and Ferris, B. (1974) J. Biol. Chem., *249*, 704.
Nachman, R.L., Hubbard, A. and Ferris, B. (1973) J. Biol. Chem., *248*, 2928.
Nakao, K. and Angrist, A. (1968) Nature, *217*, 960.
Nurden, A.T. and Caen, J.P. (1974) Brit. J. Haematol., *28*, 253.
Okumura, T. and Jamieson, G.A. (1975) J. Biol. Chem., in press.
Osler, A.G. and Siraganian, R.P. (1972) Prog. Allergy, *16*, 450.
Packham, M.A., Guccione, M.A., Chang, P-L. and Mustard, J.F. (1973) Amer. J. Physiol., *225*, 38.
Paulus, J.M.and Kinet-Denoel, C. (1973) Nouv. Rev. Franc. Haemat., *13*, 494.
Pfleger, R.C., Anderson, N.G. and Snyder, F. (1968) Biochemistry, *7*, 2826.
Phillips, D.R. (1972) Biochemistry, *11*, 4582.
Pepper, D.S. and Jamieson, G.A. (1968) Nature, *219*, 1252.
Pepper, D.S. and Jamieson, G.A. (1970) Biochemistry, *9*, 3706.
Puett, D., Wasserman, B.K., Ford, J.D. and Cunningham, L.W. (1973) J. Clin. Invest., *52*, 2495.
Rambourg, A. and Leblond, C.P. (1967) J. Cell Biol., *32*, 27.
Reddick, R.L. and Mason, R.G. (1973) Amer. J. Pathol., *70*, 473.
Roseman, S. (1970) J. Chem. Phys. Lipids, *5*, 270.
Salganicoff, L. and Fukami, M.H. (1972) Arch. Biochem. Biophys., *153*, 726.
Salganicoff, L., Hebda, P.A., Yandrasitz, J. and Fukami, M.H. (1975) Biochim. Biophys. Acta, *385*, 394.
Schick, P.K. and Yu, B.P. (1974) J. Clin. Invest., *54*, 1032.
Schulz, H. and Heipler, E. (1959) Klin. Wschr., *37*, 273.
Schulz, H. (1966) Verh. Deut. Ges. Pathol., *50*, 239.
Schulz, H. (1968) Electron Microscopy of Blood Platelets and Thrombosis, Springer Verlag, Berlin.
Seaman, G.V.F. and Vassar, P.S. (1966) Arch. Biochem. Biophys., *117*, 10.
Shulman, N.R., Marder, V.J., Hiller, M.C. and Collier, E.M. (1964) Prog. Haematol., *4*, 222.

Siegal, A., Burri, P.H., Weibel, E.R., Bettex-Galland, M. and Lüscher, E.F. (1971) Thromb. Diath. Haemorrh., *25*, 252.

Siegal, A. and Lüscher, E.F. (1967) Nature, *215*, 745.

Smith, D.F., Kosow, D.P. and Jamieson, G.A. (1975) Fed. Proc., in press.

Snyder, P.D., Desnick, R.J. and Krivit, W. (1972) Biochem. Biophys. Res. Commun., *46*, 1857.

Solatunturi, E. and Paasonen, M.K. (1966) Ann. Med. Exp. Biol. Fenn, *44*, 427.

Spaet, T.H. and Lejnieks, I. (1969) Proc. Exp. Biol. Med., *132*, 1038.

Spiro, R.G. (1975) J. Biol. Chem., *250*, 2842.

Spiro, R.G. and Spiro, M.J. (1971) J. Biol. Chem., *246*, 4899.

Stoffel, W. (1971) Ann. Rev. Biochem., *40* 57.

Stoltzner, G., Dzoga, K. and Wissler, R.W. (1972) Lab. Invest., *27*, 357.

Svejgaard, A. (1969) Iso-Antigenic Systems of Human Blood Platelets – A survey, Ser. Haematol., Vol. II, No. 3.

Tao, R.V.P., Sweeley, C.C. and Jamieson, G.A. (1973) J. Lipid. Res. *14*, 16.

Taylor, D.G. and Crawford, N. (1974) FEBS Lett., *41*, 317.

Terada, H., Baldini, M., Ebbe, S. and Madoff, M.A. (1966) Blood, *28*, 213.

Tollefsen, D.M., Feagler, J.R. and Majerus, P.W. (1974) J. Clin. Invest., *53*, 211.

Uhlenbruck, G. (1961) Z. Immunitaetsforsch. Exp. Ther., *121*, 420.

Verymylen, J., Donati, M.B., deGaetano, G. and Verstraete, M. (1973) Nature, *244*, 167.

Waechter, C.J., Lucas, J.J. and Lennarz, W.J. (1973) J. Biol. Chem., *248*, 7570.

Warren, L., Glick, M.C. and Nass, M.K. (1966) J. Cell Physiol., *68*, 269.

Winzler, R.J. (1969) in Red Cell Membrane-Structure and Function (Jamieson, G.A. and Greenwalt, T.J., eds), p. 157, J.B. Lippincott, Philadelphia, Pa.

Woolley, D.W. and Gommi, B.W. (1964) Nature, *202*, 1074.

Wolf, L.S., Breckenridge, W.C. and Shelton, P.P.C. (1974) J. Neurochem., *23*, 175.

Yankee, R. (1974) in Platelets: Production, Function, Transfusion and Storage, (Baldini, M.G. and Ebbe, S., eds), p. 313, Grune and Stratton, New York.

Yogeeswaran, G., Laine, R.A. and Hakomori, S-I. (1974) Biochem. Biophys. Res. Commun., *59*, 591.

Zimmerman, T.S. and Müller-Eberhard, H.J. (1973) Science, *180*, 1183.

Zucker, M.B. and Levine, R.U. (1963) Thromb. Diath. Haemorrh., *10*, 1.

CHAPTER 5

Platelet lipids and platelet function

DANIEL DEYKIN

Boston Veterans Administration Hospital, 150 South Huntington Avenue, Boston,
Massachusetts 02130, U.S.A.

1. Introduction

The participation of platelets in hemostasis begins when platelets adhere to subendothelial collagenous tissue exposed by vascular injury and progress through a series of events collectively termed the release reaction (see Chapter 3). During the release reaction, platelet membrane phospholipases are activated, resulting in the liberation of arachidonic acid, which is further converted by platelets to prostaglandin derivatives that are also initiators of the release reaction.

Platelets are capable of forming complex lipids from acetate, glycerol, and from preformed fatty acids. Many of the agents that induce the release reaction, for example ADP, epinephrine, and thrombin, also cause striking changes in platelet lipid synthesis. It is not yet certain whether these effects reflect the direct action of the inducers themselves, or are the consequence of the release reaction and the platelet aggregation which attends it. However, it is clear that during hemostasis extensive alterations occur in platelet lipid synthesis.

Whether initiated by adhesion to collagen or by exposure to ADP, prostaglandins, or thrombin, the release reaction is preceded by change in the platelet's shape. Because of this change the components of the surface membrane are reorganized furnishing a phospholipid matrix that accelerates the reactions between clotting factors IX and VIII and between factors X, V and prothrombin. Previously regarded as a specific factor (platelet factor 3), this clot-accelerating property is more appropriately considered an intrinsic reflection of the platelet shape change. The physical nature of the alteration in the platelet membrane which makes previously 'masked' phospholipids now available for interaction with soluble procoagulants is not understood. It is clear, however, that platelet factor 3 activity is abnormal in platelets that do not aggregate normally.

Changes in platelet lipid composition alter platelet function. Increasing platelet cholesterol content renders the platelet more sensitive to certain aggregating agents. In addition, certain patients with defects in platelet function have

Gordon (ed) Platelets in Biology and Pathology
© *Elsevier/North-Holland Biomedical Press, 1976*

abnormal fatty acids, increased lecithin and decreased phosphatidyl en-
thanolamine in their platelets. Partial digestion of platelet membrane lecithin by
phospholipase C induces the release reaction.

Therefore, because platelets are capable of synthesizing complex lipids,
because alterations in lipid metabolism and in the orientation of lipids in
membranes are integral to normal function, and because abnormalities of lipid
metabolism and composition have been associated with altered platelet function,
platelets are attractive for the study of the role of lipids in cellular function.

2. Fatty acids and prostaglandins

The definitive studies of platelet fatty acid composition were performed by
Marcus et al. (1969), who showed that neither platelet membranes nor granules
were characterized by a specific lipid or fatty acid. As in other tissues the
predominant fatty acids in the platelet phospholipids were palmitic, stearic, oleic
and arachidonic. Both platelet membrane and granule phosphatidyl-ethanolamine
and phosphatidyl-inositol were enriched in arachidonic acid, which comprised
40% of the total fatty acids present in the phosphatidyl-inositides.

Marks and his associates first showed that platelets can incorporate labeled
acetate into fatty acids (Marks et al., 1960). Their work was confirmed by Hennes
and his coworkers (1966), who showed that both the de novo and chain elongation
pathways of fatty acid synthesis exist in the platelet, and by Majerus and his
associates (1969), who demonstrated acetyl-CoA carboxylase activity in platelet
extracts. Deykin and Desser (1968), reported that fatty acids formed by de novo
synthesis exchange with plasma free fatty acids, but those formed primarily by
chain elongation did not. Deykin also showed that in platelets the synthesis of
ceramides was very active. In a subsequent study (Deykin, 1971), the lipids of
intact platelets were labeled with acetate and the distribution of radioactivity in
individual fatty acids was similar in each subcellular fraction. The rapid equilibra-
tion of newly formed lipids throughout the platelet and the absence of a highly
characteristic pattern of labeling in any one subcellular fraction discount the
probability of a localized, highly unusual lipid metabolic pool among those lipids
synthesized from acetate in the resting platelet.

The platelet uptake of free fatty acids from plasma albumin has been studied by
both Spector and his associates (Spector et al., 1970; Hoak et al. 1972), and by
Cohen et al. (1970). Fatty acids are taken up by platelets first as free fatty acids
bound to the membrane. The initial binding of the fatty acids is not energy-
dependent, but on continued incubation, free fatty acids are then transferred by
an energy-dependent mechanism to internal sites within the platelet where they
may be either oxidized or incorporated into complex lipids.

Thrombin alters platelet synthesis of fatty acids from acetate and the incorporation of fatty acids into complex lipids (Deykin, 1973). At low concentrations
thrombin does not impair overall fatty acid synthesis from acetate. Indeed, it may
actually stimulate the de novo pathway. However, the incorporation into complex

lipids of the fatty acids newly formed from acetate is impaired by thrombin. Furthermore, thrombin alters the uptake of free fatty acids from plasma (Deykin, 1973). Although the initial binding of fatty acids to the platelet membrane is not impeded, the incorporation of saturated fatty acids (palmitic, stearic) into both phospholipids and glycerides is depressed. By contrast incorporation of oleic acid into phospholipids (but not into glycerides) is enhanced by thrombin. It is probable that thrombin impairs the de novo assembly of platelet complex lipids but that the enhanced incorporation of oleic acid reflects acylation of newly exposed monoacyl receptors.

The metabolism of arachidonic acid by platelets is of particular importance, since a novel class of prostaglandins (PG) formed in platelets from arachidonic acid is now thought to play a central role in platelet function. In 1971, Smith and Willis demonstrated that thrombin-aggregated platelets form and release PGE_2 and $F_{2\alpha}$ and further showed that aspirin inhibits PG formation and release. In other studies, Kloeze (1969), and Shio and Ramwell (1972), demonstrated that although PGE_2 did not itself initiate platelet aggregation, it potentiated ADP-induced platelet aggregation. $PGF_{2\alpha}$ was shown to be inert. Willis and Weiss (1973), and Salzman et al. (1973), reported that in patients with inherited disorders of platelet function PG synthesis was impaired during aggregation. However, since PGE_2 did not induce aggregation itself, the role of prostaglandins in hemostasis remained uncertain.

An important advance was made by Willis (1974a,b), who showed that during the formation of PGE_2 and $F_{2\alpha}$ a labile intermediate appeared which did induce platelet aggregation. These findings were confirmed by Smith and coworkers (1974). Further studies of the pathways of prostaglandin formation (Hamberg et al., 1974a,b; Hamberg and Samuelsson, 1974; Malmsten et al., 1975; Hamberg et al., 1975), have shown that there are at least two classes of labile intermediates formed by platelets in response to thrombin. These intermediates, the cyclic endoperoxides and their derivatives, the thromboxanes, are far more potent than any platelet aggregating agents previously described.

As platelets aggregate, phospholipases are activated, resulting in the release of arachidonic acid from platelet phospholipids. The arachidonic acid is then converted by a platelet enzyme, cyclo-oxygenase, into prostaglandin G_2, (PGG_2) a cyclic endoperoxide that has a half-life of less than 5 min. PGG_2 is a powerful initiator of platelet aggregation, but it is further transformed to an even more potent platelet aggregating agent, thromboxane A_2. This oxane is very unstable and persists for less than 40 sec in plasma before decomposing to a stable, inert compound, thromboxane B_2.

PGG_2 may also decompose to a 17-carbon compound (called HHT) with the release of a 3 carbon fragment, malonyl dialdehyde. HHT is inert, but the release of malonyl dialdehyde may serve as a convenient marker of the formation and breakdown of PGG_2.

A third pathway of transformation of PGG_2 is the formation of the classical, stable prostaglandins PGE_2 and $F_{2\alpha}$. However, since it is now established (Hamberg et al., 1974a) that in response to thrombin at least one hundred times more PGG_2 is formed than PGE_2 and $F_{2\alpha}$, and since PGG_2 and its derivative thromboxane A_2 are far more powerful than PGE_2 and $F_{2\alpha}$, the new prostaglandin compounds are clearly more important than PGE_2 and $F_{2\alpha}$ which may be relatively trivial end products in the platelet.

In addition to transformation by cyclo-oxygenase, arachidonic acid is also metabolized by a separate enzyme, platelet lipoxygenase, which converts arachidonic acid into 12L hydroxy-5, 8, 10, 14 eicosatetraenoic acid, or HETE. This compound has no apparent effect on platelet function but it has recently been shown to be a chemoattractant for human polymorphonuclear leukocytes in vitro (Turner et al., 1975). Samuelsson and his associates have reported that aspirin and indomethacin inhibit platelet cyclo-oxygenase, but that HETE formation is actually enhanced in aspirin-treated platelets (Hamberg et al., 1974a).

The existence of two pathways of arachidonic acid metabolism has been confirmed by Russell and Deykin (1976), who studied the effect of thrombin on the uptake and incorporation of arachidonic acid into complex lipids by human platelets. They found that thrombin does not impair the initial binding of arachidonic acids by platelets, but it does reduce overall incorporation of arachidonic acid into complex lipids. They found, as had Samuelsson, that thrombin caused the release of two groups of metabolites, and that one was not inhibited by aspirin. In addition these workers noted the formation of a novel lipid, presumably a phospholipid, during the thrombin-mediated alteration of platelet arachidonic acid metabolism. Russell and Deykin found that only a limited fraction of the lipids labeled by arachidonic acid was available to the thrombin-activated phospholipases.

It is clear that thrombin causes a complex remodeling of the incorporation of fatty acids into platelet phospholipids, which does not depend exclusively on either chain length or degree of unsaturation, but rather reflects the combination of several processes which include impaired de novo formation of complex lipids, enhanced acylation of monoacyl receptors, activation of phospholipases, and transformation of liberated fatty acids into derivatives which are released from the platelet.

3. Phospholipid metabolism

Platelets are capable of incorporating both orthophosphate and glycerol into phospholipids. Lewis and Majerus (1969), were the first to describe in detail the synthesis of platelet phospholipids from glycerol. In resting platelets, the predominant lipids to be labeled were phosphatidyl-choline, phosphatidyl-inositol and phosphatidic acid, but phosphatidyl-serine and phosphatidyl-ethanolamine were labeled as well. When platelets were treated with thrombin, total incorporation of glycerol into platelet phospholipids decreased, with a marked decrease of lecithin labeling. In contrast, labeling of phosphatidyl-serine was sharply but transiently increased above basal levels. The increased rate of phosphatidyl-serine synthesis persisted for approximately 20 min and then returned to pretreatment values.

These studies were extended by Deykin (1973), who compared the effects on platelet lipid synthesis of aggregation induced by thrombin and poly-1-lysine. Incorporation of glycerol into all classes of phospholipids was inhibited by both agents, suggesting that the impaired phospholipid synthesis was not a specific thrombin-mediated event, but rather reflected the consequences of aggregation itself. In these studies, thrombin did not increase phosphatidyl-serine labeling from glycerol. Since in mammalian tissues the synthesis of phosphatidyl-serine occurs by base exchange of serine for ethanolamine or choline in phosphatidyl-ethanolamine or phosphatidyl-choline (Porcellati et al., 1971; Kanfer, 1972; Bjerve, 1973), the mechanism for the enhanced phosphatidyl-serine synthesis observed by Lewis and Majerus remains unexplained.

In a subsequent study, Snyder and Deykin (1973) examined the effect of aggregation by epinephrine on glycerol incorporation in platelets in platelet-rich plasma. In contrast to the observations made with thrombin-treated washed platelets, epinephrine produced a marked, sustained increase in phosphatidyl-inositol synthesis. The effect was not immediate but occurred only after the release reaction had been completed. Aspirin inhibited but did not completely suppress the stimulation of phosphatidyl inositol synthesis. However, the stimulation of phosphatidyl-inositol did not occur in platelets from patients with storage pool disease, in which the release reaction was absent (Hutton and Deykin, 1973).

The selective enhancement of phosphatidyl-inositol formation in epinephrine-aggregated platelets is similar to the increased phosphatidyl-inositol turnover that occurs in exocrine glands following specific stimulation. Indeed, several authors have suggested that the release reaction of platelets resembles the secretory activity of acinar glandular cells. The constituents to be released from platelets are contained in discrete storage granules. During the release reaction the contents are discharged into a canalicular system which reaches the platelet surface. Whether the granules are physically extruded has not been established, but clearly new connections between the granules and the platelet vacuolar membrane are established during aggregation. Although the parallel between the platelet and acinar cells is not exact, the similarities are sufficiently close to suggest that the factors responsible for increased phosphatidyl-inositol turnover in exocrine glands during secretion may be operative in the platelet as well. As Hokin (1969), has emphasized, new phosphatidyl-inositol formation in secretory tissues seems not to be a prerequisite for the extrusion of secretory granules, but rather it is related to the reconstitution of membranes disrupted by the passage of granules through the plasma membrane.

Lloyd et al. (1974), observed a similar increase in labeling of phosphatides of washed, thrombin-treated rabbit platelets incubated with $^{32}PO_4$. In contrast to their prior observations with ADP-aggregated platelets (Lloyd and Mustard, 1974), they found that the increase in ^{32}P content of monophosphatidyl-inositol occurred after release had begun. They also suggested that the changes in phosphatidyl-inositol synthesis are part of a membrane repair process.

Platelets contain three forms of phosphoinositides: mono-, di-, and triphosphoinositiol. Cohen and his associates (1971), found that when platelets are incubated with $^{32}PO_4$ under normal osmotic conditions, only the phosphoinositides were labeled, whereas under hypotonic conditions all platelet phospholipids were labeled. The enzymes of phosphoinositide synthesis have been studied in detail by Call and his associates (1970), who first showed that platelet extracts can form CDP-diglyceride from phosphatidic acid and CTP, and then (Lucas et al., 1970) that platelet homogenates can complete the synthesis of phosphatidyl-inositides from CDP-diglyceride and myo-inositol.

In addition, Call has also characterized the platelet enzyme system that synthesizes phosphatidyl-ethanolamine (Call and Rubert, 1975). He has found that the enzyme, ethanolaminephosphotransferase is particulate and, under the conditions of his experiments, required Mn^{2+} and detergents for maximum activation. In other experiments Okuma and his associates (Okuma et al., 1973), described a particulate platelet enzyme which can acylate sn-glycerol 3-phosphate directly to form phosphatidic acid. The enzyme was surprisingly active (but only in sonicated platelets), demonstrating 40% of the activity found in liver.

Elsbach and coworkers (1971), studied platelet metabolism of lysolecithin, using concentrations of lysolecithin that occur in plasma. They found that platelets can degrade lysolecithin to glycerolphosphorylcholine or can acylate lysolecithin to form lecithin. Both reactions occurred at high pH optima. Under the conditions used by these workers, thrombin and ADP had no effect on either pathway of lysolecithin metabolism.

No unique phospholipid nor unusual pathway of phospholipid metabolism has as yet been identified in human platelets. The major questions to be resolved concern the distribution of platelet phospholipases, their mechanism of activation and control, the regulation of phospholipid synthetic pathways, and structural information concerning the role of phospholipids in the receptor sites for the many disparate agents that initiate platelet aggregation.

4. Cholesterol

Derksen and Cohen (1973), have shown that platelets cannot synthesize cholesterol. They cannot form mevalonic acid from acetate, nor can they incorporate mevalonate into cholesterol. Therefore, platelet cholesterol content reflects the initial composition of the megakaryocyte, although exchange of cholesterol with plasma lipoproteins may result in remodeling of the endogenous platelet cholesterol content. Platelet membranes have a much lower cholesterol/phospholipid ratio (approximately 5 : 10 [Marcus et al., 1969]) than that of red cell membranes (approximately 9 : 10). Recent studies suggest that changing the cholesterol content of the platelet membrane alters the platelet response to aggregating agents. Carvalho et al. (1973) studied platelet function in 17 patients with Type II hyperbetalipoproteinemia. They found that platelets from these patients, as compared to 26 normal subjects, had an enhanced response to epinephrine, collagen, and ADP. These experiments suggest a relationship between plasma cholesterol content and platelet function, but did not establish the mechanism, since incubation of normal platelets with plasma from Type II did not confer increased sensitivity to the platelets. More direct evidence linking platelet cholesterol content to platelet function was provided by Shattil and coworkers (1975). They prepared cholesterol-lecithin liposomes which were 'cholesterol normal' (cholesterol/phospholipid ratio, 1:0), 'cholesterol rich' (cholesterol/phospholipid ratio, 2:2), or 'cholesterol poor' (devoid of cholesterol). Incubation of platelets with cholesterol rich liposomes raised the platelet membrane cholesterol. Incubation with cholesterol poor liposomes lowered platelet membrane cholesterol. Cholesterol normal liposomes did not change the platelet membrane cholesterol. The acquisition of cholesterol by platelets was associated with a 35-fold increase in sensitivity to epinephrine-induced aggregation. Reduction of platelet membrane cholesterol was associated with an 18-fold reduction in sensitivity to epinephrine.

These observations would suggest that the enhanced sensitivity to aggregating agents originally observed by Carvalho and her associates might well have reflected increased platelet cholesterol content. Indeed, Bennett et al. (1974), have reported an increased cholesterol/phospholipid ratio in patients with Type II hyperlipoproteinemia whose platelets demonstrate hypersensitivity.

5. *Glycosphingolipids*

In their study of platelet lipids formed from acetate, Deykin (1973), reported that over 40% of the acetate incorporated into complex lipids was present in long-chain saturated fatty acids in ceramides, the precursors of glycosphingolipids. Subsequently, Krevit and Hammerstrom (1972), examined the composition of free ceramides in platelets. They found that although the platelet ceramides resembled plasma ceramides in their composition, C_{24} acids predominated in platelet ceramides.

There have been two analyses of platelet gangliosides (Snyder et al., 1972; Marcus et al., 1972). Both have shown that hematoside (glucosegalactosesialic acid ratio 1:1:1) is the predominant platelet ganglioside, comprising over 92% of the total platelet gangliosides.

Although no specific function for the platelet gangliosides has yet been established, Marcus et al. (1975), have speculated that they may be involved in the initial binding of serotonin by the platelet.

6. *Conclusion*

The foregoing discussion prompts the generalization that platelet lipids–or, perhaps more precisely, changes in platelet lipids–modify or may in some instances actually determine platelet function. Such a generalization must be tempered because there is as yet no firm link between platelet lipids and any single aspect of platelet function. Whether or not the transformations in lipid metabolism that occur during aggregation are only incidental or are integral to hemostasis is not known. The relative importance of the thromboxanes in the sequence of self-perpetuating platelet aggregation is not yet established. The significance of the variation in platelet sensitivity to aggregating agents caused by manipulating platelet membrane cholesterol content is also uncertain. Safrit et al. (1972), have reported abnormal phospholipid content and an unusual fatty acid distribution in the platelets (and red cells) in one family with defective platelet release reaction, but the specificity of this intriguing observation has not been ascertained.

Another possible link between platelet lipids and platelet function has been suggested by Shick and Yu (1974), who found that limited digestion of platelet phospholipids by phospholipase C triggered the platelet release reaction. They suggest that platelet membrane phospholipids are located at or near a 'receptor' for ADP and function as the modulator for the platelet release reaction. The nature of the hypothetical receptor is not known.

Although interest in platelet lipids was initially aroused by efforts to identify the lipids responsible for the clot-accelerating activity of platelets, no unique platelet lipids have as yet been described. The elucidation of those alterations in the platelet membrane which underlie the specific contribution of lipids to the coagulation cascade remains unsolved.

Despite these limits, the initial generalization–that platelet lipids are closely linked to platelet function–remains a forceful impetus to continued investigation of platelet lipid composition and metabolism.

References

Bennett, J., Shattil, S.J., Cooper, R.A. and Colman, R.W. (1974) Blood (abst.) 44, 918.
Bjerve, K.S. (1973) Biochim. Biophys. Acta., 296, 549.
Call, F.L. and Rubert, M. (1975) J. Lipid Res., 16, 352.
Call, F.L. and Williams, W.J. (1970) J. Clin. Invest., 49, 392.
Carvalho, A.C.A., Colman, R.W. and Lees, R.S. (1973) New Eng. J. Med. 290, 434.
Cohen, P., Broekman, M.J., Verkley, A., Lisman, J.W.W. and Derksen, A. (1971) J. Clin. Invest., 50, 762.
Cohen, P., Derksen, A. and Van DenBosch, H. (1970) J. Clin. Invest., 49, 128.
Derksen, A. and Cohen, P. (1973) J. Biol. Chem., 248, 7396.
Deykin, D. (1971) J. Lipid Res., 12, 9.
Deykin, D. (1973) J. Clin. Invest., 52, 483.
Deykin, D. and Desser, R.K. (1968) J. Clin. Invest., 47, 1950.
Deykin, D. and Snyder, D. (1973) J. Lab. Clin. Med., 82, 554.
Elsbach, P., Petits, P. and Marcus, A.J. (1971) Blood, 37, 675.
Hamberg, M. and Samuelsson, B. (1974) Proc. Natl. Acad. Sci. U.S.A., 71, 3400.
Hamberg, M., Svensson, J. and Samuelsson, B. (1974a) Proc. Natl. Acad. Sci. U.S.A., 71, 3824.
Hamberg, M., Svensson, J., Wakabayaski, T. and Samuelsson, B. (1974b) Proc. Natl. Acad. Sci. U.S.A., 71, 345.
Hamberg, M., Svensson, J. and Samuelsson, B. (1975) Proc. Natl. Acad. Sci. U.S.A., 72, 2994.
Hennes, A. R., Awai, K., Hamerstrand, K. and Duboff, G. (1966) Nature, 210, 839.
Hoak, J.D., Spector, A.A., Fry, G.L. and Barnes, B.C. (1972) Blood, 40, 16.
Hokin, L.E. (1969) Ann. N.Y. Acad. Sci., 165, 695.
Hutton, R.A. and Deykin, D. (1973) Proc. 16th Annual Meeting; Am. Soc. Hematol., p. 116.

Kanfer, J.N. (1972) J. Lipid Res., *13*, 468.
Kloeze, J. (1969) Biochim. Biophys. Acta., *187*, 285.
Krevit, W. and Hammarstrom, S. (1972) J. Lipid. Res., *13*, 525.
Lewis, N. and Majerus, P.W. (1969) J. Clin. Invest., *48*, 2114.
Lloyd, J.V. and Mustard, J.F. (1974) Brit. J. Haemat., *26*, 243.
Lloyd, J.V., Nishizawa, E.E. and Mustard, J.F. (1973) Brit. J. Haemat., *25*, 77.
Lucas, C.T., Call, F.L. and Williams, W.S. (1970) J. Clin. Invest. *49*, 1949.
Majerus, P.W., Smith, M.B. and Clamon, G.H. (1969) J. Clin. Invest., *48*, 21114.
Malmsten, C., Hamberg, M., Svensson, J. and Samuelsson, B. (1975) Proc. Natl. Acad. Sci. U.S.A., *72*, 1446.
Marcus, A.J., Ullman, H.L. and Safier, L.B. (1969) J. Lipid. Res., *10*, 108.
Marcus, A.J., Ullman, H.L. and Safier, L.B. (1972) J. Clin. Invest., *51*, 2602.
Marcus, A.J., Safier, L.B. and Ullman, H.L. (1975) in Biochemistry and Pharmacology of Platelets, Ciba Foundation Symposium 35, 309.
Marks, P.A., Gellhorn, A. and Kidson, C. (1960) J. Biol. Chem., *235*, 279.
Okuma, M., Yamashita, S. and Numa, S. (1973) Blood, *41*, 379.
Porcellati, G., Arienti, G., Pirotta, M. and Giorgini, D. (1971) J. Neurochem., *18*, 1395.
Russel, F.A. and Deykin, D. (1976) Am. J. Hematol., (in press).
Safrit, W., Weiss, H.J. and Phillips, G. (1972) Lipids, *7*, 60.
Salzman, E.W., Stead, N. and Deykin, D. (1973) International Congress on Hemostasis and Thrombosis, Vienna.
Schick, P.K. and Yu, B.P. (1974) J. Clin. Invest., *54*, 1032.
Shattil, S.J., Anaya-Galindo, R., Bennett, J., Colman, R.W. and Cooper, R.A. (1975) J. Clin. Invest., *55*, 636.
Shio, H. and Ramwell, P.W. (1972) Nature, *236*, 45.
Smith, J.B., Ingerman, C., Kocsis, J.J. and Silver, M.J. (1974) J. Clin. Invest., *53*, 1468.
Smith, J.B. and Willis, A.L. (1971) Nature New Biol., *231*, 235.
Snyder, P.D., Desnick, R.S. and Krevit, W. (1972) Biochem. Biophys. Res. Comm., *46*, 1857.
Spector, A.A., Hoak, J.D., Warner, E.D. and Fry, G.L. (1970) J. Clin. Invest., *49*, 1489.
Turner, S.R., Tainer, J.A. and Lynn, W.S. (1975) Nature, *257*, 680.
Willis, A.L. (1974) Science, *183*, 325.
Willis, A.L. (1974) Prostaglandins, *5*, 1.
Willis, A.L. and Weiss, H.J. (1973) Prostaglandins, *4*, 783.

CHAPTER 6

Platelet microfilaments and microtubules

N. Crawford

University Department of Biochemistry, P.O. Box 363,
Birmingham, B15 2TT, England

1. Introduction

In the circulation, mammalian blood platelets are characteristically disc-shaped and their maintenance in this form is probably essential for their unhindered passage through small bore sections of the vascular tree. From experiments involving exposure of platelets to low temperatures, colchicine, vinblastine and certain other alkaloids, there seems little doubt that a well-organized structure of microtubules lying parallel to, and just beneath, the boundary membrane (Fig. 1) sustains the cell's discoid form and helps to prevent the formation of any surface irregularities which would encourage irreversible encounters with other platelets and vascular endothelial tissue.

As part of its haemostatic activities the platelet surface membrane can respond

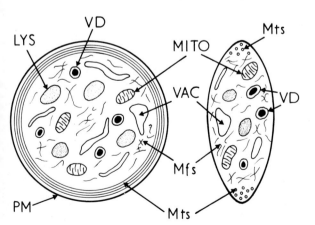

Fig. 1. Representation of platelet sectioned in (LEFT) equatorial plane and (RIGHT) in transverse plane. PM = plasma membrane; MITO = mitochondria; VAC = vacuoles; LYS = lysosomes; VD = very dense bodies (amine storage granules); Mts = microtubules; Mfs = microfilaments. Diagram modified from Behnke (1967).

Gordon (ed) Platelets in Biology and Pathology
© *Elsevier/North-Holland Biomedical Press, 1976*

to stimuli, such as thrombin and ADP, and their effect is then translated in some way to the interior of the cell to produce a well-documented sequence of events. These include firstly, a transformation from the discoid form to spheres, then spikes or pseudopodia arise from the surface and these thicken and interact with those of other platelets to form the consolidated mass known as the haemostatic plug. The progressive assembly of this plug at a site of injury in the vessel wall, eventually seals the lesion and prevents blood losses.

Many excellent electron microscope studies, notably those of White (1971), Behnke et al., (1967; 1970; 1971; 1972), Hovig (1968), Bettex-Galland and Lüscher (1960; 1965) and Zucker-Franklin (1967; 1969; 1970), have revealed that when these shape changes occur, the marginal bundle, or concentric ring, of microtubules appears to become disorganized and may even disappear altogether. Later in the process the microtubules again become prominent and are then often seen extending into the pseudopodia–indeed, they may be present throughout their length to the terminal tips (Fig. 2).

The cytoplasm of the blood platelet also contains other fibrillar elements, smaller in diameter than the microtubules, known as microfilaments (Fig. 3). In electron micrographs these filaments show more size heterogeneity than the microtubules and appear widely scattered throughout the platelet cytoplasm, often apparently intercalated between the microtubules and the inner face of the plasma membrane. The microfilaments have contractile properties and when the platelet becomes activated the filaments appear to predominate both in the pseudopodia and in the central area of the cytoplasm, where they surround and interconnect clumps of the granular organelles. It is not clearly understood if they are concerned in the formation of pseudopodia, or in the migration of the granules to the central zone by their contractile action: they could simply be found fortuitously in these regions because of prior association with the granule membranes, or with regions of plasma membrane destined to form the pseudopodia.

During the last few years these two major polymeric protein systems of the platelet have attracted considerable attention because, by analogies with other cellular systems, they could be involved as mechano-chemical mediators of the various platelet shape change phenomena, triggered by the receptor responses to surface stimuli. In addition, it is now clearly established that the blood platelet is a secreting cell and during its haemostatic activities it specifically exports from storage granules certain agents, such as the nucleoside di- and triphosphates and 5-hydroxytryptamine, which promote the platelet plug forming process by activating other adjacent platelets. The role of the microtubules and contractile microfilaments in this latter phenomenon (the 'release reaction') has not been well explored but by comparison with other secreting tissues and particularly by studies of the effects of microtubule and microfilament poisons on other secretion processes, there are strong indications that these structures may be mechanistically involved in the platelet release reaction too (see Chapter 3).

Much is now known about the appearance of the microtubules and microfilaments and the changes in their fine structure and localization which occur when

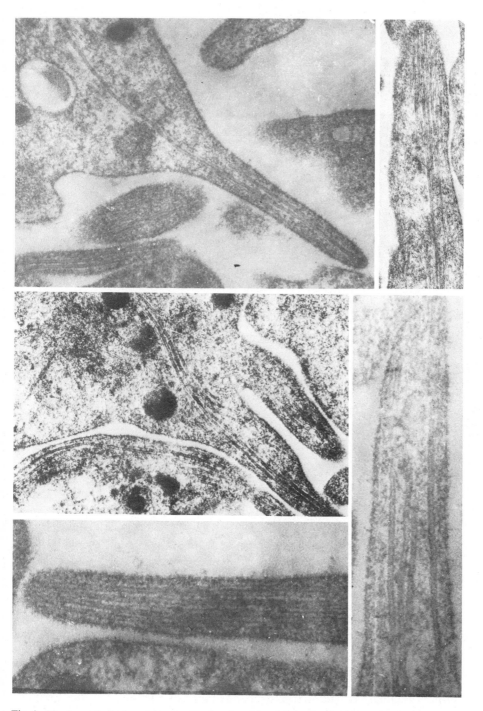

Fig. 2. Montage of electron micrographs showing microtubules in platelet pseudopodia.

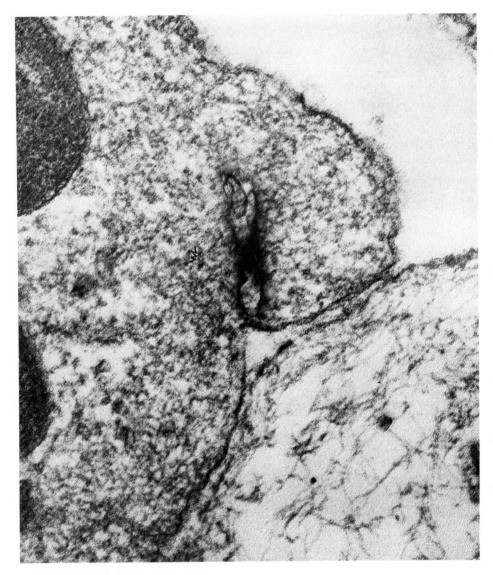

Fig. 3. Microfilaments–random distribution in cytoplasm of adjacent platelets.

the platelet is exposed to haemostatic stimuli or to agents that interact with structural proteins–for example colchicine and cytochalasin. There is, however, less information available about the molecular organisation of these structures.

In this paper I make no excuse for omitting many details of their morphology and subcellular location, since these aspects have been well reviewed in the papers of White, Behnke, Hovig, Bettex-Galland and Lüscher and Zucker-Franklin referred to earlier. What I hope to do, however, is to summarise our knowledge of the molecular organisation of these structures: in particular, the subunit proteins of which they are formed; the characteristics of the associated enzyme activities that may be involved in the energetics of assembly, interaction and function; and the similarities and differences between the platelet elements and the analogous structures of cilia, flagella and the skeletal muscle myofibril.

In a final section I have summarised some of the more significant findings from experiments using the microtubule and microfilament poisons colchicine and cytochalasin, applied both to intact cells and to isolated structural and contractile components in vitro. The relevance of these findings to the role of these polymeric protein complexes in shape-change phenomena, aggregation, and the release reaction are briefly discussed, with particular reference to the dynamic equilibria between the polymeric filaments associated with the cell membrane and the soluble subunit or monomeric pools in the cytoplasm.

It has unfortunately been necessary in this short review to be somewhat selective, in order to avoid tortuous discussion of sometimes conflicting results. I apologise in advance, therefore, if any important contributions in this now extensive field have been overlooked or inadequately presented.

2. Microfilament proteins

Since the first isolation of an actomyosin-like contractile protein complex ('thrombosthenin') from platelets by Lüscher and his colleagues (1959; 1961) and by Grette (1962), much evidence has accumulated substantiating the presence in the platelet of actin, myosin, and tropomyosin-like proteins. All of these have properties similar, though not always identical, to the corresponding components of the skeletal muscle contractile apparatus. Despite the biochemical evidence for their existence, however, the morphological identification of fibrillar structures in the platelet cytoplasm corresponding to the thick and thin filaments of the muscle myofibril has proved difficult.

Thrombosthenin represents between 15 and 20% of the total platelet protein and it can be readily isolated from the cell in a crude form by KCl extraction and low ionic strength precipitation (Bettex-Galland and Lüscher, 1961). Electron microscopic examination of partially purified preparations of this protein (Zucker-Franklin et al., 1967) has revealed a mixed population of filamentous structures between 5 and 12 nm thick, but it was not possible in these earlier studies to identify clearly the separate actinoid and myosinoid polymer species. More recently some success with platelet filament subclassification has been achieved at the whole cell level, using platelets exposed to osmotic shock (Zucker-Franklin, 1969), or after treatment with solutions containing increasing proportions of glycerol (Behnke, 1971). Using the former procedure, Zucker-Franklin found that two categories of filaments could be identified, one measuring between 5 and 7 nm and the other 8–12 nm in thickness. She suggested that these represented the actin and myosin-like filaments respectively, but the final confirmation that at least some of the smaller structures (approx. 6 nm) were similar to actin came from the later studies of Behnke and his colleagues (1971) using a heavy meromyosin (HMM) labelling technique applied to glycerol treated platelets. This procedure, originally developed by Ishikawa et al. (1969), is now regarded as almost diagnostic for actin filaments provided that suitable control studies are simultaneously carried out in which the actin-HMM complex formation is prevented by pretreatment of the HMM with ATP or pyrophosphate. Usually the HMM is prepared by mild tryptic digestion of rabbit skeletal muscle myosin and when platelet actin filaments are treated with this preparation they appear decorated with regularly spaced arrow-head complexes that show a periodicity of about 36 nm. Similar arrow-head complexes (Fig. 4) can be formed with F-actin isolated from thrombosthenin (Bettex-Galland et al., 1972) and this reaction can be inhibited by pretreatment with ATP, substantiating the view that the 6 nm filaments in the platelet cytoplasm are probably actinoid in character. The finding that these filaments are more numerous in activated platelets than in the normal cell (Bessis and Breton-Gorius, 1965) led Behnke et al. (1971) to propose that in the cytoplasm there was an equilibrium between platelet G-actin monomers and F-actin filaments, only the latter being capable of complexing with HMM.

The larger 7–12 nm filaments are generally assumed to be myosin-like but since (even with carefully controlled muscle myofibrillar preparations) the myosin filaments vary greatly in thickness depending upon the pH and ionic strength of the bathing solutions, the definitive morphological identification of platelet myosin is difficult. It is unfortunate that the small size of the platelet precludes the use of the fluorescent antibody labelling procedures which have been particularly successful for locating the individual components of the actomyosin complex in other cells (Weber and Groeschel-Stewart, 1974; Pollack et al., 1975; Clarke et al., 1975; Crawford et al., 1976).

To summarise the current view, filaments in the size range 5–7 nm which accept HMM and form arrowhead complexes are almost certainly actinoid, whereas other filaments (which in negatively stained preparations can measure between 4 and 18 nm) may be myosinoid, but require further cytochemical evidence to establish their identity.

2.1. Actin

The molecular properties of the subunit proteins constituting the platelet actomyosin complex have been studied not only by platelet enthusiasts but also by many other workers interested in cellular motile activity and the phylogenic aspects of contractile proteins. From these many studies it is clear that platelet actin, like other cytoplasmic actins, more closely resembles smooth and skeletal muscle actins than do the cell myosin and tropomyosin-like proteins resemble their counterparts in muscle tissues.

2.1.1. Physicochemical properties

Both platelet and skeletal muscle actins have closely similar molecular weights (about 43,000), migrate with the same mobility in most polyacrylamide gels (Fig.

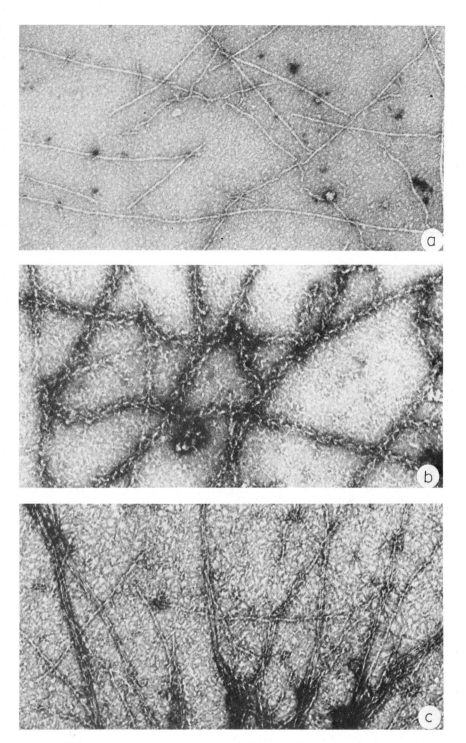

Fig. 4. Platelet actin prepared from isolated thrombosthenin: (a) untreated; (b) decorated with skeletal muscle heavy meromyosin; (c) preparation as (b), but with 2 mM ATP added to prevent the heavy meromyosin/actin interaction [Taken from Bettex-Galland et al. (1972). (Magnifications ×92,000).]

5), have almost indistinguishable amino acid analysis profiles (Fig. 6), and show similar autoradiographic patterns (Fig. 7) after one dimensional electrophoretic separation of tryptic digests iodinated with ^{125}I by the procedure of Bray and Brownlees (1973). The complete amino acid sequence data for skeletal muscle actin has now been published (Elzinga et al., 1973; Collins and Elzinga, 1975) and the residue/mol values from this data are presented in Table 1 together with our own values for pig platelet actin, leucocyte actin, and pig and rabbit skeletal muscle actins. The similarity between these actins is striking but it remains to be seen if, when a sequence study of platelet actin is performed, minor differences

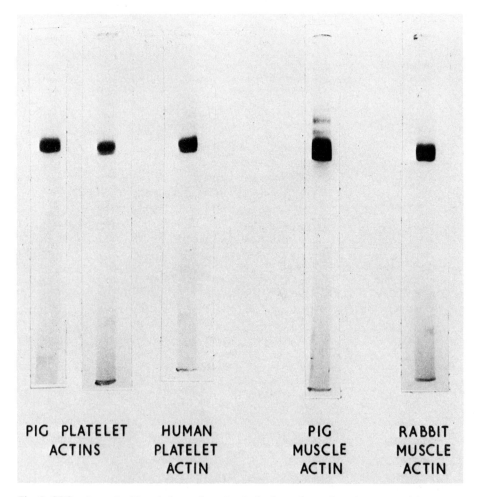

PIG PLATELET   HUMAN   PIG   RABBIT
    ACTINS   PLATELET   MUSCLE   MUSCLE
                         ACTIN   ACTIN   ACTIN

Fig. 5. SDS-polyacrylamide gel electrophoresis of platelet and muscle actins prepared from acetone powders by the procedure of Bailin and Bárány (1972). Samples treated with SDS/urea/mercaptoethanol and run in 7.5% polyacrylamide gels containing 0.1% SDS. Stained with Coomassie blue.

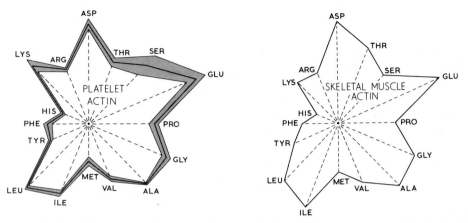

Fig. 6. Amino acid analysis profiles of platelet actin (Left) and skeletal muscle actin (Right). Radial lines are proportional to amino acid composition in moles per cent. Shaded area in platelet actin profile represents ±one standard deviation for six preparations. Muscle actin profile constructed from the sequence data for rabbit skeletal muscle protein reported by Elzinga et al. (1973).

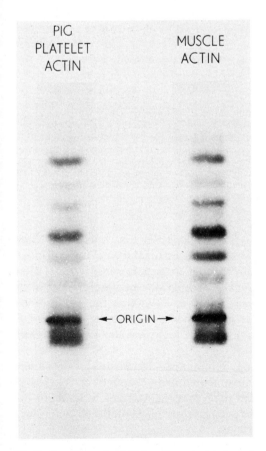

Fig. 7. One-dimensional high voltage electrophoresis of tryptic peptides of platelet and muscle actins after iodination with ¹²⁵I by the procedure of Bray and Brownlee (1973). Conditions for separation: pH 5.6; 10 kV; 9 h.

TABLE 1
Amino acid composition of various actins

Amino acid	Rabbit skeletal muscle actin (Sequence data)	Pig skeletal muscle actin	Pig platelet actins mean ± std. dev.	Human platelet actins	
	(a)	(b)	(c)	(d)	(e)
ASP	34	33.8	33.5 ± 1.7	33.4	35.5
THR	27	25.7	22.1 ± 1.4	26.1	23.3
SER	22	22.6	27.9 ± 4.4	25.1	27.1
GLU	39	46.8	39.9 ± 3.5	42.8	40.0
PRO	19	20.5	22.8 ± 1.5	19.5	22.3
GLY	28	27.4	28.5 ± 1.6	26.1	28.3
ALA	29	27.4	28.2 ± 0.4	29.8	29.2
VAL	21	21.1	19.7 ± 1.1	20.6	22.6
MET	16	16.0	12.2 ± 1.3	15.0	11.6
ILE	30	29.9	24.9 ± 1.1	27.2	23.9
LEU	26	28.3	30.0 ± 0.7	26.4	29.7
TYR	16	16.3	13.6 ± 0.9	14.4	12.2
PHE	12	11.7	14.0 ± 1.5	13.4	13.6
HIS	8	8.2	9.0 ± 0.7	8.0	7.5
3 Me-HIS	1	0.72	0.62 ± 0.08	1.0	ND
LYS	19	21.5	27.1 ± 2.5	21.8	23.9
ARG	18	17.6	19.6 ± 0.7	17.9	17.3
TRP	4	[4.0]	4.0 —	4.0	[4.0]
½-CYS	5	[5.0]	[5.0] —	[5.0]	[5.0]

All values expressed as residues/42,000 g. Results from our laboratories (columns b, c, d and e) have been derived from samples hydrolysed in duplicate for 24 and 72 h. Values in parenthesis have been assumed for the composition calculations. The tryptophan figures for pig platelet actins (c) and for human platelet actin (d) are mean values from two determinations only. ND = not determined.

(a) Data from the sequence analysis of Elzinga et al. (1973); (b) Mean value from analysis of two different preparations of pig muscle; (c) Mean and standard deviation of six different platelet actin preparations; (d) Human platelet actin sample donated by Professor Lüscher, University of Berne; (e) Platelets from Blood Transfusion Service donor–1 day after collection.

will be revealed. Gruenstein and Rich (1975) suggested that muscle and non-muscle actins are in fact different, based on two dimensional tryptic fingerprints of chicken muscle and chicken brain actins after incorporation in vivo of [³H]arginine and [³H]lysine. The brain actin lacked at least one peptide present in the muscle protein and contained six additional peptides. Whether these differences are sufficient to consider them separate gene products is not yet clear and, of course, the presence of different trypsin-insensitive regions in the molecules could possibly explain these findings.

The physico-chemical properties and amino acid compositions of several cytoplasmic actins have been recently documented in an excellent critical review by Pollard and Weihing (1974), and from their data there seems little doubt that this protein has been subject to a considerable degree of evolutionary conservation.

From the studies of Probst and Lüscher (1972) with thrombosthenin 'A' (the actin-like protein of the platelet contractile complex) it appears that within the platelet two distinct subpopulations of actin molecules may coexist each displaying slightly different properties. These workers showed that in extracts of crude platelet thrombosthenin both polymerisable and non-polymerisable forms of platelet G-actin were present but, surprisingly, both were capable of enhancing the Mg^{2+} ATPase activity of myosin and of forming superprecipitates, indicating contractile complex formation. Further evidence that two different molecular species of actin can occur in the platelet has recently been presented by Abramowitz et al. (1975), who described a second type of actin which depolymerised in conditions which would favour the polymerisation of a conventional form of G-actin–i.e., in the presence of ATP and divalent cations. Normally F-actin is depolymerised by ATP and divalent cations. They suggested that this kind of actin would be unlikely to have contractile properties, and might therefore have only a structural function, but it is not yet clear whether subunit interactions of actin and myosin without complete filament formation have any force-generating potential. This point will be discussed later in relation to the complexing of non-filamentous myosin with F-actin.

A feature of actins from both non-muscle and muscle sources is that they all contain the unusual amino acid, 3-methyl histidine. Most actins from skeletal muscle contain approximately one mol of this amino acid per mol protein, calculated on the basis of the sequence molecular weight of about 42,000 (Elzinga, 1973). Although values close to 1 mol/mol have been reported for human platelet actin (Abramowitz et al., 1975), in our own investigations using a highly sensitive short column amino acid analysis procedure with 20 different preparations of highly purified pig platelet actin we obtained a value substantially lower than this, viz. 0.62 ± 0.08 mol methyl histidine/42,000 g (Mean $\pm$ S.D.; $n = 20$). Values for brain actin as low as 0.3 mol/50,000 g have been obtained (Puszkin and Berl, 1970; 1972) and recently Jackson and Crawford (1976) found a form of actin with some properties different from F-actin which can be precipitated by Mg^{2+} from the soluble phase of guinea pig polymorphonuclear leucocytes and has a very low 3-methyl-histidine content (<0.5 mol/42,000 g). Table 2 summarises some of the values found for 3 methyl histidine in muscle and non-muscle actins.

TABLE 2
3-Methyl histidine content of various actins

Source	3-Methyl histidine content (Residues/42,000 g)	Reference
Pig platelets (mean: $\pm$S.D., $n = 20$)	0.62 ± 0.08	Own analysis
Human platelets	1.0	Own analysis
Human platelets	0.88	Booyse et al. (1973)
Rabbit skeletal muscle	0.95	Own analysis
Pig muscle	0.72	Own analysis
Bovine brain	0.28	Puszkin and Berl (1972)
Leucocyte actin	0.15	Jackson and Crawford (1976)

2.1.2. Subcellular localisation

Some electron micrographs have shown actin microfilaments in close proximity to the inner face of the platelet plasma membrane. Often they appear to form bridges between the membrane and the marginal bundle of microtubules. Actin is, of course, a notoriously 'sticky' protein (Bray, 1975) in that it readily forms complexes with several other proteins – for example, myosin, tropomyosin and the troponins of skeletal muscle and DNase 1 (Lazarides and Lindberg, 1974), spectrin (Pinder et al., 1975; Tilney and Detmers, 1975) and fibrin (Laki and Muzbeck, 1974). At present it is not clear whether this platelet membrane-associated actin is formed by polymeric assembly on G-actin monomers, intrinsic to the membrane architecture, or whether F-actin simply has transient binding affinity for some proteins of the membrane. We have recently confirmed biochemically the presence of a firmly-associated actin in isolated pig platelet membranes (Fig. 8); this survives extensive dialysis (up to 1 or 2 weeks) under conditions which would normally depolymerise F-actin (Taylor et al., 1975; Taylor et al., 1976). Moreover, after extensive dialysis of the membrane it will still enhance by 2–3-fold the Mg^{2+}-ATPase activity of muscle myosin (Fig. 9), suggesting that the membrane-bound polymer is of sufficient length and of favourable polarity for an actomyosin complex to form.

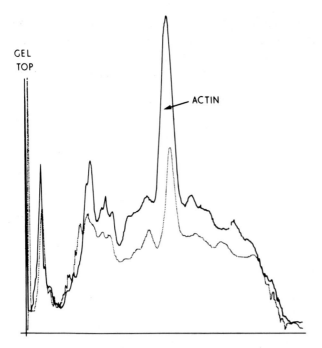

Fig. 8. Densitometer scans of SDS-solubilised pig platelet surface membrane fraction separated by SDS-polyacrylamide gel electrophoresis. Membrane polypeptides separated with (continuous line) and without (broken line) the addition of skeletal muscle actin.

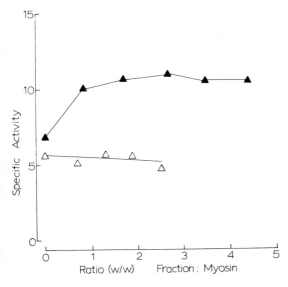

Fig. 9. Enhancement of basal Mg^{2+} ATPase activity of rabbit skeletal muscle myosin by addition of platelet membrane vesicle fraction isolated by zonal centrifugation (▲——▲). No enhancement by platelet soluble phase fraction (△——△) despite presence of 43,000 mol. wt presumptive actin band in this fraction in SDS polyacrylamide gel electrophoresis.

Some of the platelet actin is present in the soluble phase of the cell (i.e., in the supernatant after 6 million *g* min centrifugation of platelet homogenates), but this actin apparently cannot form synthetic hybrid actomyosins with muscle myosin (see Fig. 9) and may represent redundant monomeric G-actin units which have lost their contractile potential.

2.2. Myosin

As mentioned earlier, platelet myosin filaments are less easy to identify than actin and have been demonstrated convincingly only in activated platelets (Behnke et al., 1971; Zucker-Franklin and Crusky, 1972). They show more size heterogeneity (4–12 nm in thickness) than actin filaments, presumably because their tendency to form aggregates and side-to-side associations is greater under some of the fixation conditions used for electron microscopy.

2.2.1. Physicochemical properties

Platelet myosin has been isolated and partially characterised by a number of groups (Bettex-Galland et al., 1962; Booyse et al., 1970; Cohen et al., 1969; Adelstein et al., 1971; Pollard et al., 1974; Cove and Crawford, 1975; Harris and Crawford, 1975) and it is generally agreed that in dissociating conditions the major polypeptide (as in muscle) is a heavy chain component of molecular weight around 200,000. There are light chains also present (probably only 2 per heavy

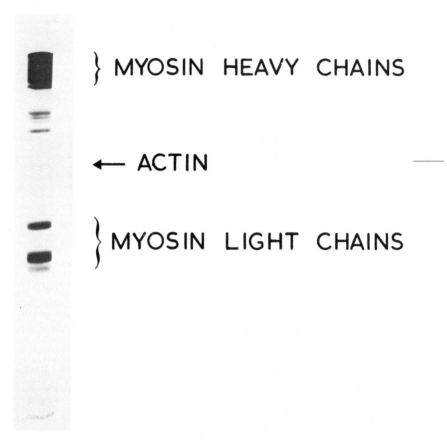

} MYOSIN HEAVY CHAINS

← ACTIN

} MYOSIN LIGHT CHAINS

Fig. 10. SDS-polyacrylamide gel electrophoresis of purified pig platelet myosin (7.5% gel containing 0.1% SDS). Separation shows the major heavy chain component (mol. wt. approx. 200,000) and the two light chain components (approx. 22,000 and 17,000). The faint band running in front of the two light chains is now considered to be a proteolytic artefact.

chain) with molecular weights around 16,000 and 20,000 (Fig. 10). In this respect platelet myosin more closely resembles the myosins of smooth muscle and heart than of striated muscle, in which three distinct light chains have now been clearly identified (Weeds, 1969; Weeds and Lowey, 1971).

Platelet myosin has a Ca^{2+}-ATPase activity which, like skeletal muscle myosin, has two pH optima (around 6 and 9) and is inhibited by Mg^{2+} ions (Fig. 11). In the presence of 3 mM Ca^{2+}, and using ATP as substrate, the enzyme is half maximally inhibited by concentrations of Mg^{2+} as low as 20–50 μM (Harris and Crawford, 1975; Crawford, 1975). The activity of platelet myosin Ca^{2+}-ATPase is lower (Pollard and Weihing, 1974) than the values recorded for skeletal muscle myosin preparations, but addition of actin from either platelet or muscle sources confers upon the molecule a Mg^{2+}-ATPase activity which at favourable myosin/actin ratios may be 8–10-fold higher than the basal Mg^{2+}-ATPase of the myosin (Fig. 12). Both the homologous and heterologous actomyosins show superprecipitation

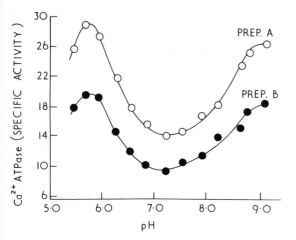

Fig. 11. pH profile of pig platelet myosin Ca^{2+}-ATPase activity. Two different preparations measured under high ionic strength (0.6 M KCl) conditions. (Specific activity – μmoles P_i/mg protein/h.)

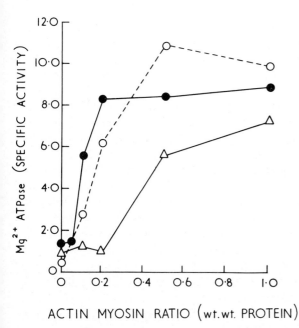

Fig. 12. Formation of synthetic actomyosins with increased Mg^{2+}-ATPase activity by combining three different preparations of platelet myosin (isolated from platelet soluble phase fractions) with rabbit skeletal muscle actin. (Specific activity – μmoles P_i/mg protein/h.)

and syneresis under low ionic strength conditions in the presence of ATP, suggesting that contractility is an inducible property of these mixtures (Cove and Crawford, 1975).

2.2.2. Subcellular localisation

Electron microscopic examination of the presumptive myosin filaments in stimulated platelets suggests that the myosin is mainly located in the cytoplasmic compartment of the cell and is not stored in significant amounts in any of the granular organelles. Some biochemical support for this soluble-phase location has been presented (Harris and Crawford, 1975; Crawford, 1975) based upon a series of studies in which the soluble phase (6 million g min supernatant from homogenates), was prepared from platelets treated by three different disruption procedures (pestle or blender homogenisation, or ultrasonication) for periods varying from a few seconds to 5 min. Under all these conditions the ratio of the content of the soluble-phase marker enzyme lactate dehydrogenase to the quantity of myosin which could be extracted from the soluble phase remained fairly constant. This suggested that the two proteins were simultaneously released from the same intracellular compartment (i.e., the cytoplasm) under these different homogenisation conditions and that this compartment may therefore represent the true intracellular localisation of at least some of the myosin.

2.2.3. Polymerisation

The fact that few myosin-like filaments have been observed in resting platelets raises the question of whether aggregation of myosin monomeric units is required for contractile activity. From our own analytical ultracentrifugation studies with both dissociated thrombosthenin and purified platelet myosin solutions it seems that monomer (5.5 S) and dimer (8.0 S) forms of myosin, as well as larger aggregates (>100 S), may all coexist even in high ionic strength conditions (Cove and Crawford, 1975; Crawford, 1975). In these sedimentation studies the ability to form larger aggregates of myosin seemed to be influenced by the presence of F-actin and ATP in the solutions; this led us to propose that a shift in the equilibrium between monomeric species and higher molecular weight aggregates may be the initiating process for myosin filament formation in the cell (Harris and Crawford, 1975). However, in a series of interesting studies Oplatka and his group (1974a,b) showed that ghost striated muscle myofibrils (that is, myofibrils from which the myosin had been completely extracted) developed isometric tension when irrigated with water soluble forms of myosin (such as polyalanyl-myosin), with myosin-free HMM, and even with the S1 head fragment isolated after mild proteolysis of myosin. Moreover, solutions of HMM placed in fine capillary tubes together with actin and ATP exhibited active streaming. One should, therefore, consider the possibility that in more primitive motile systems (such as the platelet) some form of mechanochemical coupling in the actomyosin complex could occur without full assembly of the myosin polymer to a thick filament level of organisation.

2.2.4. Regulation of contractile activity

With skeletal muscle myosins the importance of the light chain components in the contraction relaxation cycle still remains obscure and it is possible with white muscle myosin to remove one of the three light chains (the 18,000 molecular weight component) without significantly affecting enzyme activity (Lowey and Risby, 1971). Since it is this light chain in muscle that is phosphorylated by a specific protein kinase (Pires et al., 1974), it remains questionable whether this light chain has any functional importance in the muscle contractile event. In the case of platelet myosin, which has only two light chain types, the 20,000 molecular weight light chain may have a regulatory role; it can apparently be phosphorylated by an endogenous protein kinase (Adelstein et al., 1973), and recent studies have shown that this modification appears to attenuate the actin-activated Mg^{2+}-ATPase activity of the myosin (Adelstein and Conti, 1975).

Changes in Ca^{2+} flux across the sarcoplasmic reticulum are important in controlling the contraction/relaxation cycle of muscle actomyosin, apparently because Ca^{2+} influences the concerted action of the regulatory proteins (tropomyosin and the troponins) which are associated with actin at intervals along the double stranded F-actin helix. Although a tropomyosin-like protein has now been isolated and characterised from human platelets (Cohen and Cohen, 1972), and we have also confirmed its presence in pig platelets (unpublished observations), the evidence for the existence of a troponin-like complex is still somewhat circumstantial. Cohen et al. (1973) presented data which suggested that an actin-linked regulatory system exists in human platelets, and this concept was supported by the work of Thorens et al. (1973) who isolated a fraction from the soluble phase of platelets which conferred Ca^{2+} sensitivity on preparations of desensitized muscle actomyosin. Fine et al. (1975) found troponin C (the calcium binding component of the troponin system) in another non-muscle tissue (brain) by utilising the ability of troponin C to form a complex with the inhibitor protein, troponin I, in the presence of Ca^{2+}; the two proteins then run together on polyacrylamide gels but dissociate after treatment with EGTA. This technique has not yet been applied to platelets.

One finding which seems to be a common feature of non-muscle systems is that the tropomyosins have significantly lower molecular weights than skeletal muscle tropomyosin: Cohen and Cohen (1972) quoted values for human and pig platelet tropomyosins of about 30,000, our own value for pig platelet tropomyosin is 31,000, and Fine et al. (1973) quoted 30,000 for brain tropomyosin, whereas the value for skeletal muscle tropomyosin is around 35,000. Moreover, Mg^{2+} paracrystals of non-muscle tropomyosins display a shorter axial periodicity than the muscle protein–about 34 nm as against 39 nm. This finding could imply a different geometry in the association of the regulatory protein complex with actin in non-muscle actomyosin systems than exists in the skeletal muscle myofibril, but to my knowledge no comparative X-ray diffraction studies have yet been made of the two actin/tropomyosin complexes. Whether non-muscle and muscle tropomyosins are products of separate genes, or whether the former may be derived by modification of the latter, will not be known until details of their sequences beome available.

The role of Ca^{2+} as a positive allosteric effector for the platelet myosin ATPase has been recently demonstrated by Malik et al. (1974), who showed that free Ca^{2+} binds to the protein and increases the binding of ATP. Also, excess Ca^{2+} lowered the Km and Hill coefficient of the enzymes, suggesting that co-operative interactions on the globular head of the myosin molecule (the site of the ATPase activity) may have some regulatory effect, in addition to the postulated tropomyosin/troponin-like calcium regulating mechanism. Since this type of allosteric regulation has also been postulated for smooth muscle systems, this finding (like the light chain studies referred to earlier) supports the concept that the skeletal muscle myofibril is a highly specialised example, and therefore in studies of cytoplasmic actomyosins we should, perhaps, seek analogies with the less organised smooth muscle contractile apparatus.

When such comparisons are being made, it is important to consider whether the platelet contractile machinery should be regarded mainly as a 'one way system', in contrast to the finely regulated contraction/relaxation cycle of skeletal and cardiac muscle. One could postulate that the irreversibility of some platelet phenomena simply means that the intracellular ionic environment surrounding the contractile complex has been altered so that it is beyond compensatory adjustment by processes such as cytoplasmic flow and membrane ion pumping. That some form of regulatory control does exist is suggested by the finding of Cohen and de Vries (1973) who showed partial reversibility of the contraction in platelet rich plasma clots maintained under isometric conditions. This finding could imply that within the cell lies a sarcoplasmic reticulum-like pump, controlling Ca^{2+} flux changes in and out of compartments rich in the actomyosin complex. In this context, Statland et al. (1969) showed that platelet membranes have the property of accumulating Ca^{2+} in the presence of ATP, and Robblee et al. (1973) confirmed this with a more detailed study of the kinetics of the process and its ATP dependence. The rate of uptake was, however, considerably slower than with the vesicular elements of muscle, and since mixed membrane fractions were used it was not possible to determine if the pump operated at the plasma membrane or controlled the movement of ionic calcium between intracellular compartments. Further studies with well-characterised membrane subfractions should elucidate this important property of platelet membranes.

2.2.5. Summary

Platelet contractile proteins show many similarities to their counterparts in skeletal muscle but also show some significant differences. They are present in a less well ordered form than exists in the skeletal muscle myofibril and are found both in the cytosol and in association with the membrane. They show considerable variation in their level of polymeric assembly, from monomeric subunits to long filamentous forms, and the intracellular conditions which influence their transformation to the different forms obviously adds another dimension of control over their action in contractile events. However, the ease with which platelets can be harvested as a homogenous population of cells, rich in actomyosin-like proteins, makes them an ideal model system for studying non-muscle contractile activity in relation to cell motile behaviour, and such studies could yield information of both evolutionary and functional significance. Some of the ways in which these contractile proteins may be involved in platelet reactions will be discussed later.

3. Microtubule proteins

In platelets, as in many other mammalian cells, the microtubules were not clearly observed until glutaraldehyde was introduced as a fixative in electron microscopy, and some of the first demonstrations were those of Haydon and Taylor (1965), Behnke (1965), Silver (1966), Zucker-Franklin (1967), Crawford et al. (1966; 1967), Behnke and Zelander (1966), and White et al. (1966). It soon became clear that mammalian microtubules, unlike those seen in cilia and flagella, were labile polymeric assemblies and the success of these early studies was partly due to stabilisation of the assembly by the aldehyde, through its protein cross-linking action (Sabatini et al., 1963). Subsequently, the detailed electron microcope studies of Behnke (1967; 1970; 1971), White (1971), and Hovig (1968) increased our knowledge of these structures and established that in the non-activated discoid platelet the microtubules are arranged as a well ordered concentric bundle, lying subjacent to the inner face of the plasma membrane. The disassembly and rearrangement of microtubules during platelet activation was mentioned earlier in this paper.

Despite these detailed morphological studies there have been few attempts to isolate and characterise the subunit proteins of which the microtubules are composed. This is somewhat surprising, since microtubules have long been implicated in a wide variety of motile and locomotory processes in many eukaryotic cells–for example, cytoplasmic streaming, shape changes, pseudopodia formation, phagocytosis, ciliary beating, lens epithelial cell differentiation, nerve cell elongation, cell division and secretory processes. Some of these processes are closely analogous to those occurring in the activated platelet.

According to Wilson and Bryan (1974), microtubules can be subclassified into two major groups, the 'stable' and the 'labile'. Stable microtubules are typified by those seen in cilia and flagella and appear, in cross section, organised in a characteristic 9 and 2 array with the inner doublet apparently lacking the processes, or bridges, which interconnect the 9 outer doublet tubules. These microtubules can be isolated fairly intact from the organism after removal of the membrane, and they do not depolymerise readily at low temperatures or under high pressure. They are also relatively resistant to anti-mitotic agents such as colchicine, and to a number of other microtubule poisons. In contrast, however, the 'labile' microtubules, examples of which are those present in spindle fibres of dividing cells and the cytoplasmic microtubules seen in large numbers in mammalian brain and nervous tissues are extremely temperature sensitive. They also bind colchicine and interact readily with the plant alkaloids vincristine, vinblastine and podophylotoxin. Platelet microtubules appear to fall into this latter category: they become disorganised at low temperatures, they bind colchicine, and they form ordered crystalline lattices in the cytoplasm when platelets are treated with vinblastine (Behnke, 1969; White, 1968; 1969).

The mammalian microtubules studied most are those of brain, and much is now known about their 3-dimensional structure and the factors controlling assembly and disassembly. The major subunit protein of brain microtubules is a dimer with a sedimentation constant of around 6 S. This protein, known as 'tubulin' or 'neurotubulin', contains bound GTP, and as the dimer it binds colchicine with an association constant (K_a) between 2.3 and 2.5×10^6 litres/mol at 37°C (Eng et al., 1974). This property is lost, however, in the presence of denaturing agents: the dimers then split giving two non-identical monomers (the α- and β-tubulin subunits). These subunits run in SDS-polyacrylamide gels with mobilities corresponding to molecular weights of 51,000 and 53,000 (Eng et al., 1974) (or 52,000 and 55,000 in our own studies) but this mobility varies with pH, ionic strength and composition of the gel buffer systems (Wilson and Bryan, 1974). Whether each dimer is a hetero ($\alpha\beta$) dimer, or whether the microtubules are made up of a mixture of '$\alpha\alpha$' and '$\beta\beta$' dimers has not yet been satisfactorily resolved.

3.1. Isolation from platelets

The first attempts to isolate the microtubule subunit proteins from blood platelets were made by Puszkin and her colleagues (1971), who extracted from human platelets a colchicine-binding protein presumed to be the major microtubule constituent. This protein enhanced by 19–22 fold the Mg^{2+}-ATPase activity of muscle myosin. The possibility that platelet actin might have been co-purified with the colchicine binding protein was not resolved in this study, and as both proteins are similar in charge they could have co-migrated under the electrophoresis conditions used. In our own early attempts to isolate the microtubule proteins we encountered a similar difficulty: some of the established procedures for isolating brain tubulin (Weisenberg et al., 1968; Bryan and Wilson, 1971) proved inappropriate for platelets, because platelets contain a larger proportion of actin in the soluble phase than brain, and the actin co-purified with the tubulin. A procedure was eventually developed based upon the temperature dependent polymerisation method of Shelanski et al. (1973), which is now used extensively for brain tubulin isolation. By adding to the platelet polymerisation media both EDTA and EGTA the problem of actin co-polymerisation is overcome and the tubulin can be prepared relatively actin-free. This method has been described in detail elsewhere (Castle and Crawford, 1975) but a summarised flow diagram is presented in Fig. 13, together with typical gel electrophoresis separations, to illustrate the degree of purification which can be achieved by one cycle of polymerisation/depolymerisation.

3.2. *Physicochemical properties*

Analytical ultracentrifuge studies and sucrose density gradient centrifugation separations, using a colchicine binding assay revealed that the presumptive platelet tubulin had a sedimentation constant as dimer of about 6 S – similar to that of rat and bovine brain tubulins (see Figs. 14a and b). Platelet tubulin could be clearly resolved from actin by SDS polyacrylamide gel electrophoresis (Fig. 15) and the mobility of tubulin indicated a mean monomer molecular weight of $55,000 \pm 1500$ (S.D. for 8 different preparations). Actin has a mobility corresponding to a mean molecular weight of 44,000. The α- and β-monomers of tubulin co-electrophorese in this gel procedure, but in discontinuous SDS-gel systems the 55,000 molecular weight subunit can be separated into the two non-identical monomers with mobilities corresponding to 52,000 and 55,000 (Fig. 16). Table 3 shows the colchicine binding activity of the temperature polymerised platelet protein, compared with the activity of the residual soluble phase proteins after its removal. The specific activity of platelet tubulin was usually 30–50 times greater than that of the residual supernatant proteins assayed after its removal.

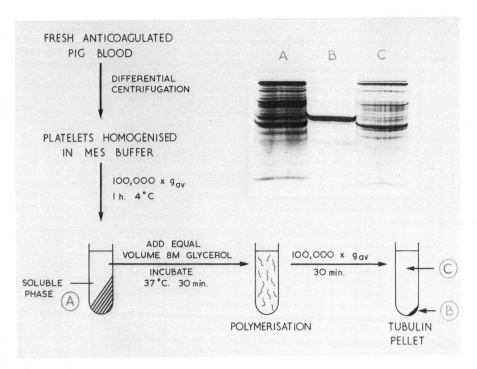

Fig. 13. Procedure for isolating tubulin from the platelet soluble phase by temperature polymerisation. (A) (B) and (C) on the slab polyacrylamide gel separations refer to samples taken at the stages marked in the flow diagram. Note that the major component (43,000 mol. wt actin) running just ahead of the tubulin in the initial soluble phase remains in the supernatant after deposition of the tubulin (55,000 mol. wt) pellet.

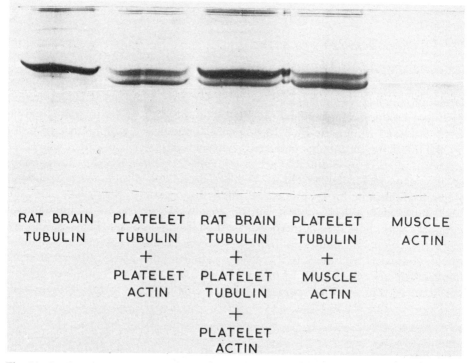

RAT BRAIN   PLATELET   RAT BRAIN   PLATELET   MUSCLE
TUBULIN   TUBULIN   TUBULIN   TUBULIN   ACTIN
               +   +   +
             PLATELET   PLATELET   MUSCLE
             ACTIN   TUBULIN   ACTIN
                            +
                         PLATELET
                         ACTIN

Fig. 14. Co-electrophoresis studies of pig platelet tubulin, rat brain tubulin and mixtures of these tubulins with purified rabbit skeletal muscle actin. All proteins treated with SDS/urea/merceptoethanol before electrophoresis in 7% SDS polyacrylamide slab gels.

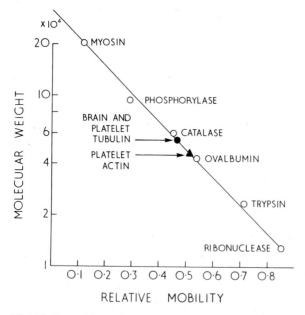

Fig. 15. Log molecular weight/mobility relationship in 7% SDS polyacrylamide gels of standard proteins and preparations of highly purified rat brain tubulin, pig platelet tubulin and pig platelet actin.

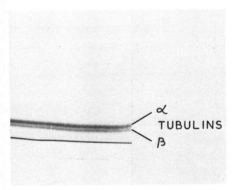

Fig. 16. Separation of pig platelet tubulin into α- and β-tubulin components by electrophoresis in discontinuous alkaline polyacrylamide gel.

TABLE 3
[^{3}H]Colchicine-binding activity of tubulin isolated from the platelet soluble phase

	Protein (mg)	Specific activity (DPM/μg)
Platelet tubulin	14.2	411.7
Supernatant after tubulin removal	238.0	11.7

Associated with the 55,000 mol. wt tubulin component in both brain and platelet preparations are small amounts of higher molecular weight (HMW) polypeptides (see also Fig. 14), some of which have molecular weights greater than 200,000. In brain, these HMW proteins have been called 'dynein-like' (Burns and Pollard, 1974; Gaskin et al., 1974) since they resemble in some of their properties the proteins of the dynein arms on the A subfibres of the outer doublet microtubules of cilia and flagella.

It is not clear yet what part these HMW proteins play, if any, in the polymeric assembly of platelet and brain microtubules, but in cilia and flagella the 'dyneins' have a divalent cation activated ATPase activity which is apparently involved in the energetics of the microtubule sliding movements during the ciliary beating and the flagella bending waves (Satir, 1968). The platelet HMW proteins can be separated from the colchicine binding 6 S tubulin on a sucrose density gradient (Fig. 17) and they too seem to have an associated ATPase which is activated by either Mg^{2+} or Ca^{2+}. It would be premature to suggest at this stage that this enzyme is involved in platelet microtubule assembly or function, but detailed studies of the characteristics of this ATPase (particularly with respect to cation dependence) and of the effect of ATPase inhibitors on tubulin polymerisation are certainly warranted. Interpretation of such studies might well be difficult, however, because of the many other divalent cation activated ATPase activities present in the blood platelet.

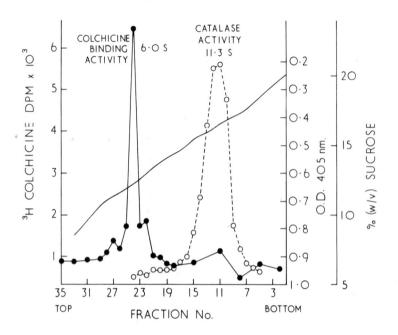

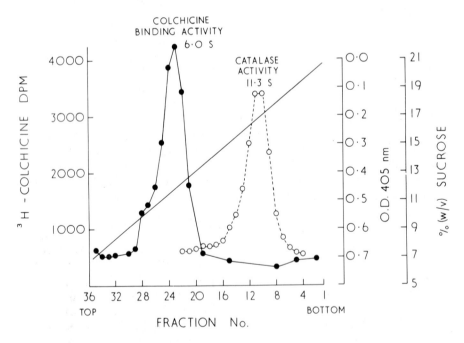

Fig. 17. Ultracentrifugation of depolymerised preparations of platelet tubulin (upper profile) and rat brain tubulin (lower profile) in sucrose density gradients (linear gradient, 7–20% w/v sucrose). Samples aspirated from bottom of tube and measured for catalase activity (included in each gradient run) O———O, and colchicine binding activity ●———● (using [³H]colchicine).

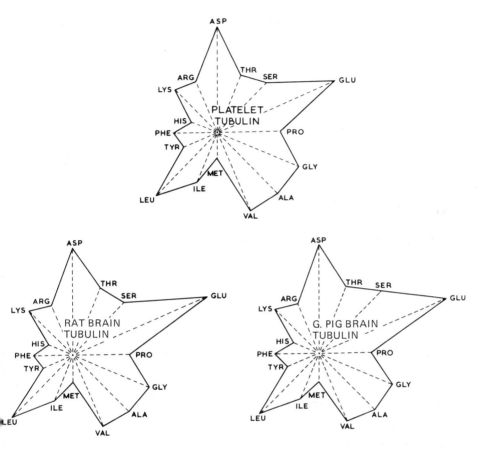

Fig. 18. Amino acid profiles of platelet tubulin (Top), rat brain tubulin (Bottom left), and guinea pig brain tubulin (Bottom right). Radial lines are proportional to amino acid composition in moles per cent.

Amino acid analyses of tubulins from pig platelet, rat brain, and guinea pig brain show striking similarities (Fig. 18). All have a high content of the acidic amino acids glutamate and aspartate. During the last few years several workers have commented on the similarities that exist between actin and tubulin: for example, the early molecular weight data, the amino acid analyses, the characteristics of polymerisation, and the presence of bound nucleotides (Mohri et al., 1967; Mohri, 1968; Stephens et al., 1967; Yamagisawa et al., 1968; Shelanski and Taylor, 1968; Weisenberg and Borisy, 1968). It is now well established, however, that the monomer molecular weights of tubulin and actin differ by about 10,000, and that the nucleotide bound to tubulin is either GTP or GDP—not the adenine nucleotides found in actin. Moreover, the unusual amino acid, 3 methyl histidine (a feature of the primary structure of both muscle and cytoplasmic actins) has not yet been detected in tubulins from any source.

In comparative studies of these two proteins, the tubulin and actin have generally been isolated either from different tissues of the same species (Stephens, 1970; Mohri and Shimomura, 1973), or from different species. Table 4 summarises some of the properties of tubulin and actin isolated from the same cells–namely, pig blood platelets. It can be seen that although there are a number of features in common, the differences between the two proteins are sufficiently significant to consider them discrete molecular entities. However, whether there is some sequence homology between tubulins and actins is still not clear: from ATPase activation studies with chicken muscle myosin and tubulin from the cilia of Tetrahymena, Alicea and Renaud (1975) suggested that some sequence homology exists, but others are sceptical. The tryptic and chymotryptic peptide maps of actin and tubulin from the scallop *Pecten* presented by Stephens (1970) suggest that large regions of homology are unlikely, and that if any homology exists at all it is probably confined to small localised sites in the molecule (perhaps the nucleotide binding sites).

TABLE 4
Comparison of properties of pig platelet tubulin and pig platelet actin

Property	Tubulin	Actin
Monomer mol. wt (from SDS polyacrylamide gel mobilities)	55,000	43,000
Sedimentation constant	6.0 S (as dimer)	2.7 S (G-actin)
Monomer heterogeneity	$\alpha + \beta$-forms	−
Colchicine binding	+ (as dimer)	−
Presence of 3-methyl histidine	−	+
Nucleotide bound	GDP/GTP	ADP/ATP
Binding to myosin (with increased Mg^{2+}-ATPase)	±	+
Arrowhead formation with heavy meromyosin	−	+
Phosphorylation (endogenous kinase + ATP)	+	−
Filament forms	Protofilaments and tubules	Double stranded helix

In our studies using antibodies to platelet actin and tubulin (Crawford et al., 1976) we found no evidence to support antigenic similarity between the two proteins, and in indirect fluorescent antibody labelling experiments with a variety of cells the two antisera complexed with morphologically different structures. Moreover, the actin antibody staining was inhibited by cytochalasin whilst the tubulin antibody staining was suppressed by pretreatment of the cells with colchicine or by exposure overnight to low temperatures. In addition, both antibodies were specifically adsorbed by the corresponding antigen, and there was no demonstrable cross reaction in immunodiffusion gel systems. Any sequence homology that exists, therefore, does not appear to involve the antigenic determinants.

3.3. Polymerisation

Electron microscopy of the platelet tubulin polymer produced by *in vitro* polymerisation procedures shows clear linear aggregation giving filaments of varying length and width with some side association (Fig. 19). So far, however, we have found no 20–30 nm structures in these polymers which are similar to the

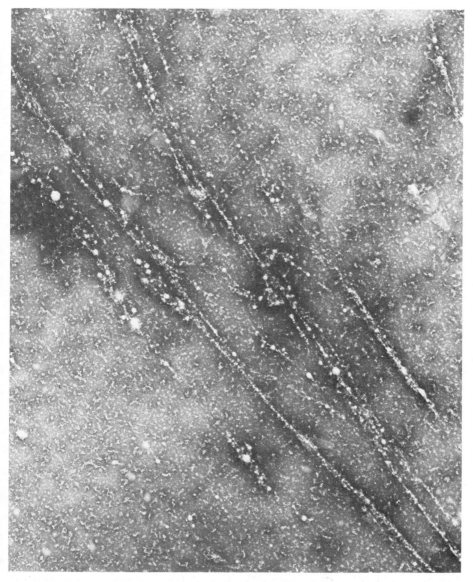

Fig. 19. Electron micrographs of once-polymerised platelet tubulin showing filamentous structures with some side-to-side association.

microtubules seen in intact platelets. Both Behnke (1967) and White (1971) described a subfilamentous structure in platelet microtubules with 6 or 7 longitudinally aligned protofilaments at centre-to-centre spacings of 5 to 6 nm. This could correspond to the helical array of 13 subunits seen in cross sections of cilia and flagella microtubules.

In our isolation procedure the conditions devised to minimise actin contamination in the tubulin preparations are perhaps not optimum for polymerisation: assembly may proceed only to the level of the protofilament intermediates. Another explanation could be that some nucleating locus is needed, like the ring structures seen in brain tubulin polymerisation experiments, or that some important co-factor which regulates the assembly is not co-purified in our procedure.

3.4. Summary

Blood platelets contain tubulin and other microtubule subunit proteins, which can be isolated from the soluble phase of the cell and show many of the properties of the microtubule subunits prepared from brain neurotubules. In vitro they assemble to form protofilaments, but fully formed microtubules have not yet been prepared from isolated tubulin/HMW protein mixtures. Polymerisation of platelet microtubule subunits in vitro, like other microtubule systems, is extremely sensitive to Ca^{++}—assembly will take place only in the presence of EGTA.

Most investigations of the changes in the form and location of platelet microtubules during haemostatic activation have been based on electron micrographic observations. Complementary studies with the isolated subunit proteins should increase our understanding of the factors and conditions which influence the polymerisation and disassembly of these structures, and the part they may play in platelet reactions.

4. Role of microtubules and microfilaments in platelet reactions

Much of our knowledge in this area has been derived from experiments in which colchicine or its analogues, vinblastine, or the fungal metabolite cytochalasin B was applied to intact cells (See Fig. 20 for molecular structures). These drugs affect cellular motile phenomena which depend on contractile forces operating within the cytoplasmic matrix or on coupled events involving the cell membrane and the structural or contractile elements lying subjacent to it.

4.1. Effect of cytochalasins

Six of these alkaloids are now known (designated A to F) but cytochalasin B, first isolated from cultures of the fungus *Helminthosporum dematioideum*, has been

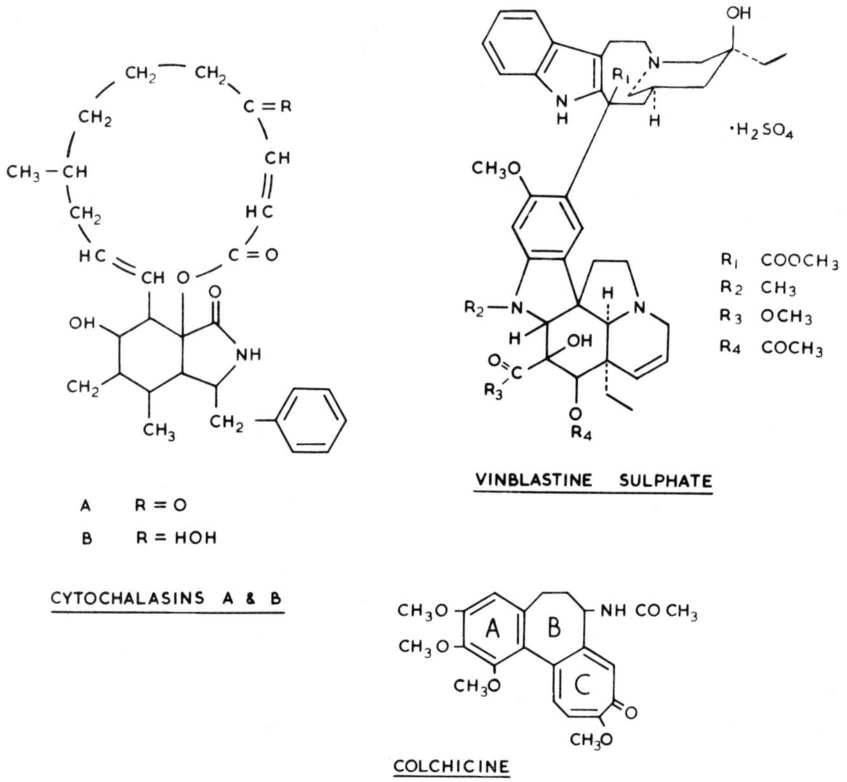

Fig. 20. Molecular structure of colchicine, vinblastine, and cytochalasins A and B.

the most widely used cytological tool. In 1971 Wessells and his colleagues listed all the cell activities known at that time which were affected by cytochalasin B. These included such diverse phenomena as axonal outgrowth of nerves, fibroblast and lymphocyte cytokinesis, fibroblast and glial cell locomotion, nuclear extrusion, cytoplasmic streaming in plants and algae, cortical contraction in *Xenopus* eggs, cardiac muscle contraction, and gut peristalsis. Since all of these processes are in some sense 'contractile', Wessells et al. (1971) suggested that they could be controlled by changes in either the competence or subcellular localisation of microfilaments.

At that time the only documented effect of cytochalasin B on blood platelets was the inhibition of clot retraction in platelet rich plasma: Wessells et al. (1971) concluded that the drug had little or no effect on the initial stages of clot formation, but that the serum was not expressed from the fibrin/platelet gel. In the same year, however, White (1971) investigated the effect of cytochalasin B on platelets in more detail, and found that although the treated platelets could still aggregate in response to ADP or thrombin, the first phase of aggregation was prolonged—presumably because the shape change and the necessary intracellular transformations were affected. In a recent scanning electron microscope study

Boyle-Kay and Fudenberg (1973) confirmed that cytochalasin prevented platelet pseudopodia formation, and showed that when pseudopodia were allowed to form before the drug was added, they could be made to disappear, indicating that this platelet motile event could be reversed by cytochalasin.

White (1971) had demonstrated that cytochalasin B consistently inhibited clot retraction in platelet rich plasma and had also explored its concentration dependence: 30 μg/ml was totally inhibitory whereas 10 μg/ml was ineffective. He noted too that the concentric bundle of microtubules was not significantly altered by the drug, either in their degree of organisation or in their close proximity to the inner face of the plasma membrane. His results in relation to the platelet release reaction were, however, much more complex: the treated cells still responded to ADP and thrombin, but although some release occurred (enough to induce some secondary aggregation) the usual migration of the granules to the centre of the cell–an event frequently observed during platelet activation–was much less evident. Since this centripetal movement of the platelet granules is normally accompanied by contraction of the microtubule ring, the implications were that cytochalasin causes some uncoupling of the microtubule/microfilament association. In a recent study using washed platelets stimulated by collagen, Haslam et al. (1975) showed that at levels of 1 μg/ml and above, cytochalasin-B inhibited the release of 5HT and other granule constituents, but at lower concentrations (0.1–0.5 μg/ml) cytochalasin actually potentiated the release reaction between 2- and 3-fold. It is difficult to see how these results could be produced by an effect on microfilaments alone, which emphasizes the current controversy about the site(s) of action of cytochalasin B.

If the assumption of Wessells et al. (1971) is made, that the many diverse cell phenomena affected by cytochalasin depend upon actin microfilament integrity and function, then one should be able to demonstrate effects on isolated actin itself, or on its reactivity with myosin, at cytochalasin concentrations which affect intact cells. Unfortunately, this has not been generally true–for example, although cytochalasin B lowers the viscosity of polymerised actin and inhibits its activation of the Mg^{2+}-ATPase of muscle heavy meromyosin (Spudich and Lin, 1972; Spudich, 1973), 50–100 μg/ml of cytochalasin or more is required—concentrations many times greater than those which affect intact cells.

These studies suggest that cytochalasin does not act by changing the integrity of pre-existing microfilaments, but they do not preclude the possibility that the intracellular equilibrium between F-actin microfilaments and G-actin monomeric units might be disturbed by cytochalasin. However, in a detailed in vitro study on the effect of cytochalasin B on the monomeric and polymeric forms of muscle actin Forer et al. (1972), concluded that G to F transformation was not affected and that the F-actin filaments formed in the presence of cytochalasin could be decorated with heavy meromyosin. They also concluded that myosin was probably the cytochalasin-sensitive component in platelets–and possibly in other cells too. This view was supported by the studies of Puszkin et al. (1973), who used radioactive cytochalasin D (a more potent analogue of cytochalasin B) and found that it bound to platelet myosin and significantly depressed the ATPase activities of platelet and muscle myosins.

These reports illustrate the controversy about the site of action of the cytochalasins, but their value as cytological tools is undisputed. More detailed investigations of their effects on platelet reactions should lead to a greater understanding of the precise roles of intracellular structural and contractile machinery.

4.2. Effects of colchicine

Unlike the cytochalasins, where the exact sites of action in the cell are still not clear, colchicine and its analogues have a well-established effect on microtubules – they have strong binding affinities for the 6S tubulin dimer. In most cells containing these structures colchicine is believed to act either by preventing the assembly process or by disrupting the formed polymer. The microtubules of cilia and flagella (which have very low turnover rates) are relatively insensitive to colchicine, apparently because they are stabilized by inter-microtubular bridges (Tilney and Gibbins, 1968). In most mammalian cells, however, a dynamic equilibrium exists between monomeric subunits and fully organised microtubules, and any modification to the tubulin subunit which inhibits assembly will shift the monomer/polymer equilibrium with a resultant disorganisation of the microtubules. Because the blood platelet is anucleate, little protein synthesis is possible, and the rapidity with which microtubules can depolymerise and reassemble suggests that this equilibrium must exist, with a substantial pool of preformed subunits.

The major microtubule subunit protein in platelets (as in brain) is tubulin, and this 110–120,000 mol. wt dimer protein can be readily isolated from the soluble phase of platelet homogenates (Castle and Crawford, 1975). At present it is not possible to ascertain how much of this soluble tubulin was originally present in the cell as a formed microtubule component and then solubilised during the homogenisation or subcellular fractionation procedures. Examination of both brain and platelet particulate elements (membrane and granular organelles) reveals that they have some colchicine binding activity which could be tubulin, but as the colchicine molecule is quite hydrophobic other membrane proteins may also bind the drug, albeit less specifically.

Platelet microtubules seem to possess cytoskeletal properties and the inhibition of shape change induced by microtubule poisons does to some extent correlate with their loss of integrity. However, platelets treated with microtubule disrupting agents such as colchicine, colcemid, and the Vinca alkaloid, vinblastine, can form pseudopodia, aggregate and apparently play a normal role in clot retraction (Boyle-Kay and Fundenberg, 1973; White, 1971). The former workers concluded from studies with the scanning electron microscope that in the presence of colcemid platelet activation could proceed as far as the pseudopodia forming step, and only the later thickening or spreading process, involving cytoplasmic flow into the pseudopodia, was suppressed.

4.3. Summary

Evidence from capping experiments with lymphocytes, indicates that microtubules and microfilaments may have a role in controlling the lateral diffusibility of intrinsic membrane proteins in the lipid layer (de Petris, 1974). This view is supported by the demonstration that membrane proteins apparently separate into low and high viscosity areas during leucocyte phagocytosis, and that this process is colchicine-sensitive (Berlin, 1975). If microtubules and microfilaments are similarly involved in the distribution of surface proteins of the platelet, then the effects of colchicine and cytochalasin could be caused by changes in the arrangement of these membrane proteins, resulting in changes in the competence of transport complexes (e.g., for Ca^{2+}), stimulatory receptor sites (e.g., for ADP or thrombin), or membrane enzymes (e.g., adenyl cyclase).

It is not clear at present exactly how contractile proteins are involved in the complex intracellular events which follow the interaction of a stimulus with the platelet membrane. Our own studies suggest that at least three equilibrium systems exist, the first two of which have been briefly referred to earlier by Behnke (1970). Firstly the equilibrium between monomeric G-actin and the polymerised F-actin, a proportion of which is tightly associated in some way with the platelet membrane elements (both the inner aspect of the boundary membrane and the membranes of the granular organelles). This will be regulated by actin-bound ATP (which is dephosphorylated during G to F transformation) and by the local ionic conditions—high ionic strength favours polymer formation and low ionic strength encourages dissociation. We found that after extensive dialysis in depolymerising conditions membrane-bound actin still enhanced the Mg^{2+}-ATPase of myosin, which suggests that the bound actin is protected in some way from depolymerisation.

The second equilibrium system is that between low molecular weight forms of myosin and the larger aggregates and filaments. In the resting cell the energetics of this equilibrium appear to favour the monomeric species but since the equilibrium is shifted in the opposite direction by F-actin and ATP, the formation of myosin filaments may also depend on local ionic conditions. Whether thick filament forms of platelet myosin are necessary for actomyosin complex formation and contractility has yet to be resolved.

The extreme lability of the platelet microtubules suggests that they exist as a third equilibrium system, in the form of fully organised microtubule structures and a tubulin subunit pool, with other higher molecular weight subunit proteins also available for completing the assembly. In the non-activated platelet the energetics of this equilibrium seem to favour the formed microtubule which must be in some way protected from disassembly by Ca^{2+}. Platelet microtubules lose their organisation during the platelet shape-change but later reassemble rapidly, though they are then more randomly distributed. These three important equilibria are summarised diagrammatically in Fig. 21.

There are still many unanswered questions about the organisation of mic-

a) ACTIN

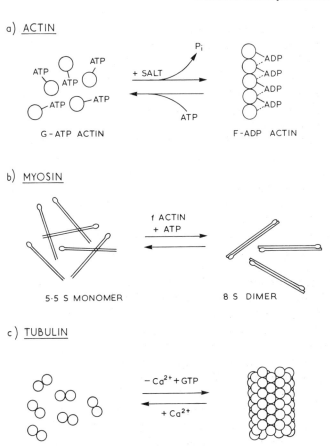

b) MYOSIN

c) TUBULIN

Fig. 21. Postulated equilibrium states existing in platelet cytosol compartment.

rotubules. For example, is the marginal bundle a single organelle, similar to a 'clock spring', or are there several concentric microtubule rings operating in association with each other? Do the microtubules have contractile or sliding potential, like those in cilia and flagella during the beating and bending waves, or are they relatively passive units of the platelet cytoskeleton? With an increasing research effort in this field, however, it is likely that these points may be resolved fairly soon.

5. Conclusions

The biochemical studies reviewed in this paper provide convincing evidence that the platelet contains actomyosin-like proteins with contractile potential, and that some of the reactions of the platelet during its haemostatic activities depend on the actions of its contractile microfilaments. However, although much is known about the morphology and distribution of microfilaments in other cells, these structures are not often seen in the cytoplasm of non-activated platelets–despite the fact that the platelet actin and myosin-like proteins will, after extraction by conventional procedures, form microfilaments in vitro. Although some of the platelet actin is apparently in a filamentous form, closely associated with the membrane, some is located in the cytosol, as is most of the myosin.

The sol/gel characteristics of the platelet cytoplasm are almost certainly regulated in part by changes in ionic strength and by the presence or absence of ATP and divalent cations, because these affect the macromolecular organisation of myosin and its ability to form complexes with F-actin filaments. Unlike the contractile proteins of the muscle myofibril, platelet cytosol actin and myosin are apparently vulnerable to proteolytic attack and modification when the structural integrity of the outer plasma membrane or the lysosomal membranes changes. Such processes could be important in the aging of platelets, and in the actions of drugs or haemostatic stimuli.

Although another contractile protein ('tropomyosin') is present in addition to actin and myosin, we do not know if this is part of a tropomyosin-troponin regulatory system (like that in muscle), since no troponin-like protein has yet been identified in the platelet. Control of contractility in platelets could be achieved through an actin-linked regulatory protein complex, and studies on the light chains of platelet myosin suggest that these may modify the ATPase active site. If so, this would be most interesting, since this form of myosin-linked regulation has so far only been identified in molluscan systems.

Platelets can be regarded as miniature muscle cells, but although research on skeletal muscle will always interest the platelet biochemist, the differences between the two systems must not be overlooked. The findings from one system should not be extrapolated to the other without taking full account of the different types of molecular organisation and, in the cytoplasmic system, the influence of a constantly changing intracellular environment. The factors which may influence the dynamic equilibrium between full organised filamentous structures and the cytoplasmic pools of contractile protein subunits are obviously important and still poorly understood, but many groups are now actively engaged in establishing model systems to investigate this question.

Our knowledge of the subunit components of platelet microtubules is still somewhat scanty: the major subunit protein ('tubulin') which is found in the microtubules of most other cells, has now been identified in, and isolated from, the platelet. How this protein is assembled into the microtubule architecture, and how the polymerisation and disassembly processes may be controlled, are points which should be resolved quite soon. The role of microtubule-bound guanine nucleotides warrants more detailed investigation, particularly with regard to phosphorylation, trans-phosphorylation and dephosphorylation mechanisms. Another worthwhile field of study would be the influence of protein kinases on the conformation of contractile proteins and hence on their subunit interactions. Some platelet protein kinases are cyclic nucleotide dependent, and since the intracellular concentrations of cAMP and cGMP change during platelet activation, these may reflect changes in the organisation of the contractile proteins.

Much of the research on platelet microtubules has been based on morphological studies with fixed, stained sections; consequently, the dynamic aspects of their organisation and function are less well appreciated. It is my hope that this review may stimulate biochemical research on these fascinating structures.

The intracellular relationship between the microtubule and microfilament systems, and their interaction with membranes may be clarified by using some of the newer physical techniques—such as fluorescence energy transfer studies with labelled subunit proteins, the use of affinity labels, and immunoperoxidase antibody procedures.

Finally, I believe that there will be increasing interest in these platelet polymeric systems, not only because of their functional importance in haemostatic and thrombotic processes, but also because the platelet has much to offer as a cell model for a whole variety of motile activities which cannot be so readily explored in other cells and tissues.

Acknowledgements

I am grateful to my colleagues Drs. David Taylor, Alan Castle and Philip Jackson for their many stimulating discussions and for their willingness to allow me to use freely some of their unpublished findings. I also acknowledge the generous financial support for our studies from the British Heart Foundation, the Cancer Research Campaign and the Medical Research Council.

References

Alicea, H.A. and Renaud, F.L. (1975) Nature, *257*, 601.
Abramowitz, J.W., Stracher, A. and Detweiler, T.D. (1975) Arch. Biochim. Biophys., *167*, 230.
Adelstein, R.S., Conti, M.A. and Anderson, W. (1973) Proc. Natl. Acad. Sci. U.S.A., *70*, 3115.
Adelstein, R.S. and Conti, M.A. (1975) Nature (London), *256*, 587.
Bailin, G. and Bárány, M. (1972) J. Mechanochem. Cell Motility, *1*, 189.
Behnke, O. (1965) J. Ultrastruct. Res., *13*, 469.
Behnke, O. and Zelander, T. (1966) Exp. Cell Res., *43*, 236.
Behnke, O. (1967) Anat. Res., *158*, 121.
Behnke, O. (1970) Int. Rev. Exp. Pathol., *9*, 1.
Behnke, O., Kristenson, B. and Engdahl, Nielson L. (1971) In: Platelet aggregation (Caen, J., ed) p. 3 Masson Paris.
Berlin, R.D. (1975) Proc. Int. Symp. on Microtubules and microtubular inhibitors. Janssen Res. Foundation. Beerse, Belgium Sept. 1975.
Bessis, M. and Breton-Gorius, J. (1965) Nouv. Rev. Franc. Hemat., *5*, 657.
Bettex-Galland, M. and Lüscher, E.F. (1959) Nature (London), *184*, 276.
Bettex-Galland, M. and Lüscher, E.F. (1960) Thromb. et Diath. Haemorrh., *4*, 178.
Bettex-Galland, M. and Lüscher, E.F. (1961) Biochim. Biophys. Acta, *49*, 536.
Boyle-Kay, M. and Fudenberg, H.H. (1973) Nature, *244*, 288.
Booyse, F.M., Hoveke, T.P. and Rafelson, Jr., M.E. (1973) J. Biol. Chem., *248*, 4083.
Bray, D. (1975) Nature, *256*, 616.
Bray, D. and Brownlee, S.M. (1973) Anal. Biochem. *55*, 213.

Burns, R.G. and Pollard, T.D. (1974) FEBS Lett., *40*, 274.
Castle, A.G., Crawford, N. (1975) FEBS Lett. *51*, 195.
Clarke, M., Schatten, G., Mazia, D. and Spudich, J.A. (1975) Proc. Natl. Acad. Sci. U.S.A., *72*, 1758.
Cohen, I. and Cohen, C. (1972) J. Mol. Biol., *68*, 383.
Cohen, I., Kaminski, E. and de Vries, A. (1973) FEBS Lett., *34*, 315.
Cohen, I. and de Vries, A. (1973) Nature, *246*, 36.
Collins, J.H. and Elzinga, M. (1975) J. Biol. Chem., *250*, 5915.
Crawford, N., Sutton, M. and Horsfield, I.G. (1966) Experimentia, *22*, 710.
Crawford, N., Sutton, M. and Horsfield, I.G. (1967) Brit. J. Haematol., *13*, 181.
Crawford, N. (1975) in Contractile proteins. FEBS Meeting, proceedings of symposium 1974 Hungarian Acad. Science p. 205.
Crawford, N., Castle, A.G., Trenchev, P. and Holborow, J.H. (1976) Cytobios. In Press.
De Petris, S. (1974) Nature, *250*, 54.
Elzinga, M., Collins, J.H., Kuehl, W.M. and Adelstein, R.S. (1973) Proc. Natl. Acad. Sci. U.S.A., *70*, 2687.
Eng, L.F., Pratt, D. and Wilson, L. (1974) Neurology, *4*, 301.
Fine, R.E., Blitz, A.L., Hitchcock, S.E. and Kahinger, R. (1973) Nature, *254*, 132.
Fine, R., Lehman, W., Head, J. and Blitz, A. (1975) Nature, *258*, 260.
Fore, A., Emmerson, J. and Behnke, O. (1972) Science, *175*, 774.
Gaskin, F., Kramer, S.B., Cantor, C.R., Adelstein, R. and Shelanski, M.L. (1974) FEBS Lett., *40*, 281.
Gruenstein, E. and Rich, A. (1975) Biochem. Biophys. Res. Comm., *64*, 472.
Haydon, G.B. and Taylor, D.A. (1965) J. Cell Biol., *26*, 673.
Hovig, T. (1968) Ser. Haematol., *1*, 3.
Ishikawa, H., Bischoff, R. and Holzer, M. (1969) J. Cell Biol., *43*, 312.
Jackson, P. and Crawford, N. (1976) Biochem. Soc. Transact. *4*, 333.
Laki, K. and Muzbek, L. (1974) Biochim. Biophys. Acta, *371*, 519.
Lazarides, E. and Lindberg, U. (1974) Proc. Natl. Acad. Sci. U.S.A., *71*, 4742.
Lowey, S. and Risby, D. (1971) Nature, *234*, 81.
Mohri, H., Murakama, S. and Maruyama, K. (1967) J. Biochem., *61*, 518.
Mohri, H. (1968) Nature, *217*, 1053.
Mohri, H. and Shimomora, M. (1973) J. Biochem. *74*, 209.
Oplatka, A., Gadasi, H. and Borejdo, J. (1974a) Biochem. Biophys. Res. Comm., *58*, 905.
Oplatka, A., Gadasi, H., Tirosh, R., Laiyed, Y., Muhlrad, A. and Liron, N. (1974b) J. Mechanochem. Cell Motility, *2*, 295.
Pinder, J.C., Bray, D. and Gratzer, W.B. (1975) Nature, *258*, 765.
Pollack, R., Osborn, M. and Weber, K. (1975) Proc. Natl. Acad. Sci. U.S.A., *72*, 994.
Pollard, T.D. (1974) CRC Critical Rev. in Biochem., *2*, 1.
Puszkin, S. and Berl, S. (1970) Nature, *225*, 558.
Puszkin, S. and Berl, S. (1972) Biochim. Biophys. Acta, *256*, 696.
Puszkin, E., Puszkin, S. and Aledort, L.M. (1971) J. Biol. Chem., *246*, 271.
Probst, E. and Lüscher, E.F. (1972) Biochim. Biophys. Acta, *278*, 577.
Robblee, L.S., Shepro, D. and Belamarich, F.A. (1973) Miciovasc. Res. *6*, 99.
Sabatini, D.D., Bensch, K.G. and Barrnett, R.S. (1963) J. Cell Biol., *17*, 19.
Satir, P. (1968) J. Cell Biol., *39*, 77.
Shelanski, M.L. and Taylor, E.W. (1968) J. Cell Biol., *38*, 304.
Silver, M.D. (1966) Nature (London), *209*, 1048.
Stephens, R.E., Renaud, F.L. and Gibbons, I.R. (1967) Science, *156*, 1606.
Stephens, R.E. (1970) Science, *168*, 845.
Spudich, J.A. and Lin, S. (1972) Proc. Natl. Acad. Sci. U.S.A., *69*, 442.
Spudich, J.A. (1973) Cold Spring Harbor. Symp. Quant. Biol., *37*, 585.
Statland, B.E., Heagan, B.M. and White, J.G. (1969) Nature, *223*, 521.
Taylor, D.G., Mapp, R. and Crawford, N. (1975) Biochem. Soc. Transact., *3*, 161.
Taylor, D.G., Williams, V.M. and Crawford, N. (1976) Biochem. Soc. Transact., in press.
Tilney, L., and Gibbins, J. (1968) Protoplasma, *65*, 167.
Tilney, L. (1974) J. Cell. Biol., *63*, 349a.
Tilney, L.G. and Detmers, P.J. (1975) J. Cell Biol., *66*, 508.
Weisenberg, R.C., Borisy, G.C. and Taylor, E.W. (1968) Biochemistry, *7*, 4466.
Wessells, N.K., Spooner, B.S., Ash, J.F., Bradley, M.O., Luduena, M.A., Taylor, E.Z., Wrenn, J.T. and Yamadaka, M. (1971) Science, *171*, 135.
Wilson, L. and Bryan, J. (1974) in Adv. in Cell & Molec. Biol. (Dupraw, E.J., ed) (Acad. Press) p. 21.

White, J.G. (1971) in Platelet Aggregation (Caen, J., ed) Masson, Paris p. 15.
White, J.G. (1968) Amer. J. Path., *53*, 447.
White, J.G. (1969) Amer. J. Path., *54*, 467.
White, J.G., Rao, G.H.R. and Gerrard, J.M. (1974) Amer. J. Pathol., *77*, 135.
Yanagisawa, T., Hasegawas and Mohri, H. (1968) Exp. Cell. Res., *52*, 86.
Zucker-Franklin, D. (1967) J. Clin. Invest., *48*, 165.
Zucker-Franklin, D. and Nachman, R.L. (1967) J. Cell Biol., *35*, 149.
Zucker-Franklin, D. (1969) J. Clin. Invest., *48*, 165.
Zucker-Franklin, D. and Grusky, G. (1972) J. Clin. Invest., *51*, 419.

Notes added in proof

(1) In a sequence study of selected cyanogen bromide peptides from human platelet actin and human cardiac muscle actin, a threonine for valine substitution was identified at position 129 in the platelet protein confirming that the synthesis of these two actins must be controlled by different genes. (Elzinga et al., 1976 Science, *191*, 94).

(2) Following the isolation and purification of the appropriate protein kinase from human platelets, Adelstein and his colleagues have now shown that phosphorylation of the 20,000 molecular weight light chain of platelet myosin results in an enhancement of the actin-activated ATPase activity. This stimulation is reversed by removal of the covalently-bound phosphate by alkaline phosphatase. Since this 20,000 molecular weight subunit is also phosphorylatable in fibroblast and chicken gizzard myosins this mechanism may be a control process common to cytoplasmic and smooth muscle myosins (Adelstein et al. in 'Proteins of Contractile Systems' ed. E.N.A. Biró Proc. 9th FEBS Meeting Budapest, North-Holland/Elsevier 37 177, 1975.)

(3) Although tubulin and actin do share some common properties such as similarity in amino acid compositions and precipitability with Vinca alkaloids, in a study of these two highly purified proteins, examined with respect to myosin ATPase activation and DNase I inhibition we have been unable to obtain evidence to support a functional homology (Castle and Crawford, 1976, FEBS Lett. in press).

CHAPTER 7

Platelet receptors

D.C.B. MILLS and D.E. MACFARLANE

*Specialised Center for Thrombosis Research,
Temple University School of Medicine, Philadelphia,
Pennsylvania 19140, U.S.A.*

1. Introduction

1.1. Receptors

The classical picture of a receptor is a component of a target cell that specifically and reversibly interacts with an effector molecule to form a complex with the special properties that initiate a train of events leading to the ultimate response of the cell. The magnitude of the response is regarded as being proportional to the concentration of the receptor–agonist complex, and as such usually exhibits the saturation kinetics characteristic of the bimolecular reaction between an enzyme and a single substrate forming an enzyme–substrate complex that undergoes a further chain of changes. In this model, the effector molecule, or agonist, can be recovered quantitatively after the reaction, or it can be changed during it. The receptor is generally regarded as being present in the plasma membrane, though it may be a soluble component of the cytosol, or located in some intracellular organelle. The physiological effects of membrane receptors can be mediated by a direct effect on the properties (e.g., permeability or polarization) of the membrane itself, or by stimulation of the formation of a secondary messenger with effects on intracellular systems. The receptor-occupancy theory implies that the agonist becomes bound to the receptor and attempts have been made to isolate stable complexes analogous to the enzyme–substrate complex. The failure of this approach in most cases suggests that the complex is generally very labile and undergoes rapid spontaneous dissociation. It has also been suggested that, in some instances, the crucial factor for a cellular response is not the concentration of the receptor–agonist complex, but its rate of dissociation. This type of mechanism has not been conclusively demonstrated as yet.

Receptor theory has developed in great measure from the study of inhibitors of drug actions. Antagonists are classified as being of two types, competitive and non-competitive, though few drugs fit this classification absolutely. Competitive antagonists act reversibly and compete with the agonist for the same combining

Gordon (ed) Platelets in Biology and Pathology
© *Elsevier/North-Holland Biomedical Press, 1976*

site on the receptor. They consequently have structural properties analogous to those of the agonist. Non-competitive antagonists should have no effect on the affinity of the receptor for the agonist; they may form reversible or irreversible complexes with the receptor, or may not react with the receptor at all, acting further along the chain of events leading to the cellular response. In some cases, however, antagonists which appear to be competitive from kinetic analysis, actually exert their effect indirectly, rather than competing with the agonist for the receptor.

The isolation and identification of receptors has been facilitated by the increasing availability of radioactively-labelled agonists and antagonists of high specific activity. The characterisation of a binding protein is, however, only a partial answer to the problem. It is also necessary to demonstrate: (1) the accessibility of the binding site to the agonist in the intact cell; (2) that the affinity, specificity and rate of binding are consistent with those observed for the interaction between the agonist and the cell, and (3) a functional relationship between the receptor–agonist complex and the physiological consequences of stimulation. In only a very few cases can all of these criteria be said to have been attained.

1.2. Scope of this discussion

Platelets interact with a large number of agents through specific receptor mechanisms. These can roughly be divided into two classes according to the size of the agonist. Considerable attention is being paid to the nature of the receptors on platelets for macromolecules such as thrombin, collagen, bovine factor VIII, antigen–antibody complexes and aggregated IgG. Interactions have also been described between platelets and components of the complement system and of the early phase of intrinsic coagulation. Although there is a great deal of information available on the nature of the platelet receptors for some of these macromolecular stimuli, we have had to limit the present discussion to receptors for low molecular weight agonists and thrombin. For the most part these will be considered under three headings: (1) receptors mediating shape change, aggregation and release; (2) receptors involved in membrane transport, and (3) receptors influencing adenylate cyclase. Possible interactions between these three types of effect will be discussed.

2. Adenosine diphosphate (ADP)

A dialysable, heat stable factor present in acid extracts of red cells and platelets was shown to cause platelet adhesion to glass (Hellem, 1960) and platelet aggregation (Øllgaard, 1961). This factor was identified as ADP by Gaarder et al. (1961). Born (1962) and O'Brien (1962) introduced the nephelometric technique for studying aggregation induced by ADP and other agents. Continuous recording of platelet aggregation at physiological temperature was first used by Cuthbertson and Mills (1963). This simple technique has formed the basis for most of the subsequent investigations into platelet pharmacology.

2.1. Activity

ADP causes aggregation which is preceded by a shape change and which may be followed by a second wave of aggregation accompanied by the release reaction (MacMillan, 1966; Mills et al., 1968) if the Ca^{2+} concentration is reduced (Mustard et al., 1975a; Macfarlane et al., 1975b). ADP also causes various biochemical changes in platelets including a small fall in the energy charge of metabolic adenine nucleotides occurring with 2 sec (Mills, 1973). This effect is accentuated by inhibitors of ATP resynthesis showing that it is due to increased ATP utilization (Mills, 1975). ADP also accelerates the turnover of phosphorus in phosphatidic acid and di- and tri-phosphoinositides (Lloyd et al., 1972, 1973). Although ADP has no measurable effects on cyclic AMP metabolism under basal conditions, it is a powerful, noncompetitive inhibitor of the activation of adenylate cyclase by PGE_1, adenosine, etc. (Haslam, 1973) and rapidly reduces previously elevated levels of platelet cyclic AMP (Cole et al., 1971; Mills and Smith, 1972). All of these effects of ADP occur in the concentration range 0.2–5 μM. Half-maximal responses are produced by the following concentrations: shape change, $\simeq 1\ \mu$M in rabbits (Born, 1970); aggregation, 0.6 μM in citrate, 0.2 μM in heparin (Mills and Roberts 1967a; Skoza et al., 1967); energy charge, 2 μM (Mills, 1975). Lloyd et al. (1973), using washed rabbit platelets, found that 0.2 μM ADP caused a half maximal increase in phosphatidic acid labelling from ^{32}P and that this effect was closely correlated with the shape change. In contrast to aggregation, shape change and the biochemical effects of ADP occur in the absence of Ca^{2+}, but there is at present no evidence to suggest that these effects are mediated by different receptors.

2.2. Specificity

The ADP receptor for aggregation has a quite remarkable degree of structural specificity. The only structural analogues that have a similar potency to ADP are those which are substituted in the 2- position of the purine ring such as 2-chloro ADP and 2-methylthio ADP; these are somewhat more active than ADP (Maguire and Michal, 1968; Gough et al., 1972). Small changes in other parts of the purine ring, or in the D-ribofuranosyl group cause marked reduction of activity (Gaarder et al., 1961). There is an absolute requirement for a pyrophosphate group in the 5' position, and the α-β methylene analogue of ADP in which the two phosphate groups are linked by a stable methylene bridge in place of the anhydride bond has less than one thousandth of the activity of ADP (Salzman et al., 1969; Horák and Barton, 1974). Other weakly active compounds are 2'-deoxy ADP, ADP 1-N oxide, 3'-deoxy ADP (cordycepin diphosphate). Adenosine 5'-tetraphosphate also causes platelet aggregation but it is not known whether this labile compound is first converted to ADP (Clayton et al., 1963; Gaarder and Laland, 1964). Reports that ATP causes aggregation (Mitchell and Sharp, 1964; Ardlie et al., 1966) probably reflect a substantial contamination of commercial ATP by ADP (Gaarder et al., 1961; Haslam, 1966).

2.3. Inhibitors

Several compounds structurally related to ADP inhibit aggregation, including adenosine (Born and Cross, 1962) and 2-substituted adenosines (Born, 1964; Born et al., 1965; Kikugawa et al., 1973a,b). It was naturally assumed that these compounds acted by competing with ADP for its receptor (Skoza et al., 1967; Born and Cross, 1963), but several observations are inconsistent with this assumption. These are: (1) inhibition by adenosine is not competitive at high inhibitor concentrations (Salzman et al., 1969; Macfarlane and Mills, 1975); (2) the inhibitory action of adenosine increases with time of exposure (Born and Cross, 1962) and (3) adenosine inhibits aggregation induced by agents other than ADP (Clayton et al., 1963; O'Brien, 1964). This fact has been wrongly used to support the notion that all aggregating agents operate through an ADP mediated step (Clayton and Cross, 1963). In contrast to adenosine, ATP is a specific antagonist of the various effects of ADP on platelets with competitive kinetics ($K_i = 20~\mu M$) and immediate onset of action (Macfarlane and Mills, 1975). It now appears likely that adenosine and 2-chloroadenosine act by stimulating adenylate cyclase to increase the intracellular cyclic AMP content. This explanation is supported by the powerful synergism seen between adenosine and inhibitors of cyclic AMP phosphodiesterase (see page 126).

Inhibition by AMP at low concentrations can be blocked by KCN, which prevents its dephosphorylation (Salzman et al., 1966b) or by adenosine deaminase which destroys any adenosine so formed (Rozenberg and Holmsen, 1968), suggesting that its action is indirect. At high concentrations AMP inhibits in its own right, probably by competition (Packham et al., 1972). Derivatives of AMP substituted in the two position, e.g., 2-methylthio AMP (Michal et al., 1969) and 2-chloro AMP (Gough et al., 1969; Kikugawa et al., 1973b) are powerful inhibitors of aggregation which may act competitively, though they have not been tested for effects on the cyclic AMP system, nor has it been shown that their inhibition is specifically directed towards ADP.

α,ω-Diadenosine 5'-polyphosphates inhibit ADP induced aggregation and the most powerful member of the series, α,ω-diadenosine 5'-pentaphosphate, has a K_i of less than $1~\mu M$ (Harrison et al., 1975). This compound is a very powerful inhibitor of adenylate kinase (K_i 2.5×10^{-9} M) with kinetics that are competitive with respect to both AMP and ATP (Lienhard and Secemski, 1973).

2.4. Binding

Several investigators have attempted to measure the binding of ADP to platelets. Born (1965) estimated the number of ADP binding sites on the assumption that adenosine binds to the same site as ADP. From the amount of adenosine bound in a rapid phase of uptake (10 min) the figure of 200,000 binding sites/cell was derived. However, no evidence was provided that any of the radioactivity associated with the platelet was actually due to intact adenosine; this is important because adenosine is rapidly phosphorylated by platelets and incorporated into their intracellular nucleotide pool (Ireland and Mills, 1966). As pointed out above, there is good reason to believe that adenosine does not bind to the ADP receptor.

Hampton and Mitchell (1966a,b) measured electrophoretic mobility of platelets in 'glass contacted' plasma. Low concentrations of ADP or noradrenaline increased the anodic mobility of platelets to the pre-contact value. Higher concentrations of ADP or noradrenaline both cause the anodic mobility to fall, as confirmed by other groups (Seaman and Vassar, 1966; Grottum, 1968). Using the maximum increase in mobility and assuming this to be due to the binding of ADP with a net increase of three negative charges per molecule bound, they obtained a figure of 85,000 ADP binding sites. This estimate cannot be regarded as realistic in the absence of adequate explanations of: (1) the effect of glass contact; (2) the biphasic dose response curve, and (3) the parallel effects of ADP and noradrenaline under conditions which preclude initiation of the release reaction.

Several authors have shown that radioactivity is taken up by platelets incubated with ^{14}C-labelled ADP (Salzman et al., 1966a; Born, 1965; Spaet and Lejnieks, 1966; Ireland and Mills, 1966; Rozenberg and Holmsen, 1968) which occurs by stepwise dephosphorylation of ADP and incorporation of the adenosine so formed. Salzman et al. (1966a) failed to show any uptake of radioactivity with ADP labelled with ^{32}P. Boullin et al. (1972) measured the radioactivity of platelet pellets prepared by centrifuging samples of PRP incubated with ^{14}C-labelled ADP. Pretreatment of the platelets with prostaglandin E_1 caused a reduction in the radioactivity found. This was interpreted as indicating that PGE_1 interferes with the binding of ADP to its receptor. Unfortunately these authors failed adequately to correct for the changes in the volume of plasma trapped in the platelet pellet when platelets change their shape and aggregate (Born, 1970).

Born and Feinberg (1975) have introduced a new and sophisticated technique for their investigation of ADP binding to platelets. A swing-out head was constructed for the Eppendorf microfuge and platelets were rapidly sedimented from plasma through a layer of silicone oil into perchloric acid. Radioiodinated albumin was included to allow a correction to be made for the volume of plasma sedimented in association with the platelets. A variety of techniques was employed to reduce the degradation of ADP or the incorporation of radioactivity into platelet nucleotides via the adenosine mechanism. They showed – in contrast to Boullin et al. (1972) – that PGE_1 did not interfere with ADP binding, and reported that only 30% of the bound radioactivity was recovered as ADP, 60% being in the form of ATP. Born and Feinberg (1975) claim to have detected 88,000 'high affinity' binding sites with K_a 5.4×10^5 M^{-1}. This is clearly an error. The Scatchard plot shown is curved and the extrapolation from the observations made at low concentrations gives $\simeq 6,000$ sites/cell. Even this figure cannot be trusted, as a wide variation in binding (0.15–0.7 pmol/10^8 platelets) is evident from the published results of different experiments using 1 μM ADP. The values reported were not corrected for the fact that only a fraction of the bound radioactivity was recovered as ADP.

Nachman and Ferris (1974) have measured the binding of ADP to membranes prepared from homogenised platelets by sucrose density gradient centrifugation. ADP was slowly bound to the membranes and a Scatchard plot of the binding characteristics was linear (K_a 6.5×10^6 M^{-1}; total binding 1.2 nmol/mg membrane protein, equivalent to 100,000 molecules bound per platelet). Binding required a divalent cation and was inhibited by sulphydryl reagents and 2-chloro adenosine, to a lesser extent by ATP and AMP, and not at all by PGE$_1$. Further studies have shown that no binding protein was present in membranes isolated from platelets disrupted by freezing and thawing, but that a soluble ADP binding protein (mol. wt. $\simeq$ 160,000) with similar characteristics to the membrane bound material, is present in platelets (Nachman, 1975). No evidence has been presented that this protein has access to ADP added to the outside of the cell. Furthermore, the slowness of the binding and its dependence on divalent cations indicate that if this material is related to the ADP receptor, its properties must have been considerably altered during extraction. A fraction of platelet metabolic ADP cannot be extracted by ethanol, suggesting that it is protein-bound (Holmsen, 1972), but the relation between this binding and that described by Nachman has not been established.

2.5. Theories of ADP action

The mechanism of action of ADP on platelets has been the subject of a considerable amount of research and even more speculation. The theories proposed fall into two main groups: (1) those in which ADP emerges unscathed from its interaction with the receptor, and (2) those in which ADP takes part in a chemical reaction. Theories of the first type include:

(a) The suggestion that ADP acts together with a divalent cation and assorted plasma proteins to form a bridge between adhering cells (Gaarder and Laland, 1964; Skalhegg et al., 1964; Clayton et al., 1963). This fails to account for the other effects of ADP or for aggregation induced by other agents.

(b) ADP could act as a competitive inhibitor of any of a number of ATPases present on the external surface of the platelet membrane, whose activity is assumed to be necessary for maintaining platelets in a nonadhesive state (Robinson et al., 1965; Salzman et al., 1966b; Chambers et al., 1967; White, 1968; Mason and Saba, 1969; Moake et al., 1970a). As ATP is not normally present in plasma, the natural substrate for such enzymes is presumably intracellular nucleotide. ADP on the outside of the cell would not therefore have access to the active site, which is in any case exposed to intracellular metabolic ADP (whose concentration is some 1000 times that required extracellularly for ADP to cause aggregation). In the case of the Na$^+$, K$^+$ activated ATPase, ADP has not been shown to inhibit the enzyme in intact cells, and ouabain, a known inhibitor, does not cause aggregation. Therefore, if ADP does regulate the activity of a membrane enzyme it must do so through a specific regulatory site rather than by the simple product inhibition so far demonstrated in fragmented membrane preparations.

One action of ADP on a membrane enzyme which does have many of the characteristics expected of an ADP receptor is its ability to inhibit the platelet adenylate cyclase. As we shall discuss below, however, this effect cannot account for the ability of ADP to induce either shape change or aggregation (see page 191).

The presence of a 'high energy' phosphate group in ADP suggests that this molecule could act as an energy source for the aggregation response (Spaet and Lejnieks, 1966). However, dephosphorylation of ADP does not appear to be essential for the induction of aggregation, as cyanide can block dephosphorylation without inhibiting aggregation (Salzman et al., 1966b).

The possibility that ADP acts as a phosphate acceptor has been suggested by the observation of Guccione et al. (1971) that ADP added to washed rabbit platelets is rapidly phosphorylated to ATP. Little AMP was formed, and this was interpreted as excluding the action of adenylate kinase. The phosphorylation of ADP was blocked by 10^{-5} M pCMBS (Guccione et al., 1971) but the effect of this concentration of pCMBS on shape change was not reported. The effect was enhanced by the addition of ATP and was attributed to the action of a nucleoside diphosphate kinase (NDPK). Nucleoside diphosphate kinase (EC 2.7.4.6) is a soluble enzyme which, unlike the ADP receptor, has low substrate specificity (Mourad and Parks, 1966) and an absolute requirement for divalent cations (Agarwal and Parks, 1971). The 5'-diphosphates of guanosine, uridine, cytosine and inosine, while they are phosphorylated by washed rabbit platelets at at least one-tenth the rate of ADP, have less than 1/10,000 of the activity of ADP as inducers of shape change (Packham et al., 1974). Likewise, the 5'-triphosphates of guanosine and cytosine are half as active as ATP as phosphate donors, but are much weaker inhibitors of platelet aggregation than ATP. NDPK is therefore an unlikely candidate for the ADP receptor. However, an enzyme capable of phosphorylating extracellular ADP at the expense of intracellular ATP might have the desired characteristics. A conformational change in the enzyme induced by the donation of a phosphate radical to ADP could mediate the diverse pharmacological effects of ADP. The net effect of such an operation would result in the formation of ^{32}P-labelled ATP in the medium when ADP acts on platelets previously labelled with ^{32}P. Evidence that transmembrane phosphorylation of ADP can indeed occur has been presented (Mustard et al., 1975b), and in view of the theoretical importance of these observations, we look forward to their extension and confirmation.

3. 5-Hydroxytryptamine (5HT)

It has been known for a long time that a vasoconstrictor substance is present in serum, and it was demonstrated some sixty years ago that this activity could be extracted from platelets (Janeway et al., 1918). Rapport et al. (1948) showed that this substance was 5-hydroxytryptamine (5HT). This discovery occurred at the same time as the identification of the substance responsible for the staining characteristics of enterochromaffin cells ('enteramine') as 5HT (Erspamer and Asero, 1952). 5HT in serum is derived from platelets, from which it is released during clotting (Rand and Reid, 1951). Interest in 5HT metabolism and pharmacology was stimulated by the suggestion that it could be a central neurotransmitter, a thesis supported by the interesting effects of the 5HT antagonist, lysergic acid diethylamide.

Platelets are aggregated by 5HT and have an avid uptake and storage mechanism for it. During the release reaction induced by thrombin and other agents, the 5HT is specifically released. The superficial resemblance between platelets and nerve endings has generated considerable pharmacological interest in the interactions of 5HT with platelets, and this topic is discussed at length in Chapter 8. Some aspects relevant to platelet receptors will, however, be summarised here.

3.1. Actions

Platelet aggregation induced by 5HT was first observed by Mitchell and Sharp (1964). In human citrated platelet-rich plasma the aggregation is usually weak and reversible, and it is preceded by a shape change. The concentrations needed are between 0.2 and 10 μM and higher concentrations have less effect (Baumgartner and Born, 1968). On occasions biphasic aggregation has been seen in human plasma (White, 1970; Besterman and Gillett, 1973) and occurs regularly with citrated platelet-rich plasma from cats (Tschopp, 1969; Mills, 1970) and in heparinized plasma from pigs (Gordon and Drummond, 1975). Rabbit platelets are not aggregated by 5HT in citrated PRP, but do aggregate when the plasma is recalcified (Mitchell and Sharp, 1964). Duck thrombocytes do aggregate with 5HT though they do not respond to ADP (Belamarich and Simoneit, 1973). When 5HT is added together with other aggregating agents, a degree of synergism is seen, but if the addition of the second agent is delayed for more than a few minutes, the second response is inhibited (Baumgartner and Born, 1968).

Born et al. (1972) compared the effects of structural analogues of 5HT with variations in the ring substituents and side chain modifications, including alpha methylation and alkylation of the amine. Of 17 compounds tested, 16 caused a shape change and 11 caused aggregation, in some cases as powerfully as 5HT. Many of the compounds were also inhibitors of 5HT induced aggregation, i.e., they were partial agonists. Clearly the 5HT receptor does not have the striking specificity characteristic of the ADP receptor or of the 5HT uptake mechanism (see below). Platelet aggregation by 5HT is powerfully and specifically inhibited by methysergide (Mitchell and Sharp, 1964), bromo LSD and chlorpromazine (Michal and Penglis, 1969), and by LSD and dibenzyline but not by morphine or cocaine (Michal, 1969).

The mechanism of the pharmacological effects of 5HT on excitable tissues is not well understood, though there is some evidence that changes in membrane permeability to K^+ or Cl^- may be involved (Douglas, 1975). Born et al. (1972) noted that replacement of Na^+ by choline in the suspending medium inhibited the shape change induced by 5HT whereas the ADP induced shape change was unaffected, suggesting that, as in many other tissues, the action of 5HT on platelets may depend upon the extracellular Na^+ concentration. This interesting possibility has not, to our knowledge, been systematically investigated.

Platelets that have been enriched in sialic acid by incubation with CMP-*N*-acetyl neuraminic acid together with a crude fraction of rat liver, containing sialotransferase, show increased rates of 5HT uptake (Szabados et al., 1975) and enhanced susceptibility to 5HT-induced aggregation (Mester et al., 1972). The increase in potassium flux associated with uptake is also enhanced (Michal et al., 1972). The suggested relationship between platelet membrane sialic acid and 5HT binding has parallels in other tissues: treatment of rat stomach strips with neuraminidase and EDTA selectively inactivates their response to 5HT (Wooley and Gommi, 1964). However, platelets from patients with the hereditary giant platelet syndrome of Bernard and Soulier have reduced amounts of total and neuraminidase susceptible sialic acid (Grottum and Solum, 1969) but take up serotonin faster than do normal platelets (Walsh et al., 1975).

3.2. *Uptake*

Human platelets normally contain a high concentration of 5HT ($\approx 3 \times 10^{-18}$ mol/platelet, or roughly 0.3 mmol/litre of platelet water) sequestered in specialized storage organelles together with nucleotides and calcium. These granules are strongly osmiophilic, inherently electron dense (White, 1969), and the heaviest of the subcellular particles separated by gradient centrifugation (Pletscher, 1968); they are consequently known as the dense granules. In contrast to the adrenal medulla, where catecholamines are stored in a constant molar ratio with ATP, the storage capacity for 5HT in normal platelets far exceeds their content. Platelets, not having tryptophan decarboxylase (Clark et al., 1954; Zucker, 1962) do not synthesize 5HT, and probably acquire the amine during their life in the circulation. When platelets are incubated in vitro with 5HT, the amine is rapidly and actively incorporated into the cell (Sano et al., 1958). Platelets labelled in this way with radioactive serotonin and reinfused into the donor retain the label for a period comparable to their life span (Heyssel, 1961; Heyssel et al., 1967), indicating the apparent irreversibility of the uptake mechanism.

Platelets from patients who do not have dense granules also take up radioactive 5HT, but the radioactivity is not retained and oxidised products are lost to the plasma (Pareti et al., 1974). Reserpine causes a similar effect in normal platelets (DaPrada et al., 1965). This is interpreted as indicating that the platelet plasma membrane has an active uptake mechanism for 5HT, and that 5HT accumulating in the cytosol is rapidly transported into the granules where it is protected from the action of the mitochondrial monoamine oxidase.

5HT uptake in vitro displays saturation kinetics, and the concentration of 5HT at which the initial rate of uptake is half maximal is about 0.2 μM (Born and Gillson, 1959; Tuomisto, 1974). In spite of this, many investigators have studied the effects of inhibitors using excessively high concentrations of 5HT, thus underestimating the potency of the specific competitive uptake inhibitors relative to the action of non-specific membrane stabilising drugs. The latter are concentrated in membranes and can cause morphological and toxic changes including 5HT leakage and lysis at comparatively low concentrations, e.g., 30 μM for propranolol (Lemmer et al., 1972). Because of the rapidity of the uptake at low 5HT concentrations, either rapid sampling techniques – e.g., using formalin to stop the reaction (Costa and Murphy, 1975) – or dilution of the platelet suspension should be used to obtain accurate initial rates. Imipramine and some of its analogues are powerful competitive inhibitors of platelet 5HT uptake (Tuomisto, 1974) at approximately the same concentrations ($\simeq 10^{-7}$ M) at which they inhibit 5HT uptake by brain synaptosomes. In contrast, LSD and methysergide are active only at concentrations around 10^{-4} M (Stacey, 1961). This clearly demonstrates the differences between the structural specificity of the uptake mechanism and that of the pharmacological receptors for aggregation and shape change.

The rate of 5HT uptake depends upon the pH (Stacey, 1961; Lingjaerde, 1969) and ionic composition of the medium, falling off with increasing pH from 6.0 to 8.0, and requiring sodium ions (DaPrada et al., 1967; Sneddon, 1969). Reduction of Na^+ concentration reduced the affinity of the uptake system for 5HT but did not change the maximal uptake rate. These kinetics do not appear to be compatible with the theory that energy for 5HT transport is provided by the movement of monovalent cations down a thermodynamic activity gradient (Sneddon, 1971). Although choline is a competitive inhibitor of 5HT uptake with $K_i = 20$ mM (Lingjaerde, 1969), it was used to replace Na^+ in these experiments which complicates their interpretation. There is evidence that Cl^- may be transported together with 5HT (Lingjaerde, 1971a,b,c), and that the affinity of the transport mechanism for Cl^- is affected by other monovalent anions, such as acetate. It has also been reported that the K^+ flux across the plasma membrane increases when platelets are incubated with 25–100 μM 5HT (Born, 1967), but it is not clear whether this effect is linked to 5HT uptake, to the action of 5HT on its receptor, or to the shape change induced by 5HT.

Born et al. (1972) showed, for a series of N-disubstituted tryptamines, that increasing chain length of the aliphatic substituents caused increasing activity as inhibitors of 5HT uptake, and decreasing activity as inhibitors of 5HT-induced aggregation. Of four derivatives of 5HT with side chain modifications, only 5-hydroxy-α-methyltryptamine was taken up to an appreciable extent. Of 12 analogues tested, 11 were powerful competitive inhibitors of 5HT uptake, but 5-methoxy-α-methyltryptamine was virtually inactive as an uptake inhibitor, though it caused shape change and aggregation. This has been confirmed with more refined techniques by Drummond and Gordon (1975) who also showed that cinanserin was 30,000 times more potent as an inhibitor of aggregation than as an uptake inhibitor. These observations clearly demonstrate that the structural specificity of the uptake acceptor differs from that of the pharmacological receptor and this is further illustrated by the inability of methysergide to block uptake (K_i against aggregation 0.03 μM; against uptake 125 μM; Born et al., 1972). This evidence clearly rules out the possibility that the receptor for aggregation and the uptake receptor are one and the same (Baumgartner, 1969; Baumgartner and Born, 1969; Born and Michal, 1975).

3.3. Binding

At low temperatures, the binding of 5HT to platelets can be distinguished from uptake. Under these conditions a concentration dependent passive diffusion into platelet water still occurs, but by extrapolation an estimate of from 6,000 to 50,000 high affinity binding sites per platelet has been obtained (Born and Bricknell, 1959). Marcus et al. (1975) have shown that 5HT is irreversibly bound to partially purified ganglioside fractions from platelets and other tissues, and that this binding was specific for 5-hydroxyindoles, and inhibited by antioxidants and by exclusion of oxygen. Calculations indicate the presence of about 10^5 molecules of ganglioside, containing N-acetyl-neuraminic acid, per platelet. Both sialic acid and gangliosides have been suggested as possible recognition sites for 5HT (Wooley and Gommi, 1964; 1965).

Drummond and Gordon (1975) have presented evidence for three different classes of binding sites, with apparent dissociation constants of 2.3×10^{-8}, 1.5×10^{-7} and 2×10^{-6} M. The specific receptor blocker cinanserin (see above) displaced 5HT by an amount corresponding to the saturation capacity of the high affinity site. A strong correlation was shown between the ability of a number of drugs to inhibit 5HT-induced shape change and to block binding to the cinanserin-sensitive site. Binding of 5-methoxy-α-methyl tryptamine was demonstrated, and since this compound neither is taken up itself, nor inhibits the uptake of 5HT, binding to the uptake site is excluded. This work, though preliminary, is exciting as it represents the first evidence for binding of 5HT to a pharmacological receptor in any tissue, and emphasises the potential of the platelet as a model tissue for this type of investigation.

4. Catecholamines

Adrenaline and noradrenaline have at least four distinct actions on human platelets. At concentrations of 10^{-8}–10^{-7} M adrenaline causes a marked potentiation of aggregation induced by ADP added simultaneously or shortly afterwards (Ardlie et al., 1966; Mills and Roberts, 1967b). At about 10^{-6} M adrenaline causes a single phase aggregation, not preceded by a shape change, which is slower and less extensive than primary aggregation caused by ADP, and does not reverse spontaneously (O'Brien, 1964). Higher concentrations of adrenaline cause primary aggregation followed after a variable delay by secondary aggregation associated with the release of nucleotides and 5HT (Mills and Roberts, 1967b). In addition to these three effects, all of which can be observed with an aggregometer, adrenaline inhibits the stimulation of platelet adenylate cyclase. This effect will be discussed below (Section 7.4.1), and more details of platelet–catecholamine interactions are given in Chapter 8.

4.1. Specificity

Few analogues of adrenaline have been examined in relation to platelet aggregation. It has been established that noradrenaline is 4–10 times less potent than adrenaline (Mitchell and Sharp, 1964; Mills and Roberts, 1967b; O'Brien, 1964; Bygdeman 1968). The naturally occurring L-form of noradrenaline is 30 times more effective than the D-form (Bygdeman and Johnsen, 1969) and isoprenaline is inactive (O'Brien, 1964; Clayton and Cross, 1963). O'Brien (1964) showed that the specific α-blocker phentolamine at 10^{-8} M inhibited the effects of adrenaline, whereas phenoxybenzamine was active only at 5×10^{-5} M. Mills and Roberts (1967b) found that both potentiation and aggregation by adrenaline were blocked by dihydroergotamine (10^{-7}–10^{-6} M) but that neither phenoxybenzamine or dibenamine (N-(2-chloroethyl)-dibenzylamine) inhibited at 5×10^{-5} M even after prolonged preincubation. Thus the aggregation of platelets by catecholamines shows some of the characteristics of effects mediated by α-receptors (Ahlquist, 1948) and this is supported by the lack of specific inhibition observed with propranolol and other β-blockers (Mills and Roberts, 1967b; Bygdeman and Johnsen, 1969). However the platelet receptor is clearly different from the classical α-receptor in its resistance to blockade by alkylating halogenoalkylamines.

Isoprenaline is a weak and variable inhibitor of the effects of other aggregating agents (Mills and Roberts, 1967b; Abdulla, 1969; Mills et al., 1970) and this inhibition is relieved by propanolol. This has been interpreted as indicating that platelets have an inhibitory β receptor for catecholamines, and it has subsequently been shown that this operates through the cyclic AMP system.

4.2. Uptake and binding

Adrenaline and noradrenaline are progressively taken up by platelets in a non-saturable, energy dependent process which is partly inhibited by reserpine and some structural analogues of adrenaline (Sano et al., 1959; Hughes and Brodie, 1959). Born and Smith (1970) found that about half of the radioactivity from tritium-labelled adrenaline taken up by platelets in 5 h was recoverable as intact adrenaline, and that half was present as an acidic metabolite that regenerated adrenaline on acid hydrolysis. Adrenaline, but not the metabolite, was released from platelets by thrombin. Formation of the metabolite was inhibited by pyrogallol and other inhibitors of catechol-O-methyltransferase. Uptake was partly inhibited by propranolol, phentolamine, phenoxybenzamine and other agents. Some rapid uptake was seen and this was partly inhibited by phentolamine but not by dihydroergotamine. Abrams and Solomon (1969) compared the activities of various drugs on the uptake and release of noradrenaline by platelets with their known effects on adrenergic neurones. Desmethylimipramine (10^{-7} M) caused 50% inhibition of uptake but, in contrast to neurones, platelets did not release amines when exposed to ephedrine (10^{-3} M).

The use of selective inhibitors of uptake and aggregation indicates that it is unlikely that the uptake process has any relevance to the interaction of adrenaline with its receptor for aggregation. For example, phentolamine (Bygdeman and Johnson, 1969) and dihydroergotamine (Barthel and Markwardt, 1974, 1975) are powerful inhibitors of aggregation but poor inhibitors of uptake, whereas des-methylimipramine is a powerful uptake inhibitor with much weaker effects on aggregation (Mills and Roberts, 1967a). Washed rabbit platelets are, incidentally, exquisitely sensitive to dihydroergotamine: adrenaline-induced aggregation was blocked at 10^{-11} M, a concentration equivalent to 15 molecules per platelet (Barthel and Markwardt, 1975), which suggests that adrenaline receptors on platelets are somewhat thinly spread.

5. Thrombin

Thrombin is one of the most important activators of platelets in haemostasis, and it is the only soluble physiological agent which can induce the release reaction directly–that is, in the absence of aggregation. Platelets themselves can catalyze the production of thrombin in several different ways (Walsh, 1974), and it is possible that sufficient thrombin may be generated within platelet aggregates to trigger the release reaction without any evidence of fibrin formation, since lower concentrations of thrombin and shorter exposures are needed to induce the full release reaction than to induce coagulation. The interactions of thrombin with platelets are fully discussed in Chapter 9, but a review of platelet receptors would not be complete without a summary of recent research on thrombin.

5.1. Activity

Like most other aggregating agents, thrombin (0.1–0.3 U/ml) induces platelet aggregation preceded by a shape change. The aggregation in citrated plasma may be biphasic (Thomas, 1967), and the second phase is associated with the release reaction. The shape change and the primary aggregation are not inhibited by ATP, demonstrating that these effects are not caused by released ADP (Macfarlane and Mills, 1975). Higher concentrations of thrombin added to plasma anticoagulated with citrate or EDTA induce coagulation, which obscures the optical record, so that most investigators use washed platelets to study the effects of thrombin on platelets. Under these circumstances platelet aggregation is frequently delayed and may in part be due to the release of the contents of the storage granules, since aggregation can be inhibited by ADP-removing systems (Haslam, 1964). Lower concentrations of thrombin are required than in plasma, probably because of the absence of antithrombins. Even in the presence of EDTA, or when platelet suspensions are not stirred, thrombin can induce the release reaction (see Holmsen et al., 1969). The effects of thrombin are potentiated by adrenaline (Thomas, 1967) and by ADP (Niewiarowski and Thomas, 1966; Packham et al., 1973), and they are inhibited by heparin in the presence of heparin cofactor (Clayton and Cross, 1963), and by hirudin. Aggregation in citrated plasma is inhibited by PGE$_1$, but release induced by high concentrations of thrombin is only incompletely inhibited (Mürer, 1971). See note 1 added in proof, page 202.

5.2. Mechanism of action

Despite an intensive study of the effects of thrombin on platelets, no generally accepted theory of the interaction of platelets with thrombin has yet emerged. Thrombin is a proteolytic enzyme with a trypsin-like specificity which normally attacks bonds between arginyl and lysyl residues embedded in polypeptide chains. It has a serine residue at the active site and its activity is irreversibly inhibited by such agents as DFP, PMSF and TLCK. Thrombin also has esterolytic activity against such substrates as TAMe, BAMe, TLMe, and BAEe (Cole et al., 1967). Acetylated thrombin has been prepared which retains its esterolytic activity but has little or no action on fibrinogen or platelets (Seegers et al., 1970). Thrombin attacks fibrinogen by removing two distinct peptides: one, fibrinopeptide A, from the N-terminal end of the A(α) chain, and the other, fibrinopeptide B, from the N-terminal end of the B(β) chain of the parent molecule. Removal of fibrinopeptide A is sufficient to allow loose clotting, though tight clot formation takes place only after removal of fibrinopeptide B.

It is reasonable to suppose that the proteolytic activity of thrombin is the basis for its action on platelets, and this has stimulated a search for evidence of a specific substrate for thrombin on the platelet surface. An alternative theory, which has received comparatively little consideration, is that thrombin may cause a distortion of a platelet membrane component by binding to it without cleaving any bonds. In this sense thrombin would be acting as a hormone rather than as an enzyme.

5.3. Platelet macromolecules affected by thrombin

5.3.1. Fibrinogen

Since fibrinogen is the natural substrate for thrombin, and since fibrin monomer (formed by the action of thrombin on fibrinogen) polymerises and so could be the basis for platelet aggregation, many investigators have studied the involvement of fibrinogen in platelet reactions.

Platelets contain substantial quantities of fibrinogen (Ware et al., 1948; Salmon and Bounameaux, 1952) which is not freely exchangeable with plasma fibrinogen (Castaldi and Caen, 1965), but whose release can be stimulated by low concentrations of thrombin for brief periods (Keenan and Solum, 1972). This intracellular fibrinogen has been isolated and characterised. It is indistinguishable from plasma fibrinogen antigenically, and has nearly identical subunit structure (Ganguly, 1972; Doolittle et al., 1974). Platelet fibrinogen is more heterogenous than its plasma counterpart, possibly because of partial digestion by platelet proteolytic enzymes, and has lower molecular weight (Ganguly, 1972) and reduced clottability by thrombin. Further studies showed that about one quarter of platelet fibrinogen was different from plasma fibrinogen, and could be separated from it and the remainder of platelet fibrinogen. It also had a different pattern of degradation by plasmin (James et al., 1975).

Well washed platelets have very little fibrinogen on their surfaces (Keenan and Solum, 1972) although they respond to thrombin. Grette (1962) showed that platelet fibrinogen was not hydrolysed by trypsin or thrombin provided the release reaction was blocked. On the other hand, Schmid et al., (1962) and Morse et al., (1965) showed that platelets treated with trypsin or thrombin to release and destroy their fibrinogen, were no longer aggregable by thrombin in serum but that they aggregated in plasma. The failure of aggregation in serum can be explained by the fact that fibrinogen is a cofactor for aggregation, and does not necessarily show that fibrinogen is required for the primary interaction of thrombin and platelets.

Davey and Lüscher (1965) compared the coagulant activity of various snake venoms with their platelet release-inducing activity, and showed that there was little correlation between their ability to clot fibrinogen and to induce release. Subsequently they showed that the venom of Trimeresurus purpureomaculata could be fractionated into a coagulant fraction with no releasing activity, and a releasing principle which neither clotted fibrinogen nor had any demonstrable enzymatic activity. The coagulant and esterase activities of these venoms were inhibited by DFP though the releasing activity was not affected (Davey and Lüscher, 1967; 1968). A similar aggregating agent was isolated from Trimeresurus okinavensis (Davey and Esnouf, 1969). Since these venom principles act by a non-proteolytic mechanism they can be used to investigate neither the mechanism of action of the proteolytic release inducers nor the possible role of fibrinogen. Neither Reptilase, a component of the venom of Bothrops atrox that releases fibrinopeptide A from platelets, nor an enzyme from Agkistrodon contortrix, which splits off fibrinopeptide B, aggregate platelets (Tangen et al., 1973).

Recent studies with anti-fibrinogen antibody (FAB) fragments show that when they are present aggregation induced by thrombin is inhibited, but thrombin induced release is not (Tollefsen and Majerus, 1975). This shows again that fibrinogen is necessary as a cofactor for aggregation, but because release is not impaired, fibrinogen does not seem to be the site of action of thrombin.

It has been suggested that local generation of thrombin on the platelet surface and the subsequent formation and polymerization of fibrin monomers is the mechanism for platelet aggregation induced by ADP (Han and Ardlie, 1974a,b; Ardlie and Han, 1974). The same authors have suggested that fibrinopeptides released in this process are responsible for the release reaction. However, neither heparin nor hirudin prevent ADP-induced aggregation or release at concentrations which block the actions of thrombin (Macfarlane et al., 1975b).

5.3.2. Fibrin stabilizing factor (Factor XIII)

Factor XIII, which causes the crosslinking of polymerised fibrin by the formation of γ-glutamyl–lysyl isopeptide bonds between α- and γ-chains of adjacent fibrin monomers, is present in plasma and platelets in an inactive form, and is activated by thrombin. Approximately 16% of the Factor XIII in PRP is in the platelets; plasma and platelet Factor XIII are antigenically similar but not identical (Kiesselbach and Wagner, 1966; Bohn, 1971). Antigenic determinants on both plasma and platelet Factor XIII are lost during incubation with 20 U/ml thrombin. Ganguly and Moore (1967) demonstrated that a high molecular weight protein (5.5S) was lost from the soluble fraction of platelets incubated with thrombin. Subsequently, Ganguly (1969), searching for the substrate for thrombin, showed that platelet homogenates incubated with 50 U/ml thrombin in the cold lost at least 3 major protein components separable by polyacrylamide gel electrophoresis, besides fibrinogen which did not enter the gel. One of these proteins was partially purified and shown to be a β-globulin without Factor XIII activity and without immunological cross-reactivity with whole serum. Using aprotinin to inhibit non-specific proteolysis this protein was later identified as the platelet Factor XIII of Kiesselbach and Wagner (Ganguly, 1971). Its molecular weight was 110,000–150,000 by gel exclusion, or about half that of plasma Factor XIII. It has since been shown that plasma Factor XIII consists of four chains (two each of α and β), and that platelet Factor XIII consists of two α-chains only. The α-chains of both zymogens are cleaved by thrombin to give the active transglutaminase (Chung et al., 1974). Platelet Factor XIII can stabilise clots formed in Factor XIII deficient plasma, suggesting that it is released during clotting. Factor XIII deficient platelets do not incorporate transfused plasma Factor XIII (McDonagh et al., 1969).

5.3.3. Platelet myosin

The contractile protein in platelets formerly known as 'thrombosthenin' can be dissociated into platelet actin and myosin (see Chapter 6). Platelet myosin (Booyse et al., 1971a) has a molecular weight of 543,000 and specific ATPase activity of 20 nmol P_i/min/mg protein at 22°C in 6 mM $CaCl_2$. Cohen et al. (1969) showed that myosin from horse platelets ('thrombosthenin M') was attacked by thrombin with the release of some small peptides (less than 2% of the total proteins) and appearance of a new C-terminal but no change in ATPase activity. This protein was immunologically distinct from equine fibrinogen, but its amino acid composition as reported was closer to that of fibrinogen than myosin. These authors also demonstrated that when platelet concentrates were incubated with 10 U/ml thrombin for 1 h at 37°C, a single protein band on 4.5% polyacrylamide gels disappeared. This band ran somewhat behind their purified platelet myosin, but was taken to be identical to it. The effect of thrombin on the electrophoretic mobility of 'thrombosthenin M' was not determined, nor were cleavage fragments demonstrated on the gel (Cohen et al., 1969). Using SDS gels, Booyse et al. (1972) showed that membranes prepared from human platelets treated with thrombin (0.5–1 U/ml for 2 min at 37°C) lost material corresponding to a molecular weight of 200,000, and that lower molecular weight bands appeared at 171,000, 85,000 and 7,800. It appears from the gels shown, however, that the material which disappears could have a molecular weight substantially higher than 200,000, as the gels were calibrated only to 130,000. Phillips and Agin (1974) also reported that a polypeptide of 200,000 molecular weight was reduced in concentration by treatment of isolated membranes with thrombin.

5.3.4. 'Thrombin sensitive protein' (TSP)

Several authors have described the disappearance of a high molecular weight protein from platelets after treatment with thrombin. Ganguly and Moore (1967) demonstrated the disappearance of a single band on 7% polyacrylamide gel of solubilised platelet protein after treatment with thrombin (50 U/ml in the cold). Similar results were obtained by Nachman (1968) who had previously demonstrated an antigen in platelet lysates which disappeared after thrombin (Nachman, 1965). Ganguly (1971) subsequently showed that two bands disappeared after treatment of platelet lysates with thrombin: the slower migrating band was similar in mobility to fibrinogen, and the faster migrating band was identified as Factor XIII (see above).

Baenziger et al. (1971) treated intact platelets with thrombin and then disrupted the platelets and solubilised the particulate fraction and showed that, on SDS polyacrylamide gels, a band with molecular weight 190,000 disappeared. They called this material Thrombin Sensitive Protein (TSP) although Ganguly (1969) had earlier used this term to refer to the disappearing band which was eventually shown to be Factor XIII (Ganguly, 1971). Thrombin treatment of the particulate fraction of disrupted platelets did not remove the TSP, but TSP was released intact from whole platelets (Baenziger et al., 1972). When the released and platelet-bound materials were isolated, and their amino acid and carbohydrate compositions determined, these were quite different from those of human plasma fibrinogen and no N-terminal amino acids were found. Under conditions in which 80% of the TSP was released, less than 5% of particulate Ca^{2+}-stimulated ATPase appeared in the supernatant. Factor XIII activity was not determined (Baenziger et al., 1972).

TSP is also released by kidney bean erythrophytohaemagglutinin and its release by thrombin is inhibited by dibutyryl cyclic AMP, theophylline or prostaglandin E_1 (Brodie et al., 1972). Phillips and Agin (1974) also demonstrated that this protein was released from platelets, but failed to find it in purified platelet membranes. It seems likely, therefore, that TSP is released from storage granules and is not the substrate for the action of thrombin.

5.3.5. Membrane glycoproteins

Electromicroscopic observations of the staining properties of platelets have indicated that there are acid glycopeptides on the external surface of the plasma membrane (Behnke, 1968). Platelets contain considerable amounts of sialic acid, of which about 60% can be digested from intact cells by neuraminidase (Grottum and Solum, 1969; Kirby and Mills, 1975). This contributes significantly to the anodic electrophoretic mobility of the cells. Three major glycopeptides of molecular weight 120,000, 22,500 and 5,000 were isolated by Pepper and Jamieson (1970) from platelets digested with trypsin. Papain or pronase also removed these glycopeptides, and they could be isolated from trypsin digests of isolated platelet membranes.

When intact platelets were iodinated on the external surface by the lactoperoxidase method, a single radioactive band was obtained on SDS gels (Barber and Jamieson, 1971). Phillips (1972), using higher radioactivities showed that three glycoproteins were labeled. Their apparent molecular weights on SDS gels were 150,000, 118,000 and 92,000. Four additional protein bands were labeled but did not stain for carbohydrate. On treatment of these surface-iodinated platelets with trypsin, all three glycoprotein bands disappeared and new peaks of both radioactivity and carbohydrate staining appeared at lower molecular weights. No appreciable radioactivity was lost from the membranes during trypsin treatment. The protein corresponding to the TSP of Baenziger et al. (1971, 1972) co-migrates with Phillip's glycoprotein I on SDS gels, but the material which purified with the membrane, while staining strongly for carbohydrate, did not stain well for protein (Phillips and Agin, 1974). A similar pattern of carbohydrate staining and radioactivity was found by Nachman et al. (1973) in SDS gels of membrane protein from iodine-labeled platelets using the glucose oxidase–lactoperoxidase technique. Neuraminidase removed most of the radioactivity from the three major glycoproteins with only a slight effect on carbohydrate staining.

Phillips and Agin (1974) showed that thrombin (10 U/ml for 15 minutes at 37°C) caused a 10–50% reduction in the radioactivity of glycoprotein II (118,000 mol. wt.) from platelets labeled with iodine on the external surface. Treatment of isolated membranes of labeled platelets with thrombin caused some loss of radioactivity from all three glycoproteins and slight reduction of apparent molecular weight. Nurden and Caen (1974) also obtained three carbohydrate positive bands on SDS gels of a particulate fraction from sonicated platelets, corresponding to molecular weights of 155,000, 135,000 and 103,000. Somewhat different patterns were obtained from abnormal platelets: in Glanzmann's thrombasthenia the band at 135,000 was absent, and in the hereditary giant platelet syndrone (Bernard-Soulier) the 155,000 band was reduced (Nurden and Caen, 1975). Low platelet sialic acid has been reported in this latter condition (Grottum and Solum, 1969), as well as defective agglutination with bovine factor VIII or ristocetin (Walsh et al., 1975; Weiss et al., 1974). Incubation of normal platelets with trypsin caused rapid loss of carbohydrate staining of the 155,000 mol. wt. band, followed by disappearance of the 135,000 mol. wt. band (Nurden and Caen, 1975).

The glycoproteins contribute in a most important way to the properties of platelet membrane, and the finding of deficiencies in thrombasthenic and Bernard-Soulier platelets is most exciting. The hydrolysis of glycoprotein II by thrombin could be important, but it must be admitted that the process is rather slow in comparison to the speed with which thrombin exerts its effects on platelets.

As this section should have made all too clear, the hypothesis that thrombin acts by hydrolysing a surface protein has received a lot of attention, and the subject is complicated and not a little confused. This is due in part to a failure to distinguish clearly between the final action of thrombin, which is to induce the release of a variety of products, and the primary interaction of thrombin with its supposed substrate. This substrate must be available to thrombin (i.e., it must be on the external surface of the platelet) and its hydrolysis should not be inhibited by agents (e.g., PGE_1) which block the release reaction by an action on the stimulus transfer pathway.

5.4. Binding of thrombin

If thrombin acts as a hormone rather than an enzyme to trigger platelet reactions, it is reasonable to suppose that there should be a finite number of sites on the platelet surface capable of binding thrombin when present in activating concentrations*. Ganguly (1974) labelled thrombin with ^{125}I and demonstrated that radioactivity was bound to platelets, but did not give an estimate of the number of binding sites. Tollefsen et al. (1974), using ^{125}I-labelled thrombin of high purity, independently demonstrated two classes of saturable binding sites. One had a dissociation constant of 0.02 U/ml (2×10^{-10} M) and a capacity of about 500 molecules/cell and the other bound 50,000 molecules with a dissociation constant of 2.9 U/ml (3×10^{-8} M). Non-saturable binding was also observed. Radioactivity was rapidly displaced by non-radioactive thrombin, and was found predominantly at the platelet plasma membrane by radioautography. In another report it was shown that prothrombin and the intermediates 1 and 2 did not bind, whereas, after full activation of the molecule to thrombin, binding did occur (Tollefsen et al., 1975). Binding was unaffected by the presence of anti-fibrinogen antibody fragments (Tollefsen and Majerus, 1975).

Both binding characteristics and the activity of thrombin to induce the release reaction are influenced by anions. Some 30-fold less thrombin is required to induce 50% release of serotonin from platelets suspended in cacodylate or acetate-containing solutions, but the affinity of platelets for thrombin was increased so that binding of 100 molecules/platelet occurred at the least concentration of thrombin required for complete release regardless of the anion present. The clotting of fibrinogen was also accelerated by these anions, but neither the esterase activity nor the cleavage of fluorescamine reacting material from fibrinogen were. Cacodylate was shown to accelerate the polymerization of fibrin monomer, and it was suggested that this effect was responsible for the shortened clotting time. However, the fibrinogen clotting time in the presence of high concentration of thrombin, in which presumably polymerization is the rate limiting step, was not shortened by cacodylate (Shuman and Majerus, 1975).

It would appear from this work that one or both of these binding sites could represent a receptor for thrombin, but this may not be the case. Ganguly (1974) and Tollefsen et al. (1974) demonstrated that thrombin inactivated by treatment with DFP binds in an identical way to platelets, and competes with active thrombin. However, even when present in large excess, inactivated thrombin did

---

* See note 2 added in proof, page 202.

not inhibit the action of active thrombin, but instead potentiated it (Phillips, 1974; Phillips and Agin, 1974). The reasons for this are not clear, although it could be due to protection of thrombin from antithrombin or adsorbant surfaces, since this potentiation was very evident in PRP, but not in a purified system (Martin et al., 1975). This topic is discussed in more detail in Chapter 9.

It can be concluded that despite the major effort that has been made to elucidate the action of thrombin on platelets, this action remains mysterious.

6. Other aggregating agents

6.1. Vasopressin

Haslam and Rosson (1972) showed that 8-arginine vasopressin causes aggregation of human platelets in heparinised plasma but that it is much less active in citrated plasma. Aggregation is preceded by a shape change, and sometimes occurs in two waves. The first wave is only slightly inhibited by the creatine kinase/phosphocreatine system which blocks ADP-mediated aggregation. 8-Lysine and 8-ornithine vasopressins were as active as the arginine compound, and 2-phenylalanine, 8-lysine vasopressin was more active at low concentrations, suggesting that the effect on platelets is more closely related to the pressor than to the antidiuretic actions of the hormone. On a molar basis, vasopressin was about 40 times as active as ADP. Platelets from rabbits and pigs did not respond to vasopressin, and dog platelets, which were only tested in citrated plasma, showed a shape change but no aggregation. That vasopressin acts directly on platelets, without involving released ADP, was confirmed by the observation that neither aggregation nor shape change was inhibited by 250 μM ATP (Macfarlane and Mills, 1975). 8-Lysine vasopressin caused a fall in the energy charge of the adenosine nucleotides similar to that caused by ADP and 5HT. This effect was seen in the presence of EDTA, so is not dependent on the availability of extracellular Ca^{2+}. Vasopressin does not inhibit prostaglandin stimulation of platelet adenylate cyclase (see Section 7.4.4). Bradykinin and angiotensin II did not cause aggregation and oxytocin was at least 50 times less active than vasopressin (Haslam and Rosson, 1972); oxytocin also selectively inhibits the effects of vasopressin (Macfarlane, 1975).

6.2. Acetylcholine

The cholinergic agents acetylcholine, carbamylcholine and acetyl-β-methylcholine cause aggregation of dog platelets and release of nucleotides and 5HT but have no effect on the platelets of man, rat or rabbit (Shermer and Chuang, 1973; Chuang et al., 1974). Release induced by 1 mM acetylcholine was blocked by an equal concentration of atropine, pilocarpine or scopolamine but not by 5 μg/ml α-bungarotoxin, suggesting a receptor of the muscarinic type; however, the very high concentrations of agonist required for an effect indicate a substantial difference between the platelet receptor and the receptor of cholinergic neurones. Aggregation induced by carbachol was preceded by a shape change, and may be associated with a substantial increase in platelet cyclic GMP (Haslam, 1975; Section 7.5).

6.3. *Prostaglandin-like aggregating agents*

Prostaglandins E_2 and $F_{2\alpha}$ are synthesized by platelets during the release reaction (Smith and Willis, 1970; Smith et al., 1973) and their synthesis is powerfully inhibited by aspirin and other non-steroidal anti-inflammatory drugs (Smith and Willis, 1971), which also inhibit secondary aggregation. Kloeze (1966) showed that low concentrations of PGE_2 potentiate the aggregation of rat platelets by ADP, though high concentrations inhibit. With human platelets, potentiation by PGE_2 is more difficult to demonstrate, and varies from one donor to another. Shio and Ramwell (1972) showed that PGE_2 at $0.3 \mu M$ inhibits the first wave and potentiates the second wave of aggregation induced by ADP in human citrated plasma. In heparinised pig plasma, PGE_2 causes aggregation directly at concentrations around 10^{-6}–10^{-5} M (MacIntyre and Gordon, 1975b). Binding of PGE_2 to human platelet membranes, which was briefly reported by Gorman (1974), revealed a high affinity binding site ($K_a = 2 \times 10^{10} M^{-1}$) with a capacity of 3.5×10^{-15} mol/mg of membrane protein. Even if all of the platelet protein (1.6–1.8 mg/10^9 cells; Marcus and Zucker, 1965) were in the membranes, this would still represent only 5 molecules bound per cell.

Fenichel et al. (1975) have shown that three synthetic analogues of PGE_2 induce aggregation of human platelets at 5–$20 \mu M$. These compounds (see Chapter 13) have a methyl group inserted in the 15 position and either a methyl group or no substituent in position 11.

Although PGE_2 can potentiate and initiate aggregation under some conditions, it cannot overcome the inhibition of secondary aggregation caused by aspirin (Shio and Ramwell, 1972), so that PGE_2 production by platelets cannot be responsible for the second phase. However, convincing evidence has recently been presented that intermediate products of arachidonic acid peroxidation are themselves powerful aggregating and releasing agents. A detailed treatment of this fascinating subject is beyond the scope of this review, as little information is available on the nature of the receptors for these compounds. Both the cyclic endoperoxide intermediates of prostaglandin synthesis, PGG_2 and PGH_2 (Hamberg et al., 1974a,b) and, more recently thromboxane A_2 (Hamberg et al., 1975) have been suggested as mediators of secondary aggregation and the release reaction. For background information on this subject the reader is referred to Smith and Macfarlane (1974) and for a more up-to-date treatment, to Chapter 13 of this volume.

7. Receptors influencing cyclic AMP metabolism

The first suggestion that cyclic AMP might be involved in the inhibition of platelet aggregation was made by Ardlie et al. (1967) who showed that the phosphodiesterase inhibitors caffeine, aminophylline and theobromine inhibited platelet aggregation induced by ADP, albeit at rather high concentrations. Since that time results from a large number of laboratories have shown that many of the most powerful inhibitors of aggregation increase the concentration of intracellular cyclic AMP in platelets, either by inhibiting phosphodiesterase, or by direct stimulation of adenylate cyclase. Several authors have discussed the overwhelming evidence for the involvement of cyclic AMP as a mediator of inhibition of aggregation, e.g., Salzman (1972), Haslam (1973), Smith and Macfarlane (1974). Several distinct receptors are involved in the control of adenylate cyclase activity. ADP and adrenaline antagonise the effects of adenylate cyclase stimulators, but the relevance of this effect to their action as aggregating agents has been disputed.

7.1. Prostaglandins

The effects of prostaglandins on many tissues are associated with increased intracellular concentrations of cyclic AMP, although it is likely that some of the diverse effects of prostaglandins may be mediated by other systems and several authors have attempted to demonstrate such systems in platelets. Abdulla and McFarlane (1971) suggested that prostaglandins E_2 and E_3 could modulate the activity of adenylate kinase in platelets, and Johnson and Ramwell (1973) also showed effects of prostaglandins on Mg^{2+} dependent, Na^+, K^+-activated ATPase. PGE_1 has also been reported to influence the activities of platelet phosphodiesterase (Amer and Marquis, 1972). Despite these activities, however, it is generally accepted that the effectiveness of prostaglandins as inhibitors of platelet aggregation is a result of their ability to stimulate adenylate cyclase.

7.1.1. PGE_1

Since the demonstration by Kloeze (1966) that PGE_1 inhibits platelet aggregation, he and a large number of other investigators have established that this prostaglandin inhibits the aggregation of platelets from both mammalian and non-mammalian species, and that it inhibits aggregation induced by virtually all primary aggregating agents.

The onset of inhibition when platelets are exposed to PGE_1 is rapid, and little further increase of inhibition of human platelets occurs after 20 sec, although the increase in other animals may continue for as long as 30 min (Kinlough-Rathbone et al., 1970). PGE_1 can inhibit shape change, aggregation and release, but the concentrations required depend on the function being examined and the nature and concentration of the stimulator (Haslam and Rosson, 1972; Macfarlane and Mills, 1975). Effects are seen in several species at concentrations as low as 30 nM (Kloeze, 1969). Aggregation induced by vasopressin is more easily inhibited by

PGE$_1$ than is aggregation by ADP or adrenaline (Haslam and Rosson, 1972). As with other inhibitors of primary aggregation, PGE$_1$ blocks secondary aggregation and the associated release reaction. Higher concentrations of PGE$_1$ ($\simeq 1\ \mu$M) are required to block the shape change caused by ADP (Kinlough-Rathbone et al., 1970; Shio et al., 1970), and release induced by high concentrations of thrombin is only partly inhibited by PGE$_1$ (Wolfe and Shulman, 1970; Mürer, 1971).

The inhibitory effects of PGE$_1$, as well as its effect on cyclic AMP levels within the platelet, are strikingly potentiated by drugs which inhibit the cyclic AMP phosphodiesterase (Mills and Smith, 1971). Theophylline (Ball et al., 1970; Mills et al., 1970; Cole et al., 1971), RA233 and papaverine (Mills and Smith, 1971), at concentrations which have little or no effect by themselves, greatly enhance the inhibition caused by PGE$_1$ added subsequently. For instance, 50 μM RA 233 alone did not inhibit aggregation induced by 100 μM ADP but caused a parallel shift in the dose response curve to PGE$_1$ corresponding to a 10-fold increase in inhibitory potency. Under similar conditions phosphodiesterase inhibitors enhance the accumulation of cyclic AMP caused by PGE$_1$. These experiments, of course, provide strong evidence that the effects of PGE$_1$ are mediated by cyclic AMP.

The effects of a large number of structural analogues of PGE$_1$ have been studied (Table 1). It can be seen that for inhibitory activity hydroxyl groups must be present on C 11 and C 15 in the correct steric configuration, and that a keto group is essential on C 9. Changes in the length of the carboxyl side chain reduce activity, but methylation or insertion of a double bond in the 2,3 position does not. The length of the methyl side chain is less critical; the activity actually increases as this chain is lengthened from 6 to 9 carbons (Kloeze, 1969). Introduction of a *cis* double bond in the 5,6 position converts PGE$_1$ to PGE$_2$ which is a weak inhibitor of shape change and aggregation, but can potentiate secondary aggregation and the release reaction (see above, Section 6.3).

Platelets incubated with PGE$_1$ and then washed and resuspended in a medium not containing PGE$_1$ aggregate normally, showing that its effects are reversible (Kinlough-Rathbone et al., 1970). The initial rate of increase in cyclic AMP levels in platelets exposed to PGE$_1$ is an hyperbolic function of PGE$_1$ concentration with a $K_a = 0.33\ \mu$M in plasma (Haslam, 1973). Since prostaglandins bind to plasma proteins (Unger, 1972) this figure may be higher than the true receptor affinity. Several investigations of the binding of PGE$_1$ to platelets have been reported. Kinlough-Rathbone et al. (1970) found less than 10^4 molecules bound per platelet. Gorman (1974) found that PGE$_1$ bound to platelet membranes to the same extent as PGE$_2$ (see Section 6.3). McDonald and Stuart (1974) found that 3×10^9 washed platelets bound 25 fmol [^{3}H]PGE$_1$ with a dissociation constant of 3 nM. This corresponds to about 5 molecules per platelet. Bound radioactivity was only partly displaced by unlabeled PGE$_1$ or PGE$_2$, but radioactivity recovered from the platelet pellet chromatographed as PGE$_1$. These authors also showed that PGE$_2$ weakly stimulated the adenylate cyclase and that PGE$_2$ is a partial agonist for the PGE$_1$ receptor.

Stimulation of adenylate cyclase in intact platelets is enhanced by the thiol reagent *N*-ethyl maleimide (NEM). NEM does not inhibit phosphodiesterase, and

TABLE 1
Structures and actions of various prostaglandins on platelets*

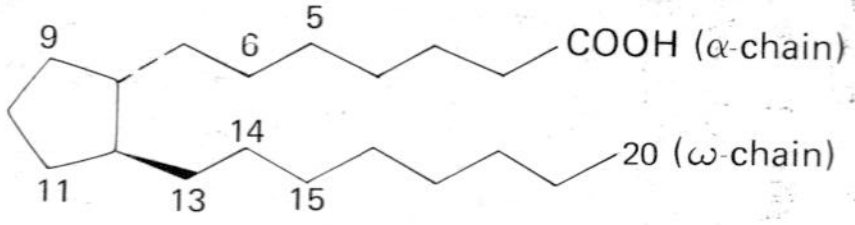

Prostaglandin carbon-numbering diagram: COOH (α-chain); (ω-chain); carbon positions labelled 5, 6, 9, 11, 13, 14, 15, 20.

Action	Name	Length of α-chain	Length of ω-chain	Position of double bonds (cis)	Substitution (α or S) 9	11	15	Relative potency (PGE₁ = 1)	Reference
Inhibitors, PGE₁ type	ω-homo PGE₁	7	9	13,14	=O	—OH	—OH	3.8	1
	2,3 trans PGE₁	7	8	13,14; 2,3 trans	=O	—OH	—OH	2.5	2
	PGE₁	7	8	13,14	=O	—OH	—OH	1	1
	PGE₁ methyl ester	7-COOCH₃	8	13,14	=O	—OH	—OH	0.86	1
	13,14 dihydro PGE₁	7	8	None	=O	—OH	—OH	0.64	1
Weak inhibitors,	α-chain homologues	5,6,8,9	8	13,14	=O	—OH	—OH	<0.02	1
	15 keto PGE₁	7	8	13,14	=O	—OH	=O	<0.01	1
No effect	PGF₁α	7	8	13,14	—OH	—OH	—OH		1
	PGF₂α	7	8	13,14; 5,6	—OH	—OH	—OH		1
	PGE₂	7	8	13,14; 5,6	=O	—OH	—OH		3
Weak inhibitor, enhances 2° phase Inhibitors, PGD₂ type	PGD₂	7	8	13,14; 5,6	—OH	=O	—OH	1.0	4
	PGD₁	7	8	13,14	—OH	=O	—OH	<0.01	5
								Approx. conc. for aggregation	
Inducers of aggregation and release	U46619	7	8	13,14; 5,6	—CH₂—	—O—	—OH	0.5 μM	6
	U44069	7	8	13,14; 5,6	—O—	—CH₂—	—OH	1.0 μM	6
	Wy-17,185	7	8	13,14; 5,6	—OH	—H	< —CH₃ / —OH	8.0 μM	7
	Wy-17,186	7	8	13,14; 5,6	=O	—H	< —CH₃ / —OH	8.0 μM	7
	Wy-16,991	7	8	13,14; 5,6	—OH	—CH₃	< —CH₃ / —OH	8.0 μM	7
	Endoperoxide (PGH₂, PGR₂, LASS)	7	8	13,14; 5,6	—O—O—		—OH	?1.0 μM	8
No action	PGG₂; 15,00H PGR₂	7	8	13,14; 5,6	—O—O—		—OOH	?2.0 μM	8
	PGH₁; PGR₁	7	8	13,14; 5,6	—O—O—		—OH	–	9

* The numbering of carbon atoms is as in the figure, and for this purpose, carbons deleted or added to alter chain lengths are ignored.

References: (1) Kloeze, 1969; (2) Van Dorp, 1971; (3) Kloeze, 1971; (4) Smith et al., 1974; (5) Macfarlane et al., 1975a; (6) Smith and Silver, 1977; (7) Fenichel et al., 1975; (8) Hamberg et al., 1974a; (9) Willis, 1974

it does not alter the time course of accumulation of cyclic AMP in the way that is characteristic of phosphodiesterase inhibition (Mills and Smith, 1972; Mills, 1974). Johnson et al. (1974,a,b) showed that the inhibitory effect of PGE_1 on aggregation was greater in the presence of NEM and suggested that a thiol group was involved in the receptor mechanism. However, MacIntyre and Gordon (1975a) showed that the inhibitory effects of NEM and PGE_1 on aggregation were merely additive. Furthermore, the thiol reagent pCMBS, which does not readily penetrate cell membranes, does not potentiate the effects of PGE_1 on adenylate cyclase although it should block any thiol group on an outward facing receptor. Both NEM and pCMBS can block the inhibition of cyclase stimulation caused by ADP (Mills, 1974). Thus, though thiol groups are clearly involved in some way in the complex control mechanisms that regulate platelet adenylate cyclase, it is unlikely that they are directly involved in the PGE_1 receptor. Johnson et al. (1974a) also reported reduction of the inhibitory effects of PGE_1 by dithiothreitol (DTT), but DTT can itself induce aggregation (MacIntyre and Gordon, 1975a) and its effects with PGE_1 were again merely additive.

Following the suggestion that opiates may exert some of their effects by blocking the stimulation of neuronal adenylate cyclase by prostaglandins (Ehren-preis et al., 1973; Collier and Roy, 1974), the effect of morphine on the ability of PGE_1 to inhibit adrenaline and ADP-induced platelet aggregation was examined by Gryglewski et al. (1975). In some donors morphine at concentrations up to $26\ \mu M$ slightly enhanced the aggregation induced in the presence of low concentrations of PGE_1 ($0.03–0.14\ \mu M$), but higher concentrations of morphine had the opposite effect. This effect cannot with certainty be attributed to an action on the PGE_1 receptor.

7.1.2. PGD_2

Smith et al. (1974) and Nishizawa et al. (1975) have recently shown that PGD_2 inhibits the aggregation of human platelets with the same potency as PGE_1, but, in contrast to PGE_1, this prostaglandin has striking species specificity. The platelets of rabbits (Smith et al., 1974) and pigs (MacIntyre and Gordon, 1975b) are weakly inhibited, and those of several other common laboratory animals are not inhibited at all (Smith et al., 1975a; Mills and Macfarlane, 1976). PGD_2 differs structurally from PGE_1 in three ways. It has a 5,6 double bond, an hydroxyl group on C 9 in place of a keto, and a keto group on C 11 in place of an hydroxyl. Prostaglandins intermediate in structure between these two, such as PGD_1, PGE_2, $PGF_{1\alpha}$ and $PGF_{2\alpha}$ have little or no inhibitory activity (Macfarlane et al., 1975a), so that it seems unlikely that PGD_2 stimulates the same receptor as PGE_1 (Mills and Macfarlane, 1974; Macfarlane et al., 1975a). Several other minor differences in the response of human platelets to PGE_1 and PGD_2 have been observed, but preliminary experiments with mixtures of PGE_1 and PGD_2 suggest that they both regulate the same adenylate cyclase (Mills and Macfarlane, 1974; 1976). The powerful antiplatelet activity of PGD_2 may have important therapeutic consequences since in many other pharmacological systems PGD_2 is relatively inert.

However, bronchoconstrictor activity has been demonstrated by Dawson et al. (1974) and pressor activity by Horton and Jones (1974).

7.2. *Adenosine*

The ability of adenosine to inhibit aggregation was discovered soon after the demonstration of ADP-induced aggregation, and for several years the mechanism of its action was disputed.

7.2.1. *Kinetics and specificity*

Adenosine (1–30 μM) inhibits aggregation induced by ADP (Born and Cross, 1962), by thrombin and adrenaline (Clayton and Cross, 1963), by 5HT (O'Brien, 1964) and by vasopressin (Haslam and Rosson, 1972). The inhibition usually increases with time of exposure (Born and Cross, 1963; Packham et al., 1969; Macfarlane and Mills, 1975) and then decreases as adenosine is removed by deamination or by uptake into platelets. When adenosine is rapidly destroyed by the addition of adenosine deaminase, the inhibition of aggregation persists for 20–30 sec after all of the adenosine has been cleared (Rozenberg and Holmsen, 1968). Adenosine inhibits or reverses shape change (Born, 1970), and is a weak inhibitor of the release reaction (Zucker and Jerushalmy, 1967).

Substantial species differences in the response of platelets to adenosine have been reported. Of the common laboratory animals, platelets of rats, guinea pigs and cats are much less inhibited by adenosine than are those of rabbits, dogs and man (Mills, 1970).

Several authors have shown that, at low concentrations ($\simeq 1\ \mu$M) adenosine has competitive kinetics (Skoza et al., 1967; Born, 1970; Michal and Born, 1971). This is not true at higher concentrations, and full inhibition does not occur (Rozenberg and Holmsen, 1968; Salzman et al., 1969; Macfarlane and Mills, 1975).

A large number of analogues of adenosine have been tested on platelets, and in general it appears that the receptor has a similar specificity for the purine moeity as the receptor for ADP (Michal, 1974). Substitutions in the 2 position can enhance potency whereas other changes usually destroy or reduce activity (see, e.g., Born et al., 1965; Kikugawa et al., 1973a). There is also a correlation between inhibition of aggregation and the ability of analogues to increase forearm blood flow on intra-arterial injection (Born et al., 1965).

The first mechanism of action proposed for adenosine was competition with ADP for the supposed ADP binding site (Born and Cross, 1963). Competition is not supported by kinetic evidence, nor does it account for the inhibition of aggregation induced by agents other than ADP, or for inhibition of the effect of thrombin on the nucleated thrombocytes of birds and reptiles, which are not aggregated by ADP (Kien et al., 1971).

Adenosine is reported to reverse the inhibition by ADP of the Na^+,K^+ dependent ATPase (Moake et al., 1970b), but since this enzyme is partly inhibited by oubain, which neither induces nor inhibits aggregation (Michal and Thorp, 1966), this is probably not relevant to its action. Adenosine also inhibits beef heart phosphodiesterase, but the effective concentration was not given (Horlington and Watson, 1970), and Mills and Smith (1971) found only 27% inhibition of platelet phosphodiesterase by 3 mM adenosine. Adenosine is rapidly phosphorylated within the platelet so that it is doubtful if platelet phosphodiesterase is exposed to high concentrations of the inhibitor, and, in any case, adenosine does not potentiate the effect of PGE_1 on intracellular cyclic AMP in platelets as do other phosphodiesterase inhibitors (Haslam and Rosson, 1975).

Rozenberg and Holmsen (1968) noted that adenosine uptake in several ways paralleled its inhibitory effect on aggregation and suggested that the uptake and subsequent phosphorylation of adenosine might deplete a pool of ATP required for aggregation. Salzman et al. (1966b) suggested the opposite, i.e. that ATP was required to maintain platelets in a non-adhesive state, and that ATP synthesised from adenosine sustained this process. Both these hypotheses require that adenosine be taken up to exert its inhibitory effect.

7.2.2. Uptake

Adenosine is taken up by platelets and rapidly phosphorylated by adenosine kinase with the formation of adenine nucleotides (Ireland and Mills, 1966; Holmsen and Rozenberg, 1968). 2-Fluoroadenosine can be incorporated in a similar fashion (Agarwal and Parks, 1975). The kinetics of uptake are complex, with a high affinity, saturable mechanism (Rozenberg and Holmsen, 1968) and a non-saturable process probably representing passive diffusion (Haslam and Rosson, 1975). There is also evidence for auto-inhibition of the high affinity system (Haslam and Rosson, 1975). The high affinity uptake system is inhibited by a number of drugs, the most powerful of which is dipyridamole, which also blocks adenosine uptake by red cells and heart muscle (Bunag et al., 1964). Dipyridamole and papaverine (Markwardt et al., 1967; Mills et al., 1970) and p-nitrophenylthioguanosine (Haslam and Rosson, 1975) block adenosine uptake by platelets without reducing its potency as an inhibitor of aggregation. This clearly indicates that the point of action of adenosine is at the cell membrane, and furthermore suggests that the uptake site and the adenosine receptor are distinct.

7.2.3. Mechanism of action

In experiments which were designed to test the ability of adenosine to inhibit aggregation when its uptake into platelets was blocked by dipyridamole (Born and Mills, 1969) it was in fact found that dipyridamole potentiated the effect of adenosine. A large number of vasodilator drugs are now known which potentiate the effects of adenosine on platelets and other tissues. Many of these also inhibit adenosine uptake, but there is no correlation between their ability to inhibit uptake and potentiate inhibition of aggregation by adenosine (Mills and Smith, 1971; Vigdahl et al., 1971; Rozenberg and Walker, 1973; Philp et al., 1973). These drugs inhibit the cyclic AMP phosphodiesterases of platelets and other tissues, and in some cases appear to be relatively specific for the enzymes in platelets (Smith and Mills, 1970; Mills, 1974; Pichard et al., 1972). The dipyridamole analogue, RA233, and papaverine are both particularly active inhibitors, compared with the methylxanthines, when the phosphodiesterase is measured at low concentrations of cyclic AMP (Mills and Smith, 1971), suggesting that RA233 and papaverine act selectively to inhibit a high affinity phosphodiesterase. RA233 potentiates the inhibition of aggregation produced by PGE_1 and isoprenaline (Mills and Smith, 1971) as well as adenosine, and it therefore seems likely that all of these agents act by stimulating adenylate cyclase. Such a stimulation has been demonstrated for adenosine and 2-chloroadenosine, both in intact platelets (Mills and Smith, 1971) and in platelet fragments (Haslam and Lynham, 1972). In the latter case the effects of adenosine are complicated, as the greatest effects of adenosine are seen at $\simeq 25 \ \mu M$, and higher concentrations of adenosine actually inhibit the stimulation of adenylate cyclase by PGE_1. In intact platelets, Haslam and Rosson (1975) found that adenosine stimulates cyclic AMP accumulation with $K_a = 1 \ \mu M$, and that its effects are strongly potentiated by papaverine. On the other hand, methylxanthines, although they inhibit phosphodiesterase, inhibit the stimulation of adenylate cyclase by adenosine. The kinetics of this inhibition are competitive, with K_i for theophylline of $25 \ \mu M$ and for caffeine of $75 \ \mu M$. This effect is therefore likely to be due to direct competition for the adenosine receptor. Thus, methylxanthines, which do not inhibit adenosine uptake (Mills and Smith, 1971; Vigdahl et al., 1971), block its effect on adenylate cyclase; whereas p-nitrophenyl thioguanosine blocks uptake without affecting cyclase stimulation. It seems clear, therefore, that the cyclase receptor for adenosine is different from the uptake site.

7.3. Isoprenaline

The β-adrenergic agent isoprenaline is a weak inhibitor of aggregation and is effective at a concentration of $0.5 \ \mu M$ (Mills and Roberts, 1967b). Abdulla (1969) and Mills et al. (1970) showed that this effect is abolished by the β-blocker propranolol and accentuated by the phosphodiesterase inhibitor theophylline. The inhibition is more obvious when collagen or thrombin is used as the aggregating agent, and is seen with rabbit as well as human platelets (Mills et al., 1970).

Abdulla (1969) showed that isoprenaline stimulates the adenylate cyclase activity of broken platelets, especially in the presence of the α-blocker phentolamine, and suggested that it exerts its effects via cyclic AMP. Mills and Smith (1971) showed that isoprenaline increases cyclic AMP synthesis in intact platelets, and that phosphodiesterase inhibitors enhance this effect. This was confirmed by Haslam and Taylor (1971a). In the absence of a phosphodiesterase inhibitor, cyclic AMP was increased by about 50% and fell back to the basal level in two minutes (Haslam, 1973). It is possible that isoprenaline also stimulates phosphodiesterase activity, for in the presence of a phosphodiesterase inhibitor the cyclic AMP concentration continues to rise at a time when it is falling in the absence of the inhibitor (Haslam, 1973). Adrenaline, which causes aggregation and inhibits the effects of PGE_1 on platelets through an α-like receptor, can also activate the β-receptor to a certain extent. In the presence of papaverine, adrenaline increased the accumulation of cyclic AMP above the level found with papaverine alone (Haslam, 1973). This effect was enhanced by the α-blocker phentolamine and inhibited by the β-blocker, propranolol.

7.4. Aggregating agents and cyclic AMP

Several aggregating agents can inhibit platelet adenylate cyclase, and since elevation of cyclic AMP inhibits aggregation, a general hypothesis has been proposed that aggregating agents induce their effects on platelets by lowering basal cyclic AMP levels (Salzman, 1972). This has been the subject of heated debate.

7.4.1. Catecholamines

Adrenaline and noradrenaline block the stimulation by PGE_1 of cyclic AMP production by intact platelets and inhibit both basal and PGE_1-stimulated adenylate cyclase in platelet lysates; these effects are blocked by phentolamine but not by propranolol (Zieve and Greenough, 1969; Robison et al., 1969; Salzman and Levine, 1971; Moskowitz et al., 1971). The inhibitory effect of adrenaline is much less pronounced in broken cell preparations than in intact platelets. When adrenaline is added to platelets after PGE_1 has already raised their cyclic AMP content, a fall in the cyclic AMP level occurs (Marquis et al., 1970; Cole et al., 1971; Haslam, 1973) which is especially rapid when no phosphodiesterase inhibitor is added (Mills and Smith, 1972).

When cyclic AMP increases are measured 10 sec after the simultaneous addition of PGE_1 and adrenaline to platelets in citrated plasma, adrenaline inhibits the stimulation non-competitively with a K_i of 0.2 μM (Macfarlane and Mills, unpublished data).

7.4.2. ADP

When ADP is added to platelets previously exposed to PGE_1 it causes a prompt reduction in cyclic AMP levels (Cole et al., 1971; Mills and Smith, 1972; Haslam, 1973). Measurement of the increase in cyclic AMP 20 sec after the simultaneous addition of ADP and PGE_1 to heparin-anticoagulated platelet-rich plasma, in the presence of caffeine, gave inhibition with non-competitive kinetics and a K_i for ADP of 0.8 μM (Haslam, 1973). We have found a similar value for the K_i using citrated platelet-rich plasma. The inhibition by ADP is relieved competively by ATP (Macfarlane and Mills, 1975) and non-competitively by the non-penetrating thiol reagent pCMBS (Mills, 1974). ADP does not appear to inhibit the adenylate cyclase of broken platelet preparations (Salzman and Levine, 1971).

7.4.3. Thrombin

Brodie et al. (1972) measured the adenylate cyclase activity of a particulate fraction of disrupted platelets. When the platelets from which this preparation was obtained had been briefly exposed to low concentrations of human thrombin, the adenylate cyclase activity was greatly reduced. The time course of this effect, and the concentrations of thrombin required, corresponded closely to the release of a 'thrombin sensitive protein' and were similar to those reported for the discharge of the dense granules (Holmsen et al., 1969); the effect was inhibited by PGE_1 and by inhibitors of the release reaction. When thrombin was added to the particulate fraction no inhibition of adenylate cyclase was found by Brodie et al. (1972), though Droller and Wolfe (1972), also using purified human thrombin, found substantial inhibition under similar conditions. Platelets treated with thrombin, and then washed to remove released ADP, responded to PGE_1 with an increase in cyclic AMP formation as large as or larger than that seen in control platelets (Mills, 1972), and thrombin added simultaneously with PGE_1 did not reduce the rate of accumulation of cyclic AMP measured in intact platelets (Macfarlane and Mills, 1975). This shows that the surface membrane adenylate cyclase of intact platelets is not irreversibly inactivated by thrombin. Haslam (1973) found that the largest proportion of the adenylate cyclase activity of platelet homogenates was associated with the granule fraction, and it is possible that the results obtained by Brodie et al. (1972) are explained by an alteration in the granules associated with the loss of their contents. No adenylate cyclase was found in the supernatant from thrombin treated cells. Platelet granules contain guanosine nucleotides (DaPrada and Pletscher, 1970) and guanosine triphosphate (GTP) is a powerful activator of platelet adenylate cyclase, especially when measured at low ATP concentrations (Krishna et al., 1972); it is therefore quite possible that the release of GTP or some other regulator during granule discharge could account for the lowered activity of adenylate cyclase observed by Brodie et al.

In contrast to the above, Droller and Wolfe (1972) showed that when platelets anticoagulated with EDTA were exposed to thrombin, their content of cyclic AMP increased, and this increase was potentiated by theophylline but not by PGE_1, suggesting activation of adenylate cyclase. Platelets synthesize prostaglandins when exposed to thrombin, and it is probable that enough PGE_2 or PGD_2 (Oelz et al., 1976) could have been formed to account for the observed increase in cyclic AMP, since the effect is blocked by aspirin (Droller, 1974).

7.4.4. 5HT and vasopressin

Adenylate cyclase in broken platelet preparations is inhibited by 5HT (Zieve and Greenough, 1969; Salzman and Levine, 1971). It is not known whether this powerful effect is blocked by specific receptor antagonists. This inhibition is not seen in intact platelets either when 5HT and PGE_1 are added simultaneously (Macfarlane and Mills, 1975) or when 5HT is added after PGE_1 (Mills, 1974).

Similarly, vasopressins have little or no effect on the adenylate cyclase of intact platelets (Haslam and Rosson, 1972; Haslam, 1973; Macfarlane and Mills, 1975), but studies with platelet fragments have not been reported. The fact that the powerful aggregating agent vasopressin does not inhibit adenylate cyclase seriously undermines the hypothesis that aggregation occurs as a consequence of lowering platelet cyclic AMP levels.

7.5. *Aggregating agents and cyclic GMP*

The occurrence in platelets of guanosine 3′,5′-cyclic monophosphate (cyclic GMP) and of the enzyme, guanylate cyclase, which catalyses its formation, were observed by Bohme and Jakobs (1973). A cyclic GMP phosphodiesterase has also been demonstrated in platelets (Hidaka et al., 1974). White et al. (1973) showed that during aggregation induced by collagen, thrombin or other agents, cyclic GMP levels were increased 2–4-fold. Jakobs et al. (1974) also showed rapid increases in cyclic GMP after platelets were exposed to aggregating agents. An early report (Glass et al., 1974) that adrenaline-induced aggregation is associated with rapid, massive increases in cyclic GMP was later shown to be due not to adrenaline but to the ascorbic acid used as an antioxidant in the adrenaline solution (Goldberg et al., 1975). Ascorbic acid neither affects the aggregation of platelets by adrenaline, nor does it cause aggregation when added by itself. Haslam and McClenaghan (1974), using a radioisotopic technique to measure the formation of [³H]cyclic GMP in platelets preincubated with [³H]guanine, found small increases in cyclic GMP in platelets exposed to collagen. This effect was not abolished by aspirin, which powerfully inhibited aggregation, but aspirin had the unexpected effect of lowering the basal cyclic GMP levels in unstimulated platelets. It was later suggested that this effect, which was also seen with sodium salicylate, sulphinpyrazone and phenylbutazone, as well as with indomethacin at high concentrations, was due to displacement of cyclic GMP from a stable, bound form, and consequent hydrolysis by phosphodiesterase (Haslam et al., 1975b). Platelet cyclic GMP levels are also raised, in heparinised blood, during ADP-induced aggregation not associated with induction of the release reaction (Haslam et al., 1975a), but these workers also showed that potentiation by cytochalasin B of the release reaction induced by collagen was not associated with any greater increase in cyclic GMP formation. The relevance of changes in cyclic GMP in human platelets to any physiological response is therefore at present somewhat unclear.

Dog platelets differ from those of most species that have been examined in that they are induced to aggregate and undergo a release reaction by cholinergic agents, including acetylcholine and carbamylcholine (Shermer and Chuang, 1973; Chuang et al., 1974). This effect has some of the characteristics of actions on muscarinic receptors, though the agonist concentrations required (0.01–1 mM) are high. With carbachol choline, cyclic GMP was increased in dog platelets in citrated plasma with a time course suggesting an association with aggregation. However, when aggregation and release were induced by acetylcholine, no increase in cyclic

GMP was seen, except in washed platelets in the presence of 0.1–1 mM calcium (Haslam, 1975). The ability of acetylcholine to cause aggregation and release with dog platelets in citrated plasma without an associated increase in cyclic GMP indicates that, even in this situation, cyclic GMP is apparently not an essential mediator of either aggregation or the release reaction.

8. Mechanisms of receptor action

In some respects the platelet is an excellent cell for investigating the interactions between receptors and drugs, as well as the mechanisms by which receptors modulate cellular responses. Platelets are easy to prepare as an almost pure suspension in their own plasma, and in this state they respond to a large number of aggregating agents and inhibitors. There is no diffusion barrier between the membrane receptors and their agonists and antagonists. The pharmacological responses are easy to study with simple apparatus, and can be correlated with several biochemical changes that occur during these responses. On the other hand, platelets occupy less than one hundredth of the volume of the plasma and there are indications that the number of receptors per platelet is not very high in some cases, so that purifying a receptor from platelets could require a large volume of starting material.

Several attempts have been made to characterize the interaction between agonists or inhibitors and platelet receptors, but some authors have failed to establish clear criteria by which specific and non-specific interactions can be distinguished. The agonists discussed in this chapter have immediate effects (within 0.5–5 sec) on platelets, either to induce shape change and a fall in adenylate energy charge, or to change the rate of cyclic AMP synthesis. The rate of interaction of these agonists with their receptors must therefore be very rapid, and the rate of dissociation probably not much slower.

8.1. Relationship between uptake and receptor action

Classical receptor theory is based on the premise that the action of the agonist on the receptor is fully reversible, so that the agonist is released unchanged, and the receptor immediately relaxes when the agonist dissociates from it. Almost identical pharmacological kinetics would result from interactions in which the agonist is the substrate for an enzyme or transport process which simultaneously acts as a receptor. Four agonists which act on platelets are indeed transported– 5HT, acetylcholine, adenosine and adrenaline. However, in at least three of these cases there is excellent evidence that transport is not relevant to the pharmacological effect. Thus, there are analogues of 5HT which induce shape change but are not transported, and drugs differ markedly in their relative efficacy as inhibitors of the two processes. Acetylcholine is also transported but little information is available relating receptor action to its uptake. Inhibitors of adenosine uptake do not block its effect on adenylate cyclase, and methyl xanthines inhibit this receptor action without influencing uptake. Adrenaline is transported slowly into platelets, and α blocking drugs do not inhibit uptake although they inhibit the pharmacological action of adrenaline.

8.2. Adenylate cyclase in the platelet

The regulatory effects of several hormones (in particular, the β-action of adrenaline) on a number of cell types is well explained by the ability of these agents to stimulate the production of cyclic AMP within the cell by activating adenylate cyclase (Robison et al., 1971), and there is little doubt that PGE_1, PGD_2, adenosine and isoprenaline inhibit platelet aggregation in this way (see Haslam, 1975; Smith and Macfarlane, 1974).

The corollary–that aggregating agents may exert their effects on platelets by lowering cyclic AMP levels–is supported by several experiments. Salzman and Neri (1969) showed that ADP and adrenaline lower the cyclic AMP level of platelet-rich plasma, but the method used to assay the cyclic AMP gave erroneously high values. Using a more specific method, a small decrease in the cyclic AMP content of platelet-rich plasma was observed after the addition of ADP or adrenaline (Salzman et al., 1972). Other authors have, however, failed to confirm this (Cole et al., 1971; McDonald and Stuart, 1973). A substantial proportion of the cyclic AMP of platelet-rich plasma is extracellular, and when phosphodiesterase is added to platelet-rich plasma to lower the blank value by destroying plasma cyclic AMP, the addition of adrenaline did not decrease the platelet cyclic AMP (Haslam, 1975). When metabolic cyclic AMP levels are measured after incubating platelets with radioactive adenine, no decrease is induced by ADP or adrenaline unless the basal level is previously elevated (Haslam and Taylor, 1971a,b; Salzman et al., 1972; Haslam, 1973; McDonald and Stuart, 1973; Haslam, 1975); indeed, adrenaline alone causes a slight increase (Haslam, 1973). Salzman et al. (1972) reported a decrease when platelets were prelabelled with adenosine rather than adenine and then exposed to aggregating agents, but this could not be confirmed by Haslam (1975). Adenosine is known to stimulate cyclic AMP synthesis, an effect inhibited by ADP and adrenaline, and this may have accounted for the fall observed by Salzman et al. (1972).

It has been suggested that the stimulation of the second phase of aggregation by PGE_2 may be caused by a reduction of cyclic AMP in platelets, which has been reported to be caused by either 3×10^{-6} M (Salzman et al., 1972) or 3×10^{-10} M PGE_1 (Salzman, 1976). Other authors have not observed such a fall (Shio et al., 1972; Bruno et al., 1974; McDonald and Stuart, 1974). All these authors do, however, find an increase in cyclic AMP induced by PGE_2 at higher concentrations, which presumably is responsible for the inhibition of shape change and the first phase of aggregation by PGE_2.

The hypothesis that aggregation is linked to a decrease in cyclic AMP is weakened by the observation that the powerful aggregating agent vasopressin does not appreciably inhibit adenylate cyclase, and nor do 5HT or thrombin at aggregating concentrations (Haslam and Taylor, 1971b; Macfarlane and Mills,

1975). Also, when platelets are treated with PGE_1 followed by an aggregating agent, aggregation may occur despite the fact that cyclic AMP is still raised (Haslam and Taylor, 1971b).

In conclusion, although some aggregating agents can inhibit platelet adenylate cyclase there is no convincing evidence that the cyclic AMP level in platelets under basal conditions can be lowered. There is evidence that some of the platelet cyclic AMP is sequestered in the dense storage granules (DaPrada et al., 1972), and it has been argued that the synthesis of cyclic AMP in different compartments of platelet may be separately regulated, so that a fraction of cyclic AMP, which may be too small to measure, might regulate both the induction and inhibition of aggregation. Such an hypothesis is, of course, difficult to disprove experimentally.

8.3. Phosphoproteins

Cyclic AMP regulates glycolysis in muscle by causing the dissociation of an inactive protein kinase into an active catalytic unit and a cyclic AMP binding unit. Cyclic AMP dependent protein kinases are widely distributed in various organs throughout the animal kingdom (see, for example, Kuo and Greengard, 1969), and it is reasonable to suppose that many of the effects of cyclic AMP are mediated through protein phosphorylation.

Several authors have described a cyclic AMP dependent kinase in platelets (Marquis et al., 1971; Salzman et al., 1972; Booyse et al., 1973; 1976; Kaulen and Gross, 1974), and in general this enzyme is similar to those extracted from other tissues. Several proteins from platelet homogenates or membranes have been described, ranging in molecular weight from 52,000 to 11,000, which are either phosphorylated by the purified kinase (Booyse et al., 1976) or by a kinase which is found in platelet membranes (Steiner, 1975). The significance of the cyclic AMP dependent system has not been clearly established. Platelets also contain cyclic AMP-independent kinases (Booyse et al., 1976; Lyons et al., 1975), and recent evidence shows that the induction of the release reaction is accompanied by the phosphorylation of two proteins in the intact platelets, one of which is a component of actomyosin.

Lyons et al. (1975) loaded intact platelets with ^{32}P and identified phosphoproteins in whole cell extracts by SDS polyacrylamide gel electrophoresis. Treatment of the platelets with thrombin before extraction resulted in a marked increase in the labelling of two proteins of molecular weights 40,000 and 20,000 respectively. This labelling was very rapid (half maximal at 10–14 sec), and required only low concentrations of thrombin. It could also be caused by a release-inducing plant lectin, and was inhibited by PGE_1 or dibutyryl cyclic AMP.

These results have been confirmed and extended by Daniel et al. (1976), who found that the 20,000 molecular weight protein copurified with one of the light chains of platelet myosin. Phosphorylation of platelet myosin light chains results in a marked increase in the Mg^{2+}-dependent ATPase activity of the actin–myosin complex, and so may be relevant to the control of contraction (Adelstein and Conti, 1975; Adelstein et al., 1975). These recent results are likely to have major implications not only for the understanding of platelet reactions controlled by contractile proteins, but also those of other tissues.

8.4. *Receptors and membrane permeability*

The function of electrically excitable cells can be modified by receptors that selectively increase the permeability of the membrane to potassium, sodium, calcium or chloride, and it seems likely that at least part of the effect of acetyl choline, 5HT and the α action of adrenaline on excitable tissues is explained by this type of action (Rang, 1973). There is evidence suggesting that some platelet responses may be similarly controlled. The action of 5HT on platelets is apparently inhibited by reducing the extracellular sodium concentration and accelerated by increasing the potassium ion concentration (Born et al., 1972); also, exposing platelets to 5HT accelerates the exchange of potassium ions across the plasma membrane (Born, 1967). Further study (for instance, with 5HT analogues and inhibitors) is required to establish whether these phenomena are related to the function of the receptor mechanism, or to non-specific effects. Thrombin releases potassium and calcium from platelets, and has been reported to increase their sodium content (Sneddon and Williams, 1973) and to increase the uptake of radioactive calcium by EDTA washed platelets (Kinlough-Rathbone et al., 1973). These effects are, however, probably the result of the release reaction rather than of the interaction between thrombin and its receptor.

ADP-induced shape change is remarkably insensitive to sodium or potassium ion concentrations (Born et al., 1972), which indicates that the shape change response probably does not depend on transmembrane ionic potentials. With the exception of vasopressin, none of the receptors we have discussed depend for their interaction on extracellular calcium or magnesium, in that similar responses (either shape change or cyclic AMP changes) can be obtained in plasma anticoagulated with heparin, citrate or EDTA.

8.5. *Intracellular calcium movements*

Many intracellular enzymes are activated or inhibited by calcium ions, and a lot of evidence indicates that the function of many cell types may be regulated by changes in the cytoplasmic calcium ion concentration. For example, calcium released from the sarcoplasmic reticulum of striated muscle enables actin to interact with myosin, to activate the myosin Mg^{2+}-ATPase and induce contraction, and several secretory cells seem to be stimulated by mobilization of calcium (see Chapter 3).

Such a regulatory system requires four components: (1) calcium pumps which move calcium either into specialized organelles inside the cell or through the plasma membrane to the exterior; (2) a mechanism for releasing stored calcium to the cytoplasm, or for increasing plasma membrane permeability to calcium; (3) a stimulus transfer pathway from the relevant receptor and (4) a calcium sensitive target which regulates cell functions.

The concentration of calcium ions in the cytosol of platelets can be inferred from the function of several systems, some of which also provide evidence that the cytosol concentration rises during the shape change and the release reaction.

First, the normal disc shape of platelets is maintained by an equatorial bundle of microtubules, composed of tubulin, and during the shape change these microtubules disappear. Polymerisation of isolated tubulin into microtubules in vitro is inhibited and reversed by calcium ions, although the concentration required under physiological concentrations of magnesium and GTP is disputed (Weisenberg, 1972, gives 6 μM whereas Borisy et al., 1974, suggest 150 μM). Secondly, the formation of blebs and spikes during the shape change must result in an increase in surface free energy, so it is likely that a contractile mechanism is involved, and, in fact, a constricting band of microfilaments appears during the shape change. Platelet actin-myosin interaction (see Chapter 6) is probably responsible for both the shape change and for the formation of these microfilaments (and, later, for clot retraction), and this interaction is activated by calcium at about 0.5 μM (Hanson et al., 1973). Thirdly, phosphorylase b of platelets is activated independently of cyclic AMP by calcium at submicromolar concentrations, and this enzyme becomes activated during ADP-induced aggregation (Gear and Schneider, 1975).

From these figures it would be reasonable to suppose that changes in the cytosolic calcium ion concentration in the range 10^{-7} to 10^{-5} M might regulate platelet functions, but providing direct evidence for this is not easy. Platelets have a calcium pump (Grette, 1963; Statland et al., 1969; Robblee et al., 1973a) as well as calcium storage sites, and release of calcium from these storage sites occurs during the release reaction (see Holmsen et al., 1969). However, this release is the result of, rather than the cause of platelet activation, and the quantity of calcium released is so big that it could obscure the small changes which might initiate the activation. If the sequestered platelet calcium were equally distributed throughout the cell water, its concentration would be about 30 mM (assuming a platelet volume of 9.5 μm^3 and a calcium concentration of 2.7×10^{-6} mol/platelet; Lages et al., 1975); this is about 100,000-fold higher than the predicted resting cytoplasmic concentration.

During the release reaction induced by thrombin and other agents, platelets may take up radioactive calcium from the medium (Kinlough-Rathbone et al., 1974; Massini and Lüscher, 1974), possibly by exchange of calcium into the storage granules (which are exposed to the exterior during the release reaction), or alternatively by uptake into the expanded canalicular system. Precipitation of calcium by pyroantimonate in thrombin-treated platelets occurred not in the cytoplasm but associated with structures resembling altered granules (Robblee et al., 1973b), which suggests that the former explanation is correct. This calcium uptake does not appear to be necessary for the action of thrombin, since thrombin can induce release in the presence of EDTA.

Several different groups of workers have used the divalent metal ionophore A23187, which forms lipid–soluble complexes with calcium and magnesium, to investigate the effects of calcium ion movements within the platelet (Feinman and Detwiler, 1974; Yuen and Macey, 1974; Massini and Lüscher, 1974; White et al.,

1974; Mürer et al., 1975; Kinlough-Rathbone et al., 1975; Feinstein and Fraser, 1975). The results of these investigations may be summarized as follows. Low concentrations of the ionophore (e.g., 0.2 μM in washed platelets, 10 μM in plasma) induce platelet aggregation and the release reaction preceded by a shape change. Shape change and aggregation depend neither on release of granule contents nor on prostaglandin synthesis since they occur with degranulated platelets in the presence of aspirin (Kinlough-Rathbone et al., 1975). Release reaction is, however, partially inhibited by drugs that inhibit prostaglandin synthesis (White et al., 1974; Feinstein and Fraser, 1975), as well as by agents that increase cyclic AMP (Feinstein and Fraser, 1975).

Although the ionophore does induce the uptake of calcium from the medium (White et al., 1974; Massini and Lüscher, 1974; Mürer et al., 1975), this is not necessary for its action – shape change and release are only slightly reduced by calcium chelators. Platelets treated with the ionophore may lose about 60% of their magnesium; this is not, however, a result of the release reaction since magnesium is not released by thrombin (Feinstein and Fraser, 1975), and is not present in the releasable granules of human platelets (Skaer et al., 1976; Lages et al., 1975). Higher concentrations of the ionophore result in toxic effects on platelet metabolism and morphology (Mürer et al., 1975), which may in part be due to this magnesium loss.

Since the ionophore activates platelets in the presence of calcium chelators its effects cannot be explained by an increase in the permeability of the plasma membrane to calcium; indeed, such an action would deplete the cytoplasm of calcium and block calcium-mediated effects. Most authors have assumed that the effect of the ionophore is to mobilize calcium from internal stores to the cytoplasm and that this effect is more rapid than the depletion of calcium to the exterior, but no evidence is yet available to support this supposition directly.

The first suggestion that platelet reactions may be regulated by calcium movements was made by Grette (1962) and this has been echoed by many writers since. The recent use of calcium ionophores provides evidence which strongly suggests, but does not prove, that intracellular calcium ion movement does indeed regulate platelet function. Better methods of measuring cytoplasmic calcium ion concentrations are, however, required to show that calcium movements are responsible for the transmission of receptor-mediated effects.

References

Abdulla, Y.H. (1969) J. Atheroscler. Res., *9*, 171.
Abdulla, Y.H. and McFarlane, E. (1971) Biochem. Pharmacol., *20*, 1726.
Abrams, W.B. and Solomon, H.M. (1969) Clin. Pharmacol. Ther., *10*, 702.
Adelstein, R.S. and Conti, M.A. (1975) Nature, *256*, 597.
Adelstein, R.S., Conti, M.A., Daniel, J.L. and Anderson, W. (1975) in Biochemistry and Pharmacology of Platelets, Ciba Foundation Symposium 35 (New Series) Elsevier, Amsterdam.
Agarwal, R.P. and Parks, R.E. (1971) J. Biol. Chem., *246*, 2258.
Agarwal, K.C. and Parks, R.E. (1975) Biochem. Pharmacol., *24*, 2239.

Ahlquist, R.P. (1948) Am. J. Physiol., 153, 586.
Amer, M.S. and Marquis, N.R. (1972) in Prostaglandins in Cellular Biology (Ramwell, P.W. and Phariss, B.B., eds), p. 93, Plenum Press, N.Y.
Ardlie, N.G. and Han, P. (1974) Br. J. Haematol., 26, 331.
Ardlie, N.G., Glew, G. and Schwartz, C.J. (1966) Nature, 212, 415.
Ardlie, N.G., Glew, G., Schultz, B.G. and Schwartz, C.J. (1967) Thromb. Diath. Haemorrh., 18, 670.
Baenziger, N.L., Brodie, G.N. and Majerus, P.W. (1971) Proc. Nat. Acad. Sci. U.S.A., 68, 240.
Baenziger, N.L., Brodie, G.N. and Majerus, P.W. (1972) J. Biol. Chem., 247, 2723.
Ball, G., Brereton, G.G., Fulwood, M., Ireland, D.M. and Yates, P. (1970) Biochem. J., 120, 709.
Barber, A.J. and Jamieson, G.A. (1971) Biochemistry, 10, 4711.
Barthel, W. and Markwardt, F. (1974) Biochem. Pharmacol., 23, 37.
Barthel, W. and Markwardt, F. (1975) Biochem. Pharmacol., 24, 1903.
Baumgartner, H.R. (1969) J. Physiol., 201, 409.
Baumgartner, H.R. and Born, G.V.R. (1968) Nature, 218, 137.
Baumgartner, H.R. and Born, G.V.R. (1969) J. Physiol., 201, 397.
Behnke, O. (1968) J. Ultrast. Res., 24, 51.
Belamarich, F.A. and Simoneit, O.W. (1973) Microvasc. Res., 6, 229.
Besterman, E.M.M. and Gillett, M.P.T. (1973) Nature, 241, 223.
Bohme, E. and Jakobs, K.H. (1973) Int. Res. Commun. Sys., 1, 30.
Bohn, H. (1971) Blut, 22, 237.
Booyse, F.M., Hoveke, T.P., Zschocke, D. and Rafelson, M.E. (1971) J. Biol. Chem., 246, 4291.
Booyse, F.M., Hoveke, T.P., Kiesielski, D. and Rafelson, M.E. (1972) Microvasc. Res., 4, 199.
Booyse, F.M., Guiliani, D., Marr, J.J. and Rafelson, M.E. (1973) Ser. Haematol., 6, 351.
Booyse, F.M., Marr, J., Yang, D-C., Guiliani, D. and Rafelson, M.E. (1976) Biochim. Biophys. Acta, 422, 60.
Borisy, G.G., Olmsted, J.B., Marcum, J.M. and Allen, C. (1974) Fed. Proc., 33, 167.
Born, G.V.R. (1962) Nature, 194, 927.
Born, G.V.R. (1964) Nature, 202, 95.
Born, G.V.R. (1965) Nature, 206, 1121.
Born, G.V.R. (1967) J. Physiol., 190, 273.
Born, G.V.R. (1970) J. Physiol., 209, 487.
Born, G.V.R. and Bricknell, J. (1959) J. Physiol., 147, 153.
Born, G.V.R. and Cross, M.J. (1962) J. Physiol., 166, 29.
Born, G.V.R. and Cross, M.J. (1963) J. Physiol., 168, 178.
Born, G.V.R. and Feinberg, H. (1975) J. Physiol., 251, 803.
Born, G.V.R. and Gillson, R.E. (1959) J. Physiol., 148, 472.
Born, G.V.R. and Michal, F. (1975) in Biochemistry and Pharmacology of Platelets, Ciba Foundation Symposium 35 (New Series), p. 287, Elsevier, Amsterdam.
Born, G.V.R. and Mills, D.C.B. (1969) J. Physiol., 202, 41.
Born, G.V.R. and Smith, J.B. (1970) Br. J. Pharmacol., 39, 765.
Born, G.V.R., Haslam, R.J., Goldman, M. and Lowe, R.D. (1965) Nature, 205, 678.
Born, G.V.R., Juengjaroen, K. and Michal, F. (1972) Br. J. Pharmacol., 44, 117.
Boullin, D.J., Green, A.R. and Price, K.S. (1972) J. Physiol., 221, 415.
Brodie, G.N., Baenziger, N.L., Chase, L.R. and Majerus, P.W. (1972) J. Clin. Invest., 51, 81.
Bruno, J.J., Taylor, L.A. and Droller, M.J. (1974) Nature, 251, 721.
Bunag, R.D., Douglas, C.R., Imai, S. and Berne, R.M. (1964) Circ. Res., 15, 83.
Bygdeman, S. (1968) Acta Physiol. Scand., 73, 28.
Bygdeman, S. and Johnsen, Ø. (1969) Acta Physiol. Scand., 75, 129.
Castaldi, P.A. and Caen, J. (1965) J. Clin. Pathol., 18, 579.
Chambers, D.A., Salzman, E.W. and Neri, L.L. (1967) Arch. Biochem. Biophys., 119, 173.
Chuang, H.Y.K., Shermer, R.W. and Mason, R.G. (1974) Res. Commun. Chem. Pathol. Pharmacol., 7, 330.
Chung, S.I., Lewis, M.S. and Folk, J.E. (1974) J. Biol. Chem., 249, 940.
Clark, C.T., Weissbach, H. and Udenfriend, S. (1954) J. Biol. Chem., 210, 139.
Clayton, S. and Cross, M.J. (1963) J. Physiol., 169, 82.
Clayton, S., Born, G.V.R. and Cross, M.J. (1963) Nature, 200, 138.
Cohen, I., Bohak, Z., De Vries, A. and Katchalski, E. (1969) Eur. J. Biochem., 10, 388.
Cole, B., Robison, G.A. and Hartmann, R.C. (1971) Ann. N.Y. Acad. Sci., 185, 477.
Cole, E.R., Koppel, J.L. and Olwin, J.H. (1967) Nature, 213, 405.
Collier, H.O.J. and Roy, A.C. (1974) Nature, 248, 24.

Costa, J.L. and Murphy, D.L. (1975) Nature, *255*, 407.
Cuthbertson, W.F.J. and Mills, D.C.B. (1963) J. Physiol., *168*, 29.
Daniel, J.L., Holmsen, H. and Adelstein, R.S. (1976) Fed. Proc., *35*, 806 (Abstr.).
Da Prada, M. and Pletscher, A. (1970) Biochem. J., *119*, 117.
Da Prada, M., Bartholini, G. and Pletscher, A. (1965) Experientia, *21*, 135.
Da Prada, M., Tranzer, J.P. and Pletscher, A. (1967) J. Pharmacol. Exp. Ther., *158*, 394.
Da Prada, M., Burkhard, W.P. and Pletscher, A. (1972) Experientia, *28*, 845.
Davey, M.G. and Esnouf, M.P. (1969) Biochem. J., *111*, 733.
Davey, M.G. and Lüscher, E.F. (1965) Nature, *207*, 730.
Davey, M.G. and Lüscher, E.F. (1967) Nature, *216*, 857.
Davey, M.G. and Lüscher, E.F. (1968) Biochim. Biophys. Acta, *165*, 490.
Dawson, W., Lewis, R.L., McMahon, R.E. and Sweatman, W.J.F. (1974) Nature, *250*, 331.
Detwiler, T.C. (1972) Biochim. Biophys. Acta, *256*, 163.
Detwiler, T.C. and Feinman, R.D. (1973a) Biochemistry, *12*, 282.
Detwiler, T.C. and Feinman, R.D. (1973b) Biochemistry, *12*, 2462.
Doolittle, R.F., Takagi, T. and Cottrell, B.A. (1974) Science, *185*, 368.
Douglas, W.W. (1975) in The Pharmacological Basis of Therapeutics (Goodman, L.W. and Gilman, A., Eds), 5th edn, p. 613, Macmillan, New York.
Droller, M.J. (1974) Clin. Res., *22*, 103A.
Droller, M.J. and Wolfe, S.M. (1972) J. Clin. Invest., *51*, 3094.
Drummond, A.H. and Gordon, J.L. (1975) Biochem. J., *150*, 129.
Ehrenpreis, S., Greenberg, J. and Belman, S. (1973) Nature New Biol., *245*, 280.
Erspamer, V. and Asero, B. (1952) Nature, *169*, 800.
Feinman, R.D. and Detwiler, T.C. (1974) Nature, *249*, 172.
Feinstein, M.B. and Fraser, C. (1975) J. Gen. Physiol., *66*, 561.
Fenichel, R.L., Stokes, D.D. and Alburn, H.E. (1975) Nature, *253*, 537.
Friedman, F. and Detwiler, T.C. (1975) Biochemistry, *14*, 1315.
Gaarder, A. and Laland, S. (1964) Nature, *202*, 909.
Gaarder, A., Jonsen, J., Laland, S., Hellem, A. and Owren, P.A. (1961) Nature, *192*, 531.
Ganguly, P. (1969) Blood, *33*, 590.
Ganguly, P. (1971) J. Biol. Chem., *246*, 4286.
Ganguly, P. (1972) J. Biol. Chem., *247*, 1809.
Ganguly, P. (1974) Nature, *247*, 306.
Ganguly, P. and Moore, R. (1967) Clin. Chim. Acta, *17*, 153.
Gear, A.R.L. and Schneider, W. (1975) Biochim. Biophys. Acta, *392*, 111.
Glass, D.B., White, J.G., and Goldberg, N.D. (1974) Fed. Proc., *33*, 611 (Abstr).
Goldberg, N.D., Haddox, M.K., Nicol, S.E., Glass, D.B., Sanford, C.H., Kuehl, F.A. and Estensen, R. (1975) Adv. Cyclic Nucleotide Res., *5*, 307.
Gordon, J.L. and Drummond, A.H. (1975) Biochem. Pharmacol., *24*, 33.
Gorman, R.R. (1974) Prostaglandins, *6*, 542 (Abstr.).
Gough, G., Maguire, M.H. and Michal, F. (1969) J. Med. Chem., *12*, 494.
Gough, G., Maguire, M.H. and Penglis, F. (1972) Mol. Pharmacol., *8*, 170.
Grette, K. (1962) Acta Physiol. Scand., *56*, Suppl. 195.
Grette, K. (1963) Nature, *198*, 488.
Gröttum, K.A. (1968) Lancet, *1*, 1406.
Gröttum, K.A. and Solum, N.O. (1969) Br. J. Haematol., *16*, 277.
Gryglewski, R.J., Szczeklik, A. and Bieron, K. (1975) Nature, *256*, 56.
Guccione, M.A., Packham, M.A., Kinlough-Rathbone, R.L. and Mustard, J.F. (1971) Blood, *37*, 542.
Hamberg, M., Svensson, J., Wakabayashi, T. and Samuelsson, B. (1974a) Proc. Nat. Acad. Sci. U.S.A., *71*, 345.
Hamberg, M., Svensson, J. and Samuelsson, B. (1974b) Proc. Natl. Acad. Sci. U.S.A., *71*, 3824.
Hamberg, M., Svensson, J. and Samuelsson, B. (1975) Proc. Natl. Acad. Sci. U.S.A., *72*, 2994.
Hampton, J.R. and Mitchell, J.R.A. (1966a) Nature, *211*, 245.
Hampton, J.R. and Mitchell, J.R.A. (1966b) Nature, *210*, 1000.
Han, P. and Ardlie, N.G. (1974a) Br. J. Haematol., *26*, 357.
Han, P. and Ardlie, N.G. (1974b) Br. J. Haematol., *27*, 253.
Hanson, J.P., Repke, D.I., Katz, A.M. and Aledort, L.M. (1973) Biochim. Biophys. Acta, *314*, 382.
Harrison, M.J., Brossmer, R. and Goody, R.S. (1975) FEBS Lett., *54*, 57.
Haslam, R.J. (1964) Nature, *202*, 765.

198 | D.C.B. Mills and D.E. Macfarlane

Haslam, R.J. (1966) in Physiology of Hemostasis and Thrombosis (Johnson, S.A. and Seegers, W., eds), C.C. Thomas, Springfield, Ill.
Haslam, R.J. (1973) Ser. Haematol., 6, 333.
Haslam, R.J. (1975) in Biochemistry and Pharmacology of Platelets. Ciba Foundation Symposium 35 (New Series) p. 121, Elsevier, Amsterdam.
Haslam, R.J. and Lynham, J.A. (1972) Life Sci., 11, 1143.
Haslam, R.J. and McClenaghan, M.D. (1974) Biochem. J., 138, 317.
Haslam, R.J. and Rosson, G.M. (1972) Am. J. Physiol., 223, 958.
Haslam, R.J. and Rosson, G.M. (1975) Mol. Pharmacol., 11, 528.
Haslam, R.J. and Taylor, A. (1971a) Biochem. J., 125, 377.
Halsam, R.J. and Taylor, A. (1971b) in Platelet Aggregation (Caen, J., ed), p. 85, Masson et Cie, Paris.
Haslam, R.J., Davidson, M.M.L. and McClenaghan, M.D. (1975a) Nature, 253, 455.
Haslam, R.J., McClenaghan, M.D. and Adams, A. (1975b) in Advances in Cyclic Nucleotide Research 5 (Greengard, P. and Robison, G.A., eds), p. 281, Raven Press, New York.
Hellem, A.J. (1960) Scand. J. Clin. Lab. Invest., 12, Suppl., 51.
Heyssel, R.M. (1961) J. Clin. Invest., 40, 2134.
Heyssel, R.M., Silver, L.J., Wasson, M. and Brill, A.B. (1967) Blood, 29, 341.
Hidaka, H., Asano, T., Shibuya, M. and Shimamoto, T. (1974) Thromb. Diath. Haemorrh., Suppl., 60, 321.
Holmsen, H. (1972) Ann. N.Y. Acad. Sci., 201, 109.
Holmsen, H., Day, H.J. and Stormorken, H. (1969) Scand. J. Haematol., Suppl., 8, p. 1.
Holmsen, H. and Rozenberg, M.C. (1968) Biochim. Biophys. Acta, 155, 326.
Horák, H. and Barton, P.G. (1974) Biochim. Biophys. Acta, 373, 471.
Horlington, M. and Watson, P.A. (1970) Biochem. Pharmacol., 19, 955.
Horton, E.W. and Jones, R.L. (1974) Br. J. Pharmacol. 52, 110p.
Hughes, F.B. and Brodie, B.B. (1959) J. Pharmacol. Exp. Ther., 127, 96.
Ireland, D.M. and Mills, D.C.B. (1966) Biochem. J., 99, 283.
Jakobs, K.H., Böhme, E. and Mocikat, S. (1974) Naunyn-Schmiedeberg's Arch. Pharmacol., Suppl., 282, R40.
James, H.L., Bradford, H.R. and Ganguly, P. (1975) Biochim. Biophys. Acta, 386, 209.
Janeway, T.C., Richardson, H.B. and Park, E.A. (1918) Arch. Intern. Med., 21, 565.
Johnson, M. and Ramwell, P.W. (1973) Prostaglandins, 3, 703.
Johnson, M., Jessup, R. and Ramwell, P.W. (1974a) Prostaglandins, 5, 125.
Johnson, M., Jessup, R., Jessup, S. and Ramwell, P.W. (1974b) Prostaglandins, 6, 543.
Kaulen, H.D. and Gross, R. (1974) Hoppe-Seyler's Z. Physiol. Chem., 355, 471.
Keenan, J.P. and Solum, N.O. (1972) Br. J. Haematol., 23, 461.
Kien, M., Belamarich, F.A. and Shepro, D. (1971) Am. J. Physiol., 220, 604.
Kiesselbach, T.H. and Wagner, R.H. (1966) Am. J. Physiol., 211, 1472.
Kikugawa, K., Suehiro, H. and Ichino, M. (1973a) J. Med. Chem., 16, 1381.
Kikugawa, K., Suehiro, H. and Ichino, M. (1973b) J. Med. Chem., 16, 1389.
Kinlough-Rathbone, R.L., Packham, M.A. and Mustard, J.F. (1970) Br. J. Haematol., 19, 559.
Kinlough-Rathbone, R.L., Cahil, A. and Mustard, J.F. (1973) Am. J. Physiol., 224, 941.
Kinlough-Rathbone, R.L., Cahil, A. and Mustard, J.F. (1974) Am. J. Physiol., 226, 235.
Kinlough-Rathbone, R.L., Cahil, A., Packham, M.A., Reimers, H.-J. and Mustard, J.F. (1975) Thromb. Res., 7, 435.
Kirby, E.P. and Mills, D.C.B. (1975) J. Clin. Invest., 56, 491.
Kloeze, J. (1966) Proc. Nobel Symp. II. Prostaglandins (Bergstrom, S. and Samuelsson, B., eds).
Kloeze, J. (1969) Biochim. Biophys. Acta, 187, 285.
Krishna, G., Harwood, J.P., Barber, A.J. and Jamieson, G.A. (1972) J. Biol. Chem., 247, 2253.
Kuo, J.F. and Greengard, P. (1969) Proc. Natl. Acad. Sci., 64, 1349.
Lages, B., Scrutton, M.C., Holmsen, H., Day, H.J. and Weiss, H.J. (1975) Blood, 46, 119.
Lemmer, B., Wiethold, G., Hellenbrecht, D., Bak, I.J. and Grobecker, H. (1972) Naunyn-Schmiedebergs Arch. Pharmacol., 275, 299.
Lienhard, G.E. and Secemski, I.I. (1973) J. Biol. Chem., 248, 1121.
Lingjaerde, O. (1969) FEBS Lett., 3, 103.
Lingjaerde, O. (1971a) Acta Physiol. Scand., 81, 75.
Lingjaerde, O. (1971b) Acta Physiol. Scand., 83, 257.
Lingjaerde, O. (1971c) Acta Physiol. Scand., 83, 309.
Lloyd, J.V., Nishizawa, E.E., Haldar, J. and Mustard, J.F. (1972) Br. J. Haematol., 23, 571.
Lloyd, J.V., Nishizawa, E.E. and Mustard, J.F. (1973) Br. J. Haematol., 25, 77.
Lyons, R.M., Stanford, N. and Majerus, P.W. (1975) J. Clin. Invest., 56, 924.

Macfarlane, D.E. (1975) Thesis, University of London.
Macfarlane, D.E. and Mills, D.C.B. (1975) Blood, *46*, 309.
Macfarlane, D.E., Smith, J.B., Mills, D.C.B. and Silver, M.J. (1975a) Blood, *44*, 947 (Abstr.).
Macfarlane, D.E., Walsh, P.N., Mills, D.C.B., Holmsen, H. and Day, H.J. (1975b) Br. J. Haematol., *30*, 457.
MacIntyre, D.E. and Gordon, J.L. (1975a) Biochem. Soc. Trans., *2*, 1265.
MacIntyre, D.E. and Gordon, J.L. (1975b) Nature, *258*, 337.
MacMillan, D.C. (1966) Nature, *211*, 140.
Maguire, M.H. and Michal, F. (1968) Nature, *217*, 571.
Marcus, A.J. and Zucker, M.B. (1965) The Physiology of Blood Platelets. Grune and Stratton, N.Y.
Marcus, A.J., Zucker-Franklin, D., Safier, L.B. and Ullman, H.L. (1966) J. Clin. Invest., *45*, 14.
Marcus, A.J., Safier, L.B. and Ullman, H.L. (1975) in Biochemistry and Pharmacology of Platelets. Ciba Foundation Symposium 35 (New Series), p. 309, Elsevier, Amsterdam.
Markwardt, F., Barthel, W., Glusa, E. and Hoffman, A. (1967) Naunyn-Schmiedeberg's Arch. Pharmak. Exp. Pathol., *257*, 420.
Marquis, N.R., Becker, J.A. and Vigdahl, R.L. (1970) Biochem. Biophys. Res. Comm., *39*, 783.
Marquis, N.R., Vigdahl, R.L. and Tavormina, P.A. (1971) Fed. Proc., *30*, 423 (Abstr.).
Martin, B.M., Feinman, R.D. and Detwiler, T.C. (1975) Biochemistry, *14*, 1308.
Mason, R.G. and Saba, S.R. (1969) Am. J. Pathol., *55*, 215.
Massini, P. and Lüscher, E.F. (1974) Biochim. Biophys. Acta, *372*, 109.
McDonagh, J., McDonagh, R.P., Delâge, J.M. and Wagner, R.H. (1969a) J. Clin. Invest., *48*, 940.
McDonald, J.W.D. and Stuart, R.K. (1973) J. Lab. Clin. Med., *81*, 838.
McDonald, J.W.D. and Stuart, R.K. (1974) J. Lab. Clin. Med., *84*, 111.
Mester, L., Szabados, L., Born, G.V.R. and Michal, F. (1972) Nature New Biol., *236*, 213.
Michal, F. (1969) Nature, *221*, 1253.
Michal, F. (1974) in Platelet Aggregation and Drugs (Caprino, L. and Rossi, E.C., eds), p. 185, Academic Press, London.
Michal, F. and Born, G.V.R. (1971) Nature New Biol., *231*, 220.
Michal, F. and Penglis, F. (1969) J. Pharmacol. Exp. Ther., *166*, 276.
Michal, F. and Thorp, R.H. (1966) Nature, *209*, 208.
Michal, F., Maguire, M.H. and Gough, G. (1969) Nature, *222*, 1073.
Michal, F., Born, G.V.R., Mester, L. and Szabados, L. (1972) Biochem. J., *129*, 977.
Mills, D.C.B. (1970) Symp. Zool. Soc. London, *27*, 99.
Mills, D.C.B. (1972) Circulation, *46*, 33.
Mills, D.C.B. (1973) Nature New Biol., *243*, 220.
Mills, D.C.B. (1974) in Platelets and Thrombosis (Sherry, S. and Scriabine, A., eds), p. 46, University Park Press, Baltimore.
Mills, D.C.B. (1975) in Biochemistry and Pharmacology of Platelets. Ciba Foundation Symposium 35 (New Series) p. 153, Elsevier, Amsterdam.
Mills, D.C.B. and Macfarlane, D.E. (1974) Thromb. Res., *5*, 401.
Mills, D.C.B. and Roberts, G.C.K. (1967a) Nature, *213*, 35.
Mills, D.C.B. and Roberts, G.C.K. (1967b) J. Physiol., *193*, 443.
Mills, D.C.B. and Smith, J.B. (1971) Biochem. J., *121*, 185.
Mills, D.C.B. and Smith, J.B. (1972) Ann. N.Y. Acad. Sci., *201*, 391.
Mills, D.C.B., Robb, I.A. and Roberts, G.C.K. (1968) J. Physiol., *195*, 715.
Mills, D.C.B., Smith, J.B. and Born, G.V.R. (1970) in Platelet Adhesion and Aggregation in Thrombosis: Countermeasures (Mammen, E.F., Anderson, G.F. and Barnhardt, M.I., eds), p. 175, Schattauer-Verlag, Stuttgart.
Mitchell, J.R.A. and Sharp, A.A. (1964) Br. J. Haematol., *10*, 78.
Moake, J.L., Ahmed, K., Bachur, N.R. and Gutfreund, D.E. (1970a) Biochim. Biophys. Acta, *211*, 337.
Moake, J.L., Ahmed, K. and Bachur, N.R. (1970b) Biochim. Biophys. Acta, *219*, 484.
Morse, E.E., Jackson, D.P. and Conley, C.L. (1965) J. Clin. Invest., *44*, 809.
Moskowitz, J., Harwood, J.P., Reid, W.D. and Krishna, G. (1971) Biochim. Biophys. Acta, *230*, 279.
Mourad, N. and Parks, R.E. (1966) J. Biol. Chem., *241*, 271.
Mürer, E.H. (1971) Biochim. Biophys. Acta, *237*, 310.
Mürer, E.H., Stewart, G.J., Rausch, M.A. and Day, H.J. (1975) Thromb. Diath. Haemorrh., *34*, 72.
Mustard, J.F., Perry, D.W., Kinlough-Rathbone, R.L. and Packham, M.A. (1975a) Am. J. Physiol., *228*, 1757.
Mustard, J.F., Perry, D.W., Guccione, M.A. and Kinlough-Rathbone, R.L. (1975b) in Biochemistry and Pharmacology of Platelets, Ciba Foundation Symposium 35 (New Series), p. 47, Elsevier, Amsterdam.

Nachman, R.L. (1968) Semin. Hematol., 5, 18.
Nachman, R.L. (1975) in Biochemistry and Pharmacology of Platelets, Ciba Foundation Symposium 35 (New Series) p. 23, Elsevier, Amsterdam.
Nachman, R.L. and Ferris, B. (1970) Biochemistry, 9, 200.
Nachman, R.L. and Ferris, B. (1972) J. Biol. Chem., 247, 4468.
Nachman, R.L. and Ferris, B. (1974) J. Biol. Chem., 249, 704.
Nachman, R.L. and Jaffe, E.A. (1975) J. Exp. Med., 141, 1101.
Nachman, R.L., Marcus, A.J. and Safier (1967a) J. Clin. Invest., 42, 1380.
Nachman, R.L., Marcus, A.J. and Zucker-Franklin, D. (1967b) J. Lab. Clin. Med. 66, 651.
Nachman, R.L., Hubbard, A. and Ferris, B. (1973) J. Biol. Chem., 248, 2928.
Niewiarowski, S. (1974) in Platelets and Thrombosis (Sherry, S. and Scriabine, A., eds), University Park Press.
Niewiarowski, S. and Thomas, D.P. (1966) Nature, 212, 1544.
Nishizawa, E.E., Miller, W.L., Gorman, R.R. and Bundy, G.L. (1975) Prostaglandins, 9, 109.
Nurden, A.T. and Caen, J.P. (1974) Br. J. Haematol., 28, 253.
Nurden, A.T. and Caen, J.P. (1975) Nature, 255, 720.
O'Brien, J.R. (1962) J. Clin. Pathol., 15, 452.
O'Brien, J.R. (1964) J. Clin. Pathol., 17, 275.
Oelz, O., Oelz, R., Knapp, H.R., Sweetman, B.J. and Oates, J.A. (1976) Clin. Res., 24, 17A.
Øllgaard, E. (1961) Thromb. Diath. Haemorrh., 6, 86.
Packham, M.A., Ardlie, N.G. and Mustard, J.F. (1969) Am. J. Physiol., 217, 1009.
Packham, M.A., Guccione, M.A., Perry, D.W., Kinlough-Rathbone, R.L. and Mustard, J.F. (1972) Am. J. Physiol., 223, 419.
Packham, M.A., Guccione, M.A., Chang, P.-L. and Mustard, J.F. (1973) Am. J. Physiol., 225, 38.
Packham, M.A., Guccione, M.A., Perry, D.W. and Mustard, J.F. (1974) Am. J. Physiol., 227, 1143.
Pareti, F.I., Day, H.J. and Mills, D.C.B. (1974) Blood, 44, 789.
Pepper, D.S. and Jamieson, G.A. (1970) Biochemistry, 9, 3706.
Phillips, D.R. (1972) Biochemistry, 11, 4582.
Phillips, D.R. (1974) Thromb. Diath. Haemorrh., 32, 207.
Phillips, D.R. and Agin, P.P. (1973) Ser. Haematol., 6, 292.
Phillips, D.R. and Agin, P.P. (1974) Biochim. Biophys. Acta, 352, 218.
Philp, R.B., Francey, I. and McElroy, F. (1973) Thromb. Res., 3, 35.
Pichard, A-L., Hanoune, J. and Kaplan, J-C. (1972) Biochim. Biophys. Acta, 279, 217.
Pletscher, A. (1968) Br. J. Pharmacol., 32, 1.
Rand, M.J. and Reid, G. (1951) Nature, 168, 385.
Rang, H.P. (1973) Drug Receptors: A Symposium. MacMillan, London.
Rapport, M.M., Green, A.A. and Page, I.H. (1948) J. Biol. Chem., 176, 1243.
Robblee, L.S., Shepro, D. and Belamarich, F.A. (1973a) J. Gen. Physiol., 61, 462.
Robblee, L.S., Shepro, D., Belamarich, F.A. and Towle, C. (1973b) Ser. Haematol., 6, 311.
Robinson, C.W., Kress, S.L., Wagner, R.H. and Brinkhous, K.M. (1965) Exp. Mol. Pathol., 4, 457.
Robison, G.A., Arnold, A. and Hartmann, R.C. (1969) Pharmacol. Res. Commun., 1, 325.
Robison, G.A., Butcher, R.W. and Sutherland, E.W. (1971) Cyclic AMP, Academic Press, New York.
Rozenberg, M.C. and Holmsen, H. (1968) Biochim. Biophys. Acta, 155, 342.
Rozenberg, M.C. and Walker, C.M. (1973) Br. J. Haematol., 24, 409.
Salmon, J. and Bounameaux, Y. (1952) Thromb. Diath. Haemorrh., 2, 93.
Salzman, E.W. (1972) N. Engl. J. Med., 286, 358.
Salzman, E.W. (1976) Advances in Prostaglandin and Thromboxane Research (Samuelsson, B. and Paoletti, R., eds), Vol. 2, p. 767, Raven Press, New York.
Salzman, E.W. and Neri, L.L. (1969) Nature, 224, 609.
Salzman, E.W. and Levine, L. (1971) J. Clin. Invest., 50, 131.
Salzman, E.W., Chambers, D.A. and Neri, L.L. (1966a) Thromb. Diath. Haemorrh., 15, 52.
Salzman, E.W., Chambers, D.A. and Neri, L.L. (1966b) Nature, 210, 167.
Salzman, E.W., Ashford, T.P., Chambers, D.A., Neri, L.L. and Dempster, A.P. (1969) Am. J. Physiol., 217, 1330.
Salzman, E.W., Kensler, P.C. and Levine, L. (1972) Ann. N.Y. Acad. Sci., 201, 61.
Sano, I., Kakimoto, Y. and Taniguchi, K. (1958) Am. J. Physiol., 195, 495.
Sano, I., Kakimoto, Y., Taniguchi, K. and Takesada, M. (1959) Am. J. Physiol., 197, 81.
Schmid, H.J., Jackson, D.P. and Conley, C.L. (1962) J. Clin. Invest., 41, 543.
Seaman, G.V.F. and Vassar, P.S. (1966) Arch. Biochem. Biophys., 117, 10.
Seegers, W.H., Diekamp, U. and McCoy, L.E. (1970) Thromb. Diath. Haemorrh. Suppl., 42, 115.

Shermer, R.W. and Chuang, H.Y. (1973) Fed. Proc., *32*, 844 (Abstr.).
Shio, H. and Ramwell, P. (1972) Nature New Biol., *236*, 45.
Shio, H., Plasse, A.M. and Ramwell, P.W. (1970) Microvasc. Res., *2*, 294.
Shio, H., Ramwell, P.W. and Jessup, S.J. (1972) Prostaglandins, *1*, 29.
Shuman, M.A. and Majerus, P.W. (1975) J. Clin. Invest., *56*, 945.
Skaer, R.J., Peters, P.D. and Emmines, J.P. (1976) J. Cell Sci., *20*, 441.
Skålhegg, B.A., Hellem, A.J. and Ödegaard, A.E. (1964) Thromb. Diath. Haemorrh., *11*, 305.
Skoza, L., Zucker, M.B., Jerushalmy, Z. and Grant, R. (1967) Thromb. Diath. Haemorrh., *18*, 713.
Smith, J.B. and Macfarlane, D.E. (1974) in The Prostaglandins (Ramwell, P.W., ed), Vol. 2, p. 293,
    Plenum Press, New York.
Smith, J.B. and Mills, D.C.B. (1970) Biochem. J., *120*, 20P.
Smith, J.B. and Silver, M.J. (1977) This volume.
Smith, J.B. and Willis, A.L. (1970) Br. J. Pharmacol., *40*, 545P.
Smith, J.B. and Willis, A.L. (1971) Nature New Biol., *231*, 235.
Smith, J.B., Ingerman, C., Kocsis, J.J. and Silver, M.J. (1973) J. Clin. Invest., *52*, 965.
Smith, J.B., Silver, M.J., Ingerman, C.M. and Kocsis, J.J. (1974) Thromb. Res., *5*, 291.
Smith, J.B., Ingerman, C.M. and Silver, M.J. (1975a) in Biochemistry and Pharmacology of Platelets.
    Ciba Foundation symposium 35 (New Series), p. 207, Elsevier, Amsterdam.
Sneddon, J.M. (1969) Br. J. Pharmacol., *37*, 680.
Sneddon, J.M. (1971) Br. J. Pharmacol., *43*, 834.
Sneddon, J.M. and Williams, K.I. (1973) J. Physiol., *235*, 625.
Spaet, T.H. and Lejnieks, I. (1966) Thromb. Diath. Haemorrh., *15*, 36.
Stacey, R.S. (1961) Br. J. Pharmacol., *16*, 284.
Statland, B.E., Heagan, B.M. and White, J.G. (1969) Nature, *223*, 521.
Steiner, M. (1975) Arch. Biochem. Biophys., *171*, 245.
Szabados, L., Mester, L., Michal, F. and Born, G.V.R. (1975) Biochem. J., *148*, 335.
Tangen, O., Wik, O.K. and Berman, H.J. (1973) Microvasc. Res., *6*, 342.
Thomas, D.P. (1967) Nature, *215*, 298.
Tollefsen, D.M. and Majerus, P.W. (1975) J. Clin. Invest., *55*, 1259.
Tollefsen, D.M., Feagler, J.R. and Majerus, P.W. (1974) J. Biol. Chem., *249*, 2646.
Tollefsen, D.M., Jackson, C.M. and Majerus, P.W. (1975) J. Clin. Invest., *56*, 241.
Tschopp, T.B. (1969) Thromb. Diath. Haemorrh., *23*, 601.
Tuomisto, J. (1974) J. Pharm. Pharmacol., *26*, 92.
Unger, W.G. (1972) J. Pharm. Pharmacol., *24*, 470.
Van Dorp, D. (1971) Ann. N.Y. Acad. Sci., *180*, 181.
Vigdahl, R.L., Mongin, J. and Marquis, N.R. (1971) Biochem. Biophys. Res. Commun., *42*, 1088.
Walsh, P.N. (1974) Blood, *43*, 597.
Walsh, P.N., Mills, D.C.B., Pareti, F.I., Stewart, G.J., Macfarlane, D.E., Johnson, M.M. and Egan, J.J.
    (1975) Br. J. Haematol., *29*, 639.
Ware, A.G., Fahey, J.L. and Seegers, W.H. (1948) Am. J. Physiol., *154*, 148.
Weisenberg, R.C. (1972) Science, *177*, 1104.
Weisenberger, H. (1973) in Erythrocytes, Thrombocytes, Leukocytes (Gerlach, E., Moser, K.,
    Deutsch, E. and Wilmans, W., eds), p. 327, Georg Thieme, Stuttgart.
Weiss, H.J., Tschopp, T.B., Baumgartner, H.R., Sussman, I.I., Johnson, M.M. and Egan, J.J. (1974)
    Am. J. Med., *57*, 920.
White, J.G. (1968) Blood, *31*, 604.
White, J.G. (1969) Blood, *33*, 598.
White, J.G. (1970) Scand. J. Haematol., *7*, 145.
White, J.G., Goldberg, N.D., Estensen, R.D., Haddox, M.K. and Rao, G.H.R. (1973) J. Clin. Invest., *52*,
    89a.
White, J.G., Rao, G.H.R. and Gerrard, J.M. (1974) Am. J. Pathol., *77*, 135.
Willis, A.L. (1974) Prostanglandins, *5*, 1.
Wolfe, S.M. and Shulman, N.R. (1970) Biochem. Biophys. Res. Commun., *41*, 128.
Wooley, D.W. and Gommi, B.W. (1964) Nature, *202*, 1074.
Wooley, D.W. and Gommi, B.W. (1965) Proc. Natl. Acad. Sci. U.S.A., *53*, 959.
Yuen, M. and Macey, R. (1974) Fed. Proc., *33*, 269 (Abstr.).
Zieve, P.D. and Greenough, W.B. (1969) Biochem. Biophys. Res. Commun., *35*, 462.
Zucker, M.B. (1962) in Progress in Hematology (Tocantins, L.M., ed), Vol. 2, p. 206, Grune and
    Stratton, New York.
Zucker, M.B. and Jerushalmy, Z. (1967) in Physiology of Haemostatis and Thrombosis (Johnson, S.A.
    and Seegers, W.H., eds), p. 249, C.C. Thomas, Springfield, Ill.

Notes added in proof

(1) Detwiler and Feinman (1973a,b) have developed methods for continuously monitoring the release of calcium and of ATP from washed platelets stimulated by thrombin or other proteases. The kinetics of calcium release were divided into 3 phases; a lag phase (≥ 10 sec), a logarithmic phase and a slow linear phase. Slightly different kinetics were seen for ATP release, which displayed a longer lag phase. Maximal rate of release of calcium occured with about 20,000 molecules of thrombin per platelet, though this figure was not independent of the platelet count. A model was proposed to account for the observed kinetics (Martin et al. 1975) of thrombin, trypsin and papain, involving reversible binding of thrombin to a receptor and reversible catalytic modification of the thrombin–receptor complex leading to platelet activation and release. Inevitably this model depends upon several assumptions, e.g. that all platelets respond equally, and that such known interactions as the potentiation of thrombin by released ADP (Packham et al. 1973) are immaterial.

(2) The number of binding sites was first estimated by Detwiler and Feinman (1973a) who found saturation at 2×10^4 molecules of the thrombin per platelet.

CHAPTER 8

Interactions of blood platelets with biogenic amines: uptake, stimulation and receptor binding

A.H. DRUMMOND

Department of Pathology, University of Cambridge, Tennis Court Road,
Cambridge, CB2, 1QP, England

1. Introduction

One of the most important problems facing the biochemical pharmacologist is the elucidation of the molecular events which accompany and follow the interaction of a drug or hormone with its cellular receptor. The understanding of the mechanisms responsible for the resultant cell activation and the termination of this event is greatly facilitated by the use of a homogeneous cell suspension. The blood platelet provides an example of such a system, and the aim of this chapter is to outline how the platelet can be applied to the study of biogenic amine-related reactions at the molecular level.

Platelets from all mammalian species so far studied contain variable amounts of 5-hydroxytryptamine (5HT, serotonin) (see Table 1). Catecholamines are also found in blood platelets, although their content is relatively (Born et al., 1958). There is some conjecture over the ability of platelets to synthesise 5HT: early work suggested that platelets lacked the necessary enzymes (Zucker and Borelli, 1958), but in recent years a number of investigators, using more sensitive techniques, have reported low activity of these enzymes in platelets (Lovenberg et al., 1968; Marmaras and Mimikos, 1971). In any case, the bulk of platelet 5HT originates in the enterochromaffin cells of the gastro-intestinal tract (see Erspamer, 1954). After release from these cells into the bloodstream, 5HT is taken up into platelets by an active transport system (see Section 2). Platelets possess monoamine oxidase (Paasonen, 1965), although under normal conditions the amount of 5HT which is degraded to its more acidic metabolites (5-hydroxyindoleacetic acid and 5-hydroxytryptophol) is relatively small (see Pletscher, 1968). Platelet 5HT is not exposed to the action of monoamine oxidase because the amine is localised in dense storage granules (Tranzer et al., 1966).

Blood platelets are stimulated by 5HT and catecholamines to undergo a series of reactions which are readily quantified by measuring continuously the optical density of anticoagulated platelet-rich plasma (PRP), stirred at 37°C in the presence of the stimulatory agent. When the spectrophotometric output is

Gordon (ed) Platelets in Biology and Pathology
© *Elsevier/North-Holland Biomedical Press, 1976*

TABLE 1
Platelet 5HT content in different animal species

Species	Content ($\mu g/10^9$ cells)
Rabbit	11.2[b]
Cow	5.0[a]
Pig	3.6[b]
Dog	1.7[a]
Rat	1.1[b]
Cat	0.9[a]
Man	0.5[b]
Guinea pig	0.35[b]

[a] Markwardt (1968)
[b] Drummond and Gordon (unpublished)

examined kinetically it reveals a number of features which can be correlated with a series of discrete alterations in platelet morphology (Born, 1962; O'Brien, 1962). The addition of micromolar 5HT concentrations to citrated human PRP results in a transient increase in optical density within approximately 1–3 sec (Fig. 1). The morphological basis for this phenomenon is a change in the shape of individual platelets from biconvex discs to spheres. Associated with this transformation is the centralisation of subcellular granules and the protrusion of spiky processes on the platelet surface (see White, 1974). The platelet shape change can be studied by a light-scattering technique (Michal and Born, 1971) or, more commonly, by adding 5 mM EDTA to the photometer cuvette: in the presence of EDTA, platelet

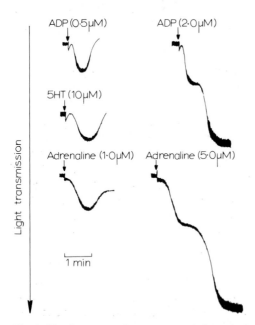

Fig. 1. Platelet aggregation responses in human citrated PRP.

aggregation does not occur. This assay is the most sensitive measure of platelet stimulation, since the cell will respond to approximately 0.1 μM 5HT or 10 nM ADP. Under normal conditions, the transient increase in optical density of the system is rapidly superseded by an increase in light transmission which is associated with the adhesion of platelets to each other; this is the process of platelet aggregation. With low concentrations of aggregating agents such as 5HT or ADP, aggregation is reversible, and a return to the basal optical density of the system is generally observed within 1–2 min; such a response is termed 'primary aggregation'. Aggregation does not readily reverse with higher ADP concentrations or with adrenaline and noradrenaline (Fig. 1), and a second increase in light transmission is often observed; this is termed 'secondary aggregation'. This latter response is associated with the selective extrusion of platelet granular constituents such as 5HT and adenine nucleotides (Mills et al., 1968) in a process known as the platelet release reaction. There are many similarities between this event and the exocytotic release processes found in other tissues such as nerve endings (Holmsen et al., 1969), and this aspect is reviewed in detail by D.E. MacIntyre in chapter 3.

Since the reader may be unfamiliar with the reactions of blood platelets, experimental variables which can affect these responses (e.g., species differences, choice of anticoagulant and calcium availability) are briefly discussed, but the main function of this review is to outline the scope of biogenic amine-platelet interactions and to emphasize their similarities with those found in other, more complex, tissues. This review does not deal comprehensively with other aspects of platelet physiology, biochemistry and pharmacology and the interested reader is referred to the following review articles: Mustard and Packham, 1970; Holmsen, 1972; Smith and Macfarlane, 1974; Weiss, 1975a,b; Mustard, 1975.

2. Uptake and storage of biogenic amines by blood platelets

Blood platelets accumulate the biogenic amines, 5HT (Humphrey and Toh, 1954; Hardisty and Stacey, 1955), adrenaline (Born et al., 1958; Sano et al., 1958) noradrenaline (Weissbach and Redfield, 1960) and dopamine (Boullin and O'Brien, 1970) against a concentration gradient at 37°C. This property and the ability of platelets to release selectively the accumulated amines have led to the proposal that blood platelets are convenient model cells for the study of various aspects of synaptic physiology and pharmacology (Paasonen 1965, 1968; Pletscher, 1968; Born, 1969; Pletscher et al., 1971). This proposal has been critically examined in an excellent review by Sneddon (1973), and readers are referred to this article for a detailed analysis of early platelet literature on the subject, as well as a discussion on the possible relationship between CNS and platelet biogenic amine-related defects. The following section briefly reviews the uptake and storage of biogenic amines by blood platelets, with particular reference to methodological considerations and to work published after 1972.

2.1. Experimental considerations

Sneddon (1973) and Tuomisto (1974) have recognized that the bulk of the early work on the uptake of biogenic amines by platelets cannot be readily compared with corresponding studies in other tissues because of the qualitative nature of the platelet work. The main criticism of this work is that the experimental conditions chosen made it impossible to measure initial uptake velocities. There are several reasons why failure to measure initial rates of uptake can lead to serious problems. The 5HT uptake system of blood platelets is not a simple process, but probably involves at least three steps; transport through the platelet plasma membrane, transport through the storage granule membrane and the formation of high molecular weight complexes with adenine nucleotides and divalent cations inside the storage granule (see Pletscher, 1968). Equilibrium studies of uptake (i.e., after long incubation periods) measure the net contribution of all three processes and consequently under those conditions inhibition of uptake by drugs or decreased uptake into defective platelets could be due to an effect on any of these steps. Investigations into the nature of the uptake process at the plasma membrane must be conducted under conditions in which it is possible to approach the measurement of initial rates of uptake. By way of an example, the uptake of 5HT by rat blood platelets should be measured over an incubation period no longer than 10 sec in order to fulfil the above criterion (Drummond and Gordon, 1976), and even under those conditions there is no justification for assuming that the measured uptake represents solely the uptake through the plasma membrane. Another problem related to the use of lengthy incubation periods is that drug potency can be severely underestimated. Buczko et al. (1975) studied the effect of chlorimipramine on the uptake of 5HT by rat blood platelets and concluded that the concentration of this drug that inhibited uptake by 50% (the IC_{50} value) was approximately 3 μM. This value was calculated on the basis of a 15 min uptake time, although in the same paper it was shown that using a 1 min uptake time, 3 μM chlorimipramine inhibited 5HT uptake by approximately 98%.

Even if the conditions chosen make it possible to apparently measure initial rates of uptake, it is important to consider the possibility that the drug under study may release endogenous 5HT. If an agent induces exocytosis of 5HT, this will result in an apparent competitive inhibition of uptake, whereas an agent such as reserpine which induces release from the storage granule into the platelet cytoplasm, will cause an apparent non-competitive inhibition of uptake. The recent discovery by Heikkila et al. (1975) that inhibition of neostriatal dopamine uptake by tricyclic antidepressants is entirely related to the releasing action of these drugs, serves to emphasise the importance of this point.

An important consideration with regard to the use of platelets in uptake studies is the medium in which the platelets are suspended. Sneddon (1973) has argued that experiments carried out in buffered artificial media may be more valid than studies in which the platelets are suspended in plasma, because plasma pH is difficult to control and may rise during the course of the experiment with a concomitant decrease in 5HT uptake (Stacey, 1961). He also points out that experiments conducted in PRP can be complicated by the adsorption of drugs to plasma proteins, leading to an underestimation of inhibitor potency. While these criticisms are certainly valid, it is equally true that it is extremely difficult to prepare platelets suspended in artificial media which have not undergone some morphological or biochemical change during the separation process. This is especially true if the medium lacks albumin and an agent (e.g., apyrase) to protect the platelets from the effects of ADP released during the washing procedure (Mustard et al., 1972; Doery et al., 1973; Mason et al., 1974; Zucker et al., 1974). In the absence of small amounts of albumin, slow release of platelet adenine nucleotides and 5HT may occur during the experiment (Doery et al., 1973; Tangen et al., 1973); such an effect would complicate the analysis of kinetic data on 5HT uptake. The importance of including apyrase in the final medium is emphasised by the recent finding that ADP is a powerful non-competitive inhibitor of 5HT uptake by rat platelets (Drummond and Gordon, 1976). If it is essential to conduct uptake studies in the absence of most plasma components, then the methods of Mustard et al. (1972), Walsh (1972) and Tangen et al. (1971) as modified by Lages et al. (1975) may be the best presently available in that results obtained with these methods appear to parallel closely the situation which prevails in PRP.

However it must be remembered that under those conditions drugs, e.g., tricyclic antidepressants will be more potent than in PRP because of the absence of most of the plasma proteins (Borga et al., 1969). It is also likely that the K_m for the 5HT transport system will be less in washed platelet suspensions than in plasma, since 5HT may also bind to plasma proteins under physiological conditions (Pignatti and Cavalli-Sforza, 1975).

2.2. Catecholamine uptake by blood platelets

2.2.1. Uptake at the plasma membrane

Although it has been known for around fifteen years that blood platelets can accumulate various catecholamines by a process which is sensitive to temperature and to metabolic inhibitors, it is still unclear whether or not an active transport system contributes to the uptake (see Sneddon, 1973). For adrenaline, noradrenaline and metaraminol, there is now mounting evidence that uptake is not a readily saturable process at physiological pH values and therefore it would appear that the system does not closely resemble that found in the adrenegic neurone (Born and Smith, 1970; Abrams and Solomon, 1969; Maclean and Potoczak, 1969; Ahtee and Saarnivaara, 1971, 1973). However there is also evidence that imipramine, desmethylimipramine and protriptyline inhibit metaraminol uptake by human platelets and that the secondary amines protriptyline and desmethylimipramine are 15–30 times more potent in this respect than the tertiary amine, imipramine (Ahtee and Saarnivaara, 1971). Although the concentrations used in the platelet study were relatively high, this latter finding is consistent with results from studies on noradrenaline uptake into peripheral or central neurones (Iversen, 1967; Carlsson et al., 1969b).

It is possible, therefore, that blood platelets contain a relatively low affinity transport system for noradrenaline, adrenaline and metaraminol, although it should be stressed that no study reported so far has attempted to investigate the kinetics of the uptake process in detail.

Another important point which remains to be resolved is whether or not the transport of these catecholamines and 5HT is mediated by a common transport carrier: it is known that noradrenaline and 5HT can utilise the same carrier for transport in the CNS (Shaskan and Snyder, 1970) and in the choroid plexus (Tochino and Shankar, 1965). Two criteria which are useful in establishing the existence of separate carriers are the sensitivity of the two uptake processes to drugs and the Na^+-dependence of the transport mechanism. Few studies have attempted to differentiate between the uptake of catecholamines and 5HT by means of drugs. Ahtee and Saarnivaara (1971) reported that the inhibitory potencies of a range of tricyclic antidepressants against metaraminol uptake did not parallel their activity against 5HT uptake; imipramine was much more active at inhibiting 5HT uptake than metaraminol uptake and in contrast, protriptyline was slightly more active against metaraminol uptake. These results, which are similar to those reported for CNS uptake systems (Carlsson et al., 1969a; Carlsson et al., 1969b), would suggest that discrete carriers exist for catecholamines and 5HT in blood platelets; however, it remains to be seen whether these results can be substantiated in studies with the recently-developed, more selective inhibitors such as Lilly 110140 (Wong et al., 1974) and FG 4963 (Buus Lassen et al., 1975). Recently Bruinvels (1975) has studied the uptake of radiolabelled 5HT, noradrenaline and dopamine by a synaptosomal preparation and has shown that by reducing the Na^+ content of the medium to 25 mM, uptake of dopamine and noradrenaline can be almost completely abolished, while 5HT uptake remains normal. Experiments of this type should be useful in determining whether or not 5HT and catecholamines share an identical carrier mechanism in platelets.

In contrast to the other catecholamines, there is reasonable support for the hypothesis that dopamine accumulates in blood platelets by a saturable energy-dependent process (Boullin and O'Brien, 1970; Solomon et al., 1970; Trenchard et al., 1975). Dopamine transport by platelets occurs against a concentration gradient and can reach accumulation ratios as high as 120 (Boullin and O'Brien, 1970). In his review, Sneddon (1973) suggested that platelets do not possess a selective dopamine carrier mechanism and that the amine utilises the platelet 5HT carrier. However the recent finding by Trenchard et al. (1975) that concentrations of chlorimipramine which completely abolish 5HT uptake by platelets have no marked effect on platelet dopamine transport suggests that Sneddon's conclusion may have been premature.

A survey of the literature on this aspect of platelet biogenic amine uptake indicates that certain definitive kinetic experiments, using low substrate concentrations and short incubation times, are lacking. It should also be borne in mind that, in vivo, platelets are rarely exposed to concentrations of catecholamines above 50 nM (Roizen et al., 1975) and therefore the possibility that platelets contain a very high-affinity catecholamine transport system should be considered. With radiolabelled catecholamines of high-specific activity now available, it should be possible to test this hypothesis.

2.3. Uptake of 5HT by blood platelets

2.3.1. Uptake of 5HT at the level of the plasma membrane

The uptake of 5HT by blood platelets can be dissected into two components, (a) passive transfer, and (b) active transport (Born and Gillson, 1959; Born and Bricknell, 1959; Pletscher, 1968).

(a) *Passive transfer.* Blood platelets can accumulate 5HT by a process of passive diffusion: that is, by a process which is not linked to an energy-requiring carrier mechanism. This system is thought to operate when the external 5HT concentration is greater than 10 μM. In this case, the accumulation of 5HT is directly proportional to the concentration of 5HT in the external medium and the uptake process is not saturated at concentrations approaching 1 mM (Pletscher, 1968). The passive diffusion of 5HT, like the active transport, depends on the incubation temperature; decreasing the temperature from 37°C to 32°C results in a 50% decrease in passive transfer (Pletscher et al., 1965). The passive uptake of 5HT is unaffected by agents such as chlorpromazine and desmethylimipramine, which are potent inhibitors of active transport (Fuks et al., 1964).

(b) *Active transport.* When the concentration of 5HT in the external medium is less than about 5 μM, active transport by the platelet is the dominant process. Since, under normal conditions in vivo, it is unlikely that plasma 5HT concentrations exceed this value, active transport is the process which operates physiologically to regulate plasma 5HT levels.

Studies in vitro have indicated that the active uptake of 5HT shows the following general characteristics:

(1) It occurs against a considerable concentration gradient between the platelet and the medium (e.g., 1000:1) and is a saturable process. The relationship between the initial rate of uptake and the substrate concentration obeys Michaelis-Menten kinetics (Humphrey and Toh, 1954; Hardisty and Stacey, 1955; Zucker and Borelli, 1956; Brodie et al., 1957; Born and Gillson, 1959; Hughes and Brodie, 1959).

(2) The process shows structural specificity, since the uptake of tryptamine and 5-hydroxy N',N'-dimethyltryptamine (bufotenine) is less than 5HT, proportional to the substrate concentration, and does not reach saturation (Hughes and Brodie, 1959; Stacey, 1961). Specificity is not, however, absolute since 5-hydroxy α-methyltryptamine and 5,6-dihydroxytryptamine appear to be accumulated by the platelet in almost exactly the same manner as 5HT itself (Lessin et al., 1965; Born et al., 1972; Da Prada et al., 1973).

(3) The uptake process shows an absolute dependence upon the extracellular concentration of Na$^+$ ions (Sneddon, 1969; Lingjaerde, 1969). In the absence of Na$^+$, there is no net 5HT transport, but as the Na$^+$ is added back to the medium, 5HT uptake is stimulated. Sneddon (1969) carried out a kinetic analysis of this

effect and found that Na^+ reduces the K_m value for the transport of 5HT. He also showed that a linear relationship existed between Na^+ concentration and the initial rate of uptake and suggested that Na^+ functions as a co-substrate with 5HT in the transport process. In keeping with theories which had been proposed for the transport of various sugars and amino acids (Crane, 1965; Kipnis and Parrish, 1965), Sneddon (1973) proposed that the uptake of 5HT proceeds by way of a mobile carrier which transverses the membrane. An essential feature of this theory is that the intracellular Na^+ concentration must be maintained at a low level relative to K^+. If the internal Na^+ rises, it will interfere with an Na^+–K^+ exchange process at the inner face of the platelet plasma membrane and the 5HT will remain bound to the carrier. Platelets, like the majority of cells, maintain low internal Na^+ levels by a Na^+ pump related to a Mg^{2+}-dependent $Na^+ + K^+$-stimulated ATPase which transports Na^+ outward and K^+ inward against a concentration gradient.

(4) The uptake of 5HT by platelets is decreased by metabolic inhibitors such as fluoride, dinitrophenol, cyanide and iodoacetate (Sano et al., 1958; Born and Gillson, 1959; Weissbach and Redfield, 1960). Efforts have been made to determine whether the bulk of the energy required for active transport is derived from the glycolytic cycle or from oxidative phosphorylation. Campbell and Todrick (1973) concluded that glycolysis was more important in this respect, but Sneddon (1971) has suggested that the link between cellular metabolism and uptake is indirect. He showed that ouabain and inhibitors of ATP production inhibited Na^+ extrusion from the cell by blocking the Na^+ pump, so tending to raise internal Na^+ levels and lowering K^+ levels. As mentioned above, such an alteration of the asymmetric ion balance across the platelet membrane would tend to inhibit 5HT-uptake. Drummond and Gordon (1976) have suggested that a transient alteration of this ion imbalance induced by ADP is responsible for the powerful inhibitory action of this compound on 5HT uptake by rat blood platelets. Of some interest in this respect is the recent work of McCoy et al. (1974), who studied platelets from patients with Down's Syndrome (Trisomy 21). It has been known for several years that the platelet content of 5HT in this disease is reduced (Rosner et al., 1965; Tu and Zellweger, 1965), but until recently no hypothesis had been proposed which adequately explained this defect. However, McCoy et al. (1974) have shown that the decreased uptake of 5HT in platelets from Down's Syndrome patients is associated with decreased platelet Mg^{2+}-dependent $Na^+ + K^+$-stimulated ATPase activity and a markedly reduced K^+/Na^+ ratio. These workers propose that the decreased ATPase activity could cause decreased Na^+ efflux, resulting in a rise in platelet Na^+ levels, with a subsequent inhibitory effect on 5HT uptake and reduced 5HT content.

(5) A characteristic of the plasma membrane active transport system for 5HT is its susceptibility to inhibition by low concentrations of tricyclic antidepressants such as imipramine (Marshall et al., 1960; Stacey, 1961; Yates, Todrick and Tait, 1964). In accord with results obtained with other tissues (Carlsson, 1970; Shaskan and Snyder, 1970), tertiary amines of the imipramine-type are more potent than secondary amines as inhibitors of platelet 5HT uptake (Todrick and Tait, 1969; Tuomisto, 1974): a similar structure–activity relationship is found with antidepres-

sants of the amitriptyline series (Todrick and Tait, 1969). Several non-tricyclic compounds, e.g., Lilly 110140, have recently been described, which are potent inhibitors of 5HT uptake in the CNS (Wong et al., 1974; Wong et al., 1975). The secondary amine, 3-(p-trifluoromethyl-phenoxy)-N-Methyl-3-phenylpropylamine (Lilly 110140), and its primary amine metabolite, Lilly 103947 are also inhibitors of 5HT uptake by blood platelets (Fig. 2), being almost equipotent in this respect with the most active tricyclic compound, chlorimipramine (Drummond and Gordon, 1975b). The competitive nature of the inhibition caused by Lilly 110140 and Lilly 103947 (Fig. 2), is similar to that found with various tricyclic antidepressants (Stacey, 1961; Ahtee and Saarnivaara, 1971; Tuomisto, 1974), and this suggests that these drugs compete with 5HT for binding to the proposed transport carrier. Further evidence in accord with this hypothesis has been reported from studies using a direct binding technique (Drummond and Gordon, 1975b), and this is outlined in Section 4.

Various 5HT analogues are also competitive inhibitors of 5HT uptake by blood platelets (Lessin et al., 1965; Born et al., 1972). Some of these (e.g., 5-hydroxy α-methyltryptamine) are also substrates for the transport system, while others (e.g., tryptamine) are not. Interestingly, slight alterations in the structure of some tryptamine derivatives can alter the pattern of inhibition from competitive to uncompetitive; 5-methoxy- and 5-chloro-α-methyltryptamine are uncompetitive

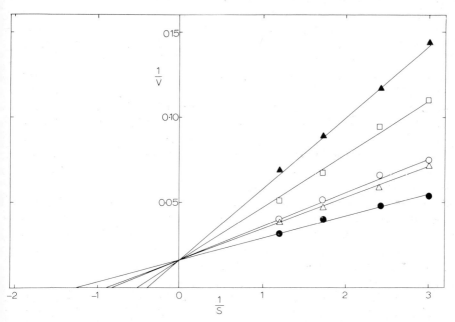

Fig. 2. Effect of Lilly 110140 and Lilly 103947 on 5HT uptake by rat blood platelets. Initial velocity of uptake (V) is expressed in units of pmoles/10 sec/10^8 cells. [^{3}H]5HT concentrations (S) used were in the range $4-9 \times 10^{-7}$ M. Additions (1 min; 37°C prior to [^{3}H]5HT) were: (●–●), saline; (△–△). Lilly 103947 (9.3×10^{-8} M); (□–□), Lilly 103947 (4.5×10^{-7} M); (○–○), Lilly 110140 (9.3×10^{-8} M); (▲–▲), Lilly 110140 (4.5×10^{-7} M).

inhibitors of 5HT uptake by human and rat platelets (Born et al., 1972; Drummond and Gordon, unpublished). The indole imino nitrogen atom appears to be important for inhibition of uptake, since the 5HT isosteres 3-(2-aminoethyl)-5-hydroxyindene and 3-2-(aminoethyl)-5-hydroxybenzofuran are respectively 7.5 and 50 times less potent in this respect than 5HT itself (Fig. 3).

Many other drugs in relatively high concentrations also inhibit 5HT uptake by blood platelets. These include α- and β-adrenoceptor blockers, 5HT antagonists, β-phenylethylamine derivatives, narcotic analgesics, coronary dilators, amantidine and –SH blockers (Stacey, 1961; Lingjaerde, 1970; Grobecker and Lemmer, 1971; Lemmer et al., 1972; Lemmer, 1973; Ahtee and Saarnivaara, 1973; de Clerck and Reneman, 1973; Richter and Smith, 1974; Harbury and Schrier, 1974; Buczko et al., 1975; Drummond and Gordon, 1975a; Ahtee, 1975). The type of inhibition observed with these drugs is generally non-competitive, and in most cases the effects on 5HT uptake are unrelated to other pharmacological actions of the drugs. Non-specific effects such as membrane-stabilization, inhibition of cellular metabolism and induction of 5HT release are most probably responsible for most of these effects. Some studies have attributed the releasing action of a particular drug to its effect on 5HT re-uptake, implying that the releasing effect is a direct consequence of uptake inhibition. Under most conditions in vitro this proposition is untenable, since the tricyclic antidepressants, which are the most potent uptake inhibitors known, require around 100-fold higher concentrations to induce release of endogenous 5HT. Moreover, the structure–activity relationships for these com-

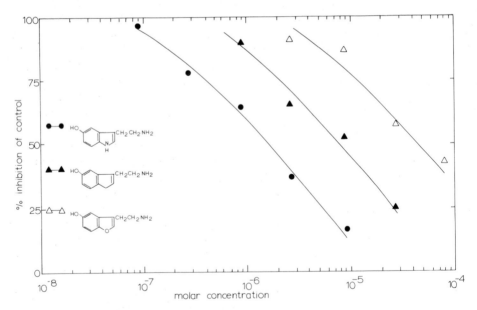

Fig. 3. Effect of 5HT isosteres; 5HT (●–●); 3-(2-aminoethyl)-5-hydroxyindene (▲–▲); 3-(2-aminoethyl)-5-hydroxybenzofuran (△–△), on the uptake of [³H]5HT (4.15×10^{-7} M) by rat blood platelets. Drugs were added simultaneously with [³H]5HT.

pounds as uptake inhibitors differ from those found when these drugs are considered as releasing agents (Ahtee et al., 1968). With a number of exceptions, e.g., reserpine, the induction of endogenous platelet release by a drug signifies the onset of non-specific effects; Lemmer et al. (1972) have proposed that blood platelets are a good model for the investigation of these nonspecific effects.

In a series of publications, Tuomisto and his colleagues have attempted to investigate the active conformation of 5HT at the platelet receptor by studying the effect of conformationally-restricted analogues on 5HT uptake (Tuomisto, 1973; Tuomisto et al., 1974; Tuomisto and Walaszek, 1974). The results obtained with tranylcypromine and its cisoid isomer demonstrated that 5HT uptake was a stereo-selective process; however, in general, this work has been hampered by the low activity of these analogues as inhibitors of 5HT uptake. This has made it difficult to differentiate between specific drug-receptor interactions and non-specific effects due to the increased lipid solubility of the analogues relative to 5HT. Studies using much more potent, stereo-selective inhibitors such as the 4-phenyl-1-aminotetralines (Sarges et al., 1974) may therefore yield more une-quivocal results regarding the active conformation of 5HT at its proposed transport carrier.

2.3.2. *Uptake of 5HT at the granule membrane level*

After transport through the platelet plasma membrane, 5HT is stored intracellu-larly at a site which renders the compound inaccessible to the enzyme monoamine oxidase (Paasonen, 1965). Tranzer et al. (1966), using rabbit and guinea pig platelets, have provided considerable evidence that 5HT is stored in intracellular organelles, which, after double fixation with glutaraldehyde and osmium tetrox-ide, appear on electron micrographs as dense osmiophilic granules. These organelles can be obtained as a homogeneous suspension by centrifugation of platelet homogenates in a continuous Urografin gradient (Da Prada et al., 1967; Da Prada et al., 1972). There is considerable similarity between these platelet granules and the more extensively studied catecholamine-containing chromaffin granules of the adrenal medulla (see Sneddon, 1973), and it is likely that common mechanisms of amine uptake are shared by both types of organelles.

The platelet dense granule is surrounded by a single membrane (Da Prada et al., 1967), and contains mainly 5HT and 5'-di- and tri-phosphonucleotides (Pletscher, et al., 1971; Goetz et al., 1971). Bivalent metals (especially Mg and Ca) are also present, although soluble proteins occur to only a minor extent (Da Prada and Pletscher, 1968; Pletscher et al. 1971). This latter point is in marked contrast to the chromaffin granule, which contains appreciable amounts of soluble proteins, among them the chromagranins (Smith, 1968). Isolated platelet granule mem-branes from rabbits contain a Mg^{2+}-stimulated ATPase, which is inhibited by N-ethylmaleimide and Na^+ (Heinrich et al., 1972). This enzyme differs from that found in the platelet plasma membrane in that it is insensitive to ouabain. Interestingly, it also appears to be dissimilar to the enzyme found in the chromaffin granule membrane, since while the platelet enzyme is inhibited by

Ca^{2+}, the chromaffin granule enzyme is stimulated. When isolated platelet storage organelles are incubated at 37°C for short time periods (1 h) with radiolabelled 5HT and mono-, di- and tri-phosphonucleotides, there is accumulation of 5HT, but no appreciable uptake of the nucleotides (Da Prada and Pletscher, 1968; Da Prada and Pletscher, 1970), suggesting that the granule membrane is selectively permeable to 5HT. Recent work indicates, however, that when longer incubations are used, some radioactive nucleotides are found in the storage organelles (Da Prada and Pletscher, 1970; Reimers et al., 1975). The uptake of 5HT is temperature-dependant, but is unaffected by metabolic inhibitors (such as fluoride, iodoacetate or ouabain) or by the depletion of glucose in the medium, indicating that the uptake may not be an active process (Da Prada and Pletscher, 1969a). Uptake of 5HT into these granules is, however, inhibited by reserpine (Da Prada and Pletscher, 1968). Although the exact mode of action of this drug remains open to question, it has been shown to accumulate irreversibly in the membranes of these 5HT-containing granules (Da Prada and Pletscher, 1969b; Enna et al., 1974), and by analogy with its action on the granular storage of catecholamines, it has been proposed that the drug binds to an amine transport carrier in the granule membrane, which is involved in the uptake process (Slotkin, 1973). There is, however, no definitive evidence in support of this hypothesis.

As well as 5HT, platelet granules can accumulate several other biogenic amines such as dopamine, noradrenaline, adrenaline and metaraminol (Da Prada and Pletscher, 1969a; Born and Smith, 1970; Ahtee and Saarnivaara, 1971), as well as a number of basic drugs (Da Prada and Pletscher, 1975). The elucidation of the mechanisms involved in the uptake of biogenic amines into the platelet storage granules has progressed less rapidly than the corresponding studies using the more readily available chromaffin granule, because isolated platelet granule membranes have not yet been widely used. It is therefore not known whether the work of Da Prada et al. (1975a) on reserpine-sensitive and -insensitive uptake of amines by chromaffin granule membranes is directly applicable to the platelet granules. Similarly, the work of Phillips (1974a,b) showing that ATP hydrolysis is a pre-requisite for amine transport but that uptake is not linked to the bulk ATPase activity of the chromaffin granule membrane remains to be proven for the platelet. It is known, however, that high molecular weight complexes are formed between 5HT and ATP inside the platelet storage granule (Berneis et al., 1969) and recent work from the Basel group (Berneis et al., 1974; Da Prada et al., 1975b) suggests that as well as providing a storage mechanism for 5HT, this interaction may also be involved in the development of a concentration gradient across the granule membrane which, in turn, stimulates the granular uptake of biogenic amines.

3. Platelet stimulation induced by biogenic amines

3.1. Catecholamines

3.1.1. The platelet shape change

Early studies indicated that adrenaline and noradrenaline did not induce human platelets to change in shape (Bull and Zucker, 1965; MacMillan, 1966; Mills and Roberts, 1967b; O'Brien and Woodhouse, 1968; Seaman and Brooks, 1969). Mustard and Packham (1970), arguing for the role of ADP in catecholamine-induced platelet stimulation (see Section 3.3), suggested that these results did not stand up to critical examination. However, Mills (1973) using human platelets, has provided convincing evidence on the basis of biochemical studies of ATP consumption, that adrenaline, in contrast to 5HT and ADP, neither induces the platelet shape change nor causes the shape change-associated decrease in the platelet adenylate energy charge. Ahtee and Michal (1972) have reported that adrenaline (0.2 μM), noradrenaline (20 μM), and dopamine (200 μM) induce rabbit platelets suspended in citrated plasma to change in shape.

3.1.2. Primary platelet aggregation

Adrenaline and noradrenaline in low concentrations ($<1 \mu$M) cause primary aggregation of human platelets in citrated or heparinised plasma (Clayton and Cross, 1963; O'Brien, 1963; Mitchell and Sharp, 1964; O'Brien et al., 1969). This aggregation differs from that induced by 5HT or ADP in that it does not readily reverse. O'Brien et al. (1969) have shown that primary aggregation is increased in human heparinised plasma relative to citrated plasma. This effect may be due to the decreased ability of adrenaline to induce the platelet release in human heparinised plasma (see below). Loeb and Mackey (1973) have reported that catecholamines can also induce primary platelet aggregation in certain species of sub-human primates, but with the exception of rabbits, platelets from other animal species are generally insensitive to the aggregatory actions of adrenaline and noradrenaline (Constantine, 1966; Sinakos and Caen, 1967; Mills, 1970; Tschopp, 1970; Klein, Szentivanyi and Fishel, 1974; see Table 2). Several investigators have found that rabbit platelets in citrated plasma do not aggregate in response to catecholamines (Mitchell and Sharp, 1964; Sinakos and Caen, 1967; Baumgartner, 1969), although others (Ahtee and Michal, 1972) have reported positive results. Baumgartner (1969) indicated that although no aggregation occurred with freshly prepared plasma, adrenaline was active when the platelet count had fallen during storage. These results, and the findings of Ahtee and Michal (1972), may be related to the known action of adrenaline to potentiate aggregation induced by other agents (see Section 3.1.4). Interestingly, Barthel and Markwardt (1974) have found that catecholamines can induce primary aggregation of washed rabbit platelets suspended in Tyrode's solution. Such a finding may also be explained by adrenaline's potentiatory effect on the action of platelet constituents (e.g., ADP, 5HT) released during the washing

TABLE 2
Species differences in platelet stimulation responses to 5HT and adrenaline (ADR)

Species	Compound	Shape change	Primary aggregation	Secondary aggregation	Potentiation
Man	5HT	+	+	− (+)	+
	ADR	−	+	+	+
Rabbit	5HT	+	+	−	+
	ADR	− (+)	− (+)	−	+
Pig	5HT	+	+	+	+
	ADR	−	−	−	−
Rat	5HT	+	−	−	+
	ADR	−	−	−	+
Guinea pig	5HT	−	−	−	−
	ADR	−	−	−	−
Cat	5HT	− (+)	+	+	+
	ADR	−	−	−	+
Mouse	5HT	+	+	−	+
	ADR	−	−	−	+

+ = responsive; − = unresponsive; (+) = occasionally responsive

procedure, although other explanations are also conceivable (e.g., the presence of a natural inhibitor in plasma).

With human platelets, the aggregatory actions of catecholamines are believed to be mediated by an α-adrenoceptor; isoprenaline does not induce aggregation, and propanolol is a relatively weak, non-stereospecific antagonist (Mills and Roberts, 1967b; Rysanek et al., 1968; Bygdeman and Johnsen, 1969). The inhibitory effects of these high concentrations of propanolol have been ascribed to an imipramine-like membrane-stabilizing action; this is compatible with the findings of Rysanek and co-workers (1968) who observed non-competitive inhibition of the second phase of adrenaline-induced platelet aggregation by propanolol (see Mills and Roberts, 1967a). In contrast, the α-antagonists dihydroergotamine and phentolamine are potent competitive inhibitors of both phases of aggregation (Mills and Roberts, 1967b; Rysanek et al., 1968). There is some controversy over the ability of the irreversible blockers (β-haloalkylamines, dibenamine and phenoxybenzamine) to inhibit catecholamine-induced platelet stimulation: Mills and Roberts (1967b) suggested that at concentrations up to 50 μM these compounds were not inhibitory, but Bygdeman and Johnsen (1969) demonstrated that although phenoxybenzamine was inactive at 10 μM, it inhibited almost totally at 100 μM. The relative lack of potency of these agents in PRP is at least partly related to the extensive binding of these compounds to plasma proteins and other non-receptor material (Graham, 1964), since Barthel and Markwardt (1974) observed more potent inhibitory effects with dibenamine in washed platelets suspended in plasma-free medium.

3.1.3. Secondary platelet aggregation and the release reaction

O'Brien (1963) reported that adrenaline in comparatively low concentrations could induce biphasic aggregation of human platelets suspended in citrated plasma, and this was confirmed by MacMillan (1966), who also showed that an 'ADP-like' substance was released from blood platelets during secondary aggregation. Mills, Robb and Roberts (1968) provided direct biochemical evidence for this by demonstrating the release of platelet 5HT, ATP, and ADP by adrenaline. Other platelet constituents such as acid-phosphatase, β-glucuronidase and adenylate kinase were not released. These workers also showed that release and the second phase of aggregation began simultaneously and that once the second phase was underway, phentolamine was no longer an effective inhibitor. The inference from this work is that secondary aggregation is mediated, not by adrenaline, but by released agents (e.g., ADP), and there is now abundant evidence from many different laboratories suggesting that this conclusion is correct (Haslam, 1967; Rossi and Levin, 1973; Macfarlane, 1974).

Unlike the primary response induced by catecholamines, secondary aggregation and the release reaction in human heparinised PRP are less than in citrated plasma (O'Brien, et al., 1969; Zucker, 1972; Gordon and Mitchinson, personal communication: see Table 3). Similar effects were observed with aggregation induced by ADP in human plasma (Mills and Roberts, 1967a), and for this case it was proposed that the biphasic aggregation observed in citrated plasma is an experimental artifact caused by the unphysiologically low levels of divalent cations (Kinlough-Rathbone et al., 1974; Mustard et al., 1975). The catecholamine-induced platelet release reaction may not, therefore, be physiologically important.

3.1.4. Platelet aggregation induced by other agents: potentiation by catecholamines

Ardlie et al. (1966) first demonstrated that adrenaline, noradrenaline and (to a lesser extent) dopamine could, in concentrations much lower than those which caused platelet aggregation, enhance platelet aggregation induced by ADP. Mills and Roberts (1967b) confirmed these findings and also showed that isoprenaline, in contrast, could only inhibit ADP-induced aggregation. Potentiation is not restricted to ADP: platelet responses to 5HT, thrombin and collagen are also enhanced

TABLE 3
The release of human platelet 5HT and adenine nucleotides (AN) in response to catecholamines: effect of anticoagulant.

Addition	5HT (ng/10^9 cells)[a]		AN (nmoles/10^8 cells)[b]	
	Heparin	Citrate	Heparin	Citrate
Saline	572	603	11.2	12.0
Adrenaline (1 μM)	503 (−12%)	301 (−50%)	9.41 (−16%)	6.9 (−42%)
Noradrenaline (1 μM)	520 (−9%)	307 (−49%)	10.0 (−11%)	7.8 (−35%)

Anticoagulant concentrations were trisodium citrate; 1:9 (by vol.) 3.8% citrate:whole blood, heparin; 1:9 (by vol.) 50 U/ml heparin:whole blood. Values shown are means of eight observations (Gordon and Mitchinson, unpublished results).
[a]   Drummond and Gordon (1974a)
[b]   Gordon and Drummond (1974)

(Baumgartner and Born, 1968; Thomas, 1968). Although platelet aggregation induced by catecholamines appears to be restricted to a few species, the potentiatory effects of these amines are more widespread (Sinakos and Caen, 1967; Baumgartner, 1969; Mills, 1970; Klein et al., 1974; see Table 2). The most extensive investigations into the nature of the adrenergic receptor mediating platelet stimulation by catecholamines have been made using the potentiatory effects of these amines as the experimental assay. α-Adrenergic receptor blockers are potent inhibitors of the process (Mills and Roberts, 1967b), although phenoxybenzamine is a non-stereoselective antagonist on platelets (Berry and Miller, 1974), in contrast to its action on other tissues (Portoghese et al., 1971). Ahtee and Michal (1972), using rabbit platelets, showed that the α-agonists phenylephrine and naphazoline potentiated ADP-induced aggregation at concentrations around 1 μM. From this and other evidence, these workers concluded that an α-adrenoceptor was responsible for the potentiatory action of adrenaline. Berry and Miller (1974) using rat platelets, take the view that the platelet receptor for catecholamines does not have all the usual characteristics of either the α- or β-adrenergic receptor, since although they found naphazoline (1 μM) active, other α-agonists such as synephrine and phenylephrine did not potentiate at concentrations up to 100 μM. Further work carried out in the absence of plasma proteins is necessary to resolve this question.

3.2. 5-Hydroxytryptamine

3.2.1. The platelet shape change

The ability of 5HT to alter the shape of human blood platelets was first recognised by O'Brien and Heywood (1966). In contrast to catecholamines, platelet aggregation induced by 5HT is invariably preceded by a shape change, although aggregation does not necessarily occur as a consequence of this event. Several analogues of 5HT, such as 5-hydroxy-$N'N'$-dimethyltryptamine, have been studied which induce the platelet shape change without causing platelet aggregation to occur (Born et al., 1972). Similarly, rat platelets undergo a shape change in response to 5HT without any ensuing aggregation (Drummond and Gordon, 1975a). Holmsen et al. (1974) have suggested that the platelet shape change, aggregation and the release reaction are all manifestations of one biochemical event, namely ATP catabolism, and Born et al. (1972) proposed that a single 5HT receptor controls both the 5HT-induced shape change and 5HT-induced platelet aggregation. On the basis of these theories the finding that 5-hydroxy-$N'N'$-dimethyltryptamine can induce the platelet shape change but not aggregation may be explained if this compound is acting as a partial agonist. Since a partial agonist is thought to bind to a receptor without having the capability to induce the full physiological response, the structural requirements for such an action would be less rigorous than for a full agonist: Born et al. (1972) concluded that platelet aggregation by 5HT analogues required greater structural specificity than was required for the production of the shape change. With the exception of guinea pig and horse, the shape change response induced by 5HT is ubiquitous among animal species (O'Brien and Heywood, 1966; Baumgartner and Born, 1968; Klein et al., 1974; Drummond and Gordon, 1975a; Drummond and Gordon, unpublished; see Table 2). Mills (1973) has shown that, like ADP, 5HT induces a rapid decrease in the platelet adenylate energy charge which appears to be associated with the change in platelet shape.

3.2.2. Primary platelet aggregation

Human platelets suspended in either citrated or heparinised plasma are aggregated by micromolar concentrations of 5HT (O'Brien, 1963; Mitchell and Sharp, 1964; O'Brien, 1964; O'Brien et al., 1969). This aggregation is generally small and reversible (see below) and higher concentrations are self-inhibitory (Baumgartner and Born, 1968). With the exceptions of guinea pig, horse and rat, platelets from all animal species so far studied can be aggregated by 5HT (see Table 2). However, this last statement must be qualified by the fact that aggregation responses to 5HT are notoriously more inconsistent than those to ADP. This variability may be partly due to a desensitization of platelet 5HT receptors which has occurred during the preparation of PRP. Platelet 5HT receptors are rapidly desensitized by exposure to low concentrations of 5HT (Baumgartner and Born, 1968; Baumgartner, 1969), and it is possible that these levels could have accumulated extracellularly by the action on platelets of thrombin, generated during centrifugation or as the result of a traumatic venepuncture.

Another characteristic of platelet aggregation induced by 5HT is its marked calcium dependence. In 1964, Mitchell and Sharp demonstrated that the addition of 2 mM calcium chloride to rabbit citrated PRP increased the platelet's sensitivity to 5HT one hundred fold. Since the addition of this concentration of calcium chloride partially restores normal in vivo levels of ionised calcium, this observation was of some physiological importance. One consequence of this finding is that, since most platelet function tests are carried out in citrated PRP, these tests will tend to underestimate any effects due to 5HT. We have examined the platelet aggregation response to 5HT in heparinised, citrated and partially recalcified citrated PRP from various animal species in an effort to assess the importance of this experimental variable (Drummond and Gordon, unpublished). While our results do not suggest that the role of 5HT in haemostasis (as measured by the photometric technique) has been seriously overlooked, they nevertheless emphasise that variations in ionised calcium levels can, under certain conditions, have dramatic effects on the platelet's responsiveness to 5HT.

In confirmation of the results of O'Brien et al. (1969), the sensitivity of human platelets to 5HT is not greatly affected by ionised calcium concentration; addition of 2 mM $CaCl_2$ to human citrated PRP increases the initial velocity of 5HT-induced primary aggregation by about 60% without altering the 5HT concentration which causes the half-maximal response. Also, there is no qualitative change in the pattern of the aggregation response; at all concentrations aggregation is, in general, reversible and there is no release of platelet adenine nucleotides.

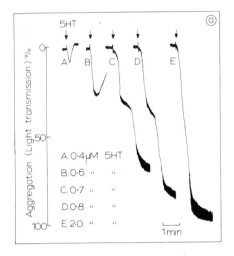 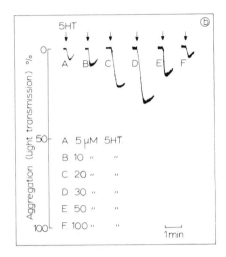

Fig. 4. Platelet aggregation responses to 5HT in (a) pig heparinised PRP and (b) pig citrated PRP.

Addition of calcium chloride to either guinea pig or rat citrated PRP does not enhance platelet sensitivity to 5HT at all, but in contrast, pig platelets become extremely responsive to 5HT in the presence of normal calcium levels (Drummond and Gordon, 1974b; Gordon and Drummond, 1975). Figure 4 shows the response of platelets to various 5HT concentrations in pig citrated and heparinised plasma. In citrated plasma, the classical platelet 5HT dose–response curve is seen; aggregation in response to all 5HT concentrations is small and reversible and higher concentrations ($>30 \mu M$) are self-inhibitory. However, in heparinised PRP, 5HT induces reversible aggregation at 0.2–0.6 μM, biphasic aggregation at around 1 μM and monophasic, irreversible aggregation at all higher concentrations up to 100 μM (the highest tested). This effect is not due to the presence of heparin since the addition of calcium chloride to citrated PRP results in a similar enhancement of responses to 5HT (Fig. 5).

5HT-induced platelet aggregation is readily inhibited by 5HT antagonists such as d-LSD, brom-LSD and methysergide, while atropine and morphine are much less potent (Mitchell and Sharp, 1964; Michal and Penglis, 1969; Michal, 1969). The platelet 5HT receptor appears, therefore, to resemble the 'D'-receptor for 5HT described by Gaddum and Picarelli (1957) on the basis of studies with the guinea pig ileum. There appears, however, to be a much greater heterogeneity amongst 5HT receptors in different tissues than is allowed by the classification of Gaddum and Picarelli (see Section 4). The phenothiazine tranquillizer chlorpromazine and its metabolites are also potent inhibitors of 5HT-induced responses in vitro (Mills and Roberts, 1967a; Michal and Penglis, 1969; Boullin et al., 1975a) but psychiatric patients receiving chlorpromazine therapy surprisingly show a specific increase in 5HT aggregation compared with normal controls or psychiatric patients not receiving the drug (Boullin et al., 1975). This effect of chronic chlorpromazine treatment appears to be due to a specific platelet

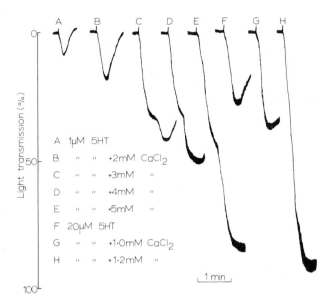

Fig. 5. Platelet aggregation responses to 5HT in recalcified pig citrated PRP. Samples containing calcium chloride concentrations in excess of 2 mM were lightly heparinised (0.4 U/ml).

alteration which, in view of its long duration of action, may arise in the megakaryocyte prior to platelet production (Boullin et al., 1975b). Enhancement of 5HT-induced aggregation is not seen after chronic ingestion of other 5HT antagonists such as methysergide and ergotamine; on the contrary, these agents are inhibitory both in vitro and ex vivo (Hilton, 1974). The Oxford group have recently found that patients with iron-deficiency anaemia also have enhanced 5HT-induced platelet aggregation (Boullin et al., 1975), but the mechanisms responsible for these results await clarification.

3.2.3. Secondary platelet aggregation and the release reaction

5HT-induced platelet aggregation in human samples is generally reversible (Baumgartner and Born, 1968), but platelets from approximately 10% of human volunteers undergo irreversible biphasic aggregation in response to 5HT (White, 1970; Besterman and Gillett, 1973; Boullin et al., 1975). Our own results indicate that this effect is not consistently observed in replicate blood samples from one subject and that biphasic aggregation in response to 5HT is usually associated with enhanced platelet sensitivity to other aggregating agents, which raises the possibility that this effect is dependent upon the potentiatory action of 5HT on aggregation induced by ADP or thrombin, generated during the preparation of PRP. In contrast, cat platelets suspended in citrated plasma consistently undergo biphasic, irreversible aggregation in response to 5HT (Baumgartner et al., 1969; Tschopp, 1970), and this reaction is associated with the release of platelet adenine nucleotides (Mills, 1970). As indicated above (Section 3.2.2.), pig platelets undergo biphasic aggregation in response to 5HT in the presence of adequate levels of ionised calcium, and, under those conditions, about 25% of platelet adenine nucleotides are released (Gordon and Drummond, 1975). An interesting finding from this work was that all of the released nucleotides were recovered in the supernatant plasma. During the release reaction induced by other agents (e.g., collagen) a percentage of platelet ATP is converted irreversibly to IMP, inosine and hypoxanthine (Holmsen and Day, 1971). The fluorescence assay used to measure total adenine compounds in PRP during the platelet release reaction (Gordon and Drummond, 1974) is sensitive enough to detect this conversion to nonadenine compounds and in pig heparinised PRP collagen decreases the total adenine content of PRP by about 20% during the release reaction (Drummond and Gordon, unpublished). The fact that 5HT does not apparently convert platelet ATP to non-adenine compounds during the release reaction raises the possibility that the mechanism responsible for the releasing action of 5HT is different from that which mediates the effect of other releasing agents.

3.2.4. Potentiation and inhibition of platelet aggregation induced by other agents

Baumgartner and Born (1968) showed that low concentrations of 5HT could potentiate platelet aggregation induced by ADP or adrenaline. This effect was most marked when 5HT and the other aggregating agent were added simultaneously, and inhibition of aggregation occurred when 5HT was preincubated with PRP for longer times (10–20 min) prior to the addition of the second agent. These workers proposed that this inhibitory effect was due to an imipramine-like membrane stabilization effect, although the primary phase of aggregation induced by adrenaline was also markedly inhibited (see Mills and Roberts, 1967a). Michal and Motamed (1975) have recently shown that both the stimulatory and inhibitory effects of 5HT are methysergide-sensitive, which suggests that a more specific effect of 5HT is responsible. The synergistic effects of 5HT and ADP are extremely marked in pig heparinised plasma: maximal platelet aggregation results from the simultaneous addition of 5HT and ADP in concentrations which induce only a change in platelet shape when added separately (Drummond and Gordon, unpublished). At present the mechanism which is responsible for this synergism is unclear.

3.3. Platelet stimulation induced by biogenic amines: mechanisms

Two main lines of evidence suggested that primary platelet aggregation induced by biogenic amines was mediated by ADP: firstly, the ADP analogue, adenosine, is a powerful inhibitor of aggregation induced by ADP, 5HT or adrenaline (Born and Cross, 1963; O'Brien, 1964) and secondly, ADP-consuming systems inhibit aggregation induced by all three agents (Haslam, 1964, 1967). However, in the past five years a number of observations have been reported which are not readily accommodated within this scheme. Firstly, adenosine was originally thought to be a specific competitive inhibitor of ADP-induced aggregation (Born and Cross, 1963; Skoza et al., 1967) but is now believed to act, not by competing with ADP for its receptor, but by increasing the level of adenosine-3,5-cyclic monophosphate (cyclic AMP) in platelets (Haslam and Lynham, 1973; Haslam and Rosson, 1975). This inhibits the platelet aggregation response to all aggregating agents (Mills and Smith, 1971; Haslam, 1973; Smith and Macfarlane, 1974). Secondly, agents which are specific ADP antagonists, e.g., 2-methylthioAMP, nitrofurantoin, 2-*n*-amyl-thioAMP and ATP (Michal et al., 1969; Rossi and Levin, 1973; Kikugawa et al., 1973; Macfarlane, 1974) do not affect primary aggregation induced by 5HT or adrenaline (Michal, 1971; Rossi and Levin, 1973; Macfarlane, 1974). Figure 6 shows that 100 μM 2-*n*-amylthioAMP substantially inhibits aggregation induced by 3 μM ADP with little effect on that induced by the same concentration of 5HT. Thirdly, duck thrombocytes do not aggregate in response to ADP but are aggregated by 5HT (Belamarich and Simoneit, 1973). Also, after platelets have been made unresponsive to ADP by prior exposure to this nucleotide the platelets will still aggregate in response to adrenaline or 5HT (O'Brien, 1965; Evans and Gordon, 1974). The bulk of the recent experimental evidence therefore suggests that biogenic amines stimulate platelets not by the formation or release of ADP but by a specific interaction of the amine with a cellular receptor which, in turn, initiates a series of events culminating in the production of the physiological response.

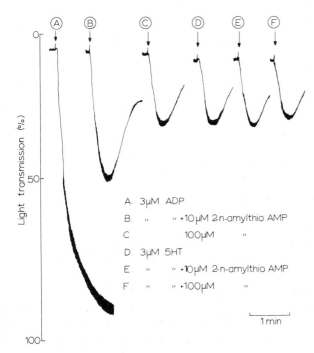

A. 3µM ADP
B. "   " +10 µM 2-n-amylthio AMP
C.   100µM   "
D. 3µM 5HT
E. "   " +10µM 2-n-amylthio AMP
F. "   " +100µM   "

1 min

Fig. 6. Effect of 2-*n*-amylthioAMP on platelet aggregation responses to ADP and 5HT in human citrated PRP.

It has been proposed that platelet stimulation by catecholamines or 5HT is mediated by the same receptors on the platelet membrane which are involved in the active transport of these amines (Baumgartner and Born, 1968, 1969; Baumgartner, 1969; Born and Smith, 1970), but Bygdeman and Johnsen (1969) showed that there was no correlation between inhibition of catecholamine uptake and inhibition of aggregation for several α-blockers, suggesting that the uptake of adrenaline and noradrenaline is separate from the induction of platelet aggregation. In the case of 5HT a similar lack of correlation exists for antagonists and uptake inhibitors (Cumings and Hilton, 1971; Born et al., 1972; Drummond and Gordon, 1975a). In addition, Born et al. (1972) showed that analogues of 5HT such as 5-methoxy α-methyltryptamine are potent platelet stimulants but are not substrates for the active transport system. These findings suggest that separate receptors exist on the platelet membrane to mediate the two different responses, and preliminary work on the characterisation of these receptors supports this concept (Drummond and Gordon, 1975b). A more detailed account of this work is given in Section 4.

The steps between binding of 5HT or catecholamines to their receptors and production of the platelet shape change or aggregation remain open to question. The most obvious intracellular mediators in the platelet, as in other cells, are cyclic AMP, guanosine-3',5'-cyclic monophosphate (cyclic GMP) and calcium, and the possible involvement of these agents in platelet responses is discussed at length in Chapter 7.

4. Platelet receptors for biogenic amines

The general characteristics of biogenic amine receptors on blood platelets were discussed briefly in Section 3 and the following section will review the studies which have attempted to elucidate the molecular characteristics of these receptors. Although platelets are well suited for such hormone-receptor studies, (see below) their potential remains at present largely unrecognised.

4.1. Catecholamines

In general, studies on platelet catecholamine receptors have taken second place to studies on their indoleamine counterparts. Platelet stimulation by adrenaline and noradrenaline appears to be mediated by an α-adrenoceptor (see Section 3), and several observations suggest that this receptor is associated with the platelet contractile protein, thrombosthenin. Firstly, Levy-Toledano (1971) reported that adrenaline and noradrenaline could protect isolated thrombosthenin from the inhibitory effects of N-ethylmaleimide (NEM). Both thrombosthenin super-precipitation and ATPase activity were inhibited by NEM, but this effect was abolished by prior incubation with relatively high concentrations of the catecholamines. This protective effect was inhibited by phentolamine but not by propranolol, suggesting α-adrenoceptor involvement. Secondly, Berry and Miller (1975) showed that radiolabelled phenoxybenzamine binds irreversibly to rat platelet thrombosthenin but not to several other platelet proteins. Because of the various non-receptor interactions which have been reported for this drug, (Graham, 1964), the work of Berry and Miller is difficult to evaluate in terms of the platelet α-adrenoceptor. These two observations, however, bring to mind the studies concerning the action of phorbol myristate acetate (PMA) on platelets. Like adrenaline (Bull and Zucker, 1965), PMA induces platelet aggregation which is not preceded by a change in platelet shape (Zucker et al., 1974; Estensen and White, 1974). Moreover, PMA is also known to interact with platelet actomyosin: in low concentrations this agent stimulates superprecipitation and ATPase activity (Puszkin and Zucker, 1973). These findings, together with the reported surface localisation of thrombosthenin (Booyse et al., 1971) and the postulated relationship between the platelet ADP receptor and thrombosthenin (Nachman and Ferris, 1974) suggest that it would be unwise to dismiss the results of Levy-Toledano (1971) and Berry and Miller (1975) as simply non-specific effects. However, definitive evidence that thrombosthenin or some associated macromolecule is related to the platelet α-adrenoceptor remains to be reported.

Human blood platelets also contain β-adrenoceptors, which, on stimulation by catecholamines, mediate an increase in platelet adenylate cyclase activity (Abdulla, 1969; Mills and Smith, 1971), but it is not yet known whether this β-adrenoceptor is similar to that in adipose tissue and cardiac muscle (β_1) or that in tracheal and uterine smooth muscle (β_2) (Lands et al., 1967). However, since procedures are now available for determining the number and distribution of β-receptors on cells (Lefkowitz et al., 1974; Levitzki et al., 1974; Aurbach et al., 1974), it would be of interest to use these techniques on platelets.

4.2. 5-Hydroxytryptamine

The receptor mediating the stimulatory effects of 5HT on the platelet has many similarities to the classical 'D'-5HT receptor (see Section 3). A number of workers have used platelets to test the hypothesis that the 5HT receptor is a sialic acid-containing ganglioside (Woolley, 1958; Gielen, 1965). Mester et al. (1972) showed that when the platelet membrane is enriched in sialic acid, 5HT-induced aggregation is enhanced while ADP-induced aggregation is diminished. In contrast, however, two groups of workers reported that by decreasing the amount of platelet sialic acid with neuraminidase, 5HT- and ADP-induced aggregation are similarily enhanced (Davis et al., 1972; Greenberg et al., 1975). Since sialic acid is predominantly responsible for the net negative charge on platelets (Madoff et al., 1964), it is likely that the enhanced aggregation response after neuraminidase treatment is due, at least in part, to decreased repulsive forces between neighbouring platelets. The measurement of a biochemical parameter (e.g., guanylate cyclase) which is not dependent on cell–cell contact would help to clarify this point. One problem associated with the use of enzymes and other agents as membrane receptor probes is that since glycoproteins are free to interact and to move laterally in the plane of the membrane, the biological effect of such probes may be indirect, due to glycoprotein redistribution, rather than a direct effect on a particular membrane constituent. One way of addressing this problem would be to isolate a membrane protein which specifically binds the ligand in question, and this approach was used by Marcus, Safier and Ullman (1975) who isolated a 5HT-binding ganglioside from platelets. A detailed study of the binding reaction showed, however, that the ganglioside had relatively low affinity for 5HT and did not fulfill the criteria of reversibility or specificity expected of a physiological receptor.

Recently, techniques have been developed for studying the binding of reversible ligands to their receptors (for review, see Snyder, 1975), and our group used a high-speed centrifugation binding assay to investigate the interactions between 5HT and its receptors on intact rat blood platelets (Drummond and Gordon, 1975a,b). Rat platelets were chosen for this study because they are stimulated by 5HT to undergo a photometrically-measurable change in shape (see Section 3) and they also accumulate 5HT by active transport (see Section 2). The receptor binding experiments were carried out at 4°C because at 37°C the active transport system for 5HT makes it impossible to measure a small amount of specific receptor-bound 5HT against a background of intracellular radioactivity. At 4°C, active transport does not occur, and the binding appears to be restricted to the external membrane.

Binding of high specific activity [³H]5HT to rat platelets was rapid and readily reversible (Fig. 7). Specific binding was also directly proportional to the number of platelets in the preparation and corresponded to greater than 90% of the platelet-bound radioactivity. Scatchard analysis of the binding of 5HT to platelets within the 5HT concentration range 1 nM–10 μM gave a curvilinear relationship from which three sites could be resolved. The apparent dissociation constants for these sites and their number per cell are shown in the inset (Fig. 8). The resolution of three separate sites from a curvilinear Scatchard plot is a slightly hazardous

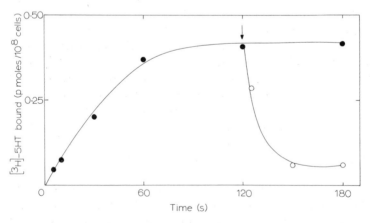

Fig. 7. Time course of the specific binding of [³H]5HT to intact rat blood platelets at 4°C. [³H]5HT was used at a concentration of 16 nM. At 120 sec, saline (●–●); or unlabelled 5HT (8 μM) (○–○), was added.

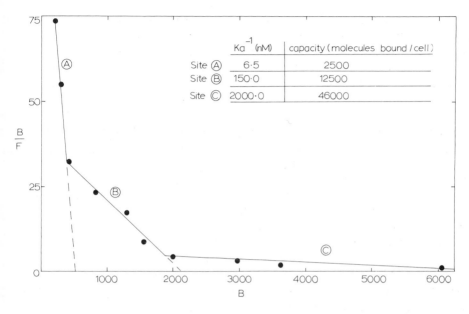

Fig. 8. Scatchard analysis of the binding of [³H]5HT to intact rat blood platelets at 4°C. [³H]5HT in the concentration range 0.001–10 μM was incubated with 0.1 ml portions of rat citrated PRP containing 0.1 mM 5HT (unlabelled) or an equivalent volume of isotonic saline for 120 sec at 4°C. The amount of [³H]5HT binding to platelets under both conditions was measured and the value obtained in the presence of 0.1 mM 5HT (unlabelled) was subtracted to give specific binding. B, amount of specifically bound 5HT (fmoles/10⁸ cells); F, free concentration of 5HT (nM).

procedure, since there could be other explanations for such a pattern (e.g., negative cooperativity). We found, however, that low concentrations of 5HT antagonists (e.g., d-LSD) inhibited binding to the highest affinity site without affecting either the affinity or capacity of the two other sites (Fig. 9). Since d-LSD is a powerful inhibitor of the 5HT-induced platelet shape-change, we compared the potencies of a range of 5HT-antagonists against both high-affinity [³H]5HT binding and the 5HT-induced shape-change. There was high correlation between drug concentrations which inhibited binding and the shape-change (Table 4). Pizotifen and cyproheptadine, which are structurally related anti-5HT and anti-histamine drugs, were amongst the most powerful tested, inhibiting both the high-affinity binding of [³H]5HT and the shape-change at concentrations around 1 nM. An unexpected finding was that both the d- and l-isomers of LSD were highly active against both parameters. Atropine, which is a 5HT 'M'-receptor antagonist according to the classification of Gaddum and Picarelli (1957), was around one thousand times less active than LSD or pizotifen.

Inhibitors of 5HT uptake can also inhibit the platelet shape-change induced by 5HT (Born et al., 1972; Drummond and Gordon, 1975a). When these compounds were tested for their ability to inhibit [³H]5HT binding, we found that they could abolish the binding to both the high- and middle-affinity sites. In order to calculate their potencies against the two sites individually, experiments of the type shown

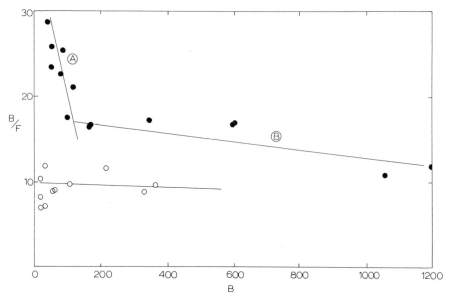

Fig. 9. Scatchard analysis of the effect of d-LSD on the specific binding of [³H]5HT to intact rat blood platelets at 4°C. Details of the experiment were as described in Fig. 8. Additions: (●–●), saline; (○–○), 80 nM d-LSD (1 min at 4°C prior to 5HT).

in Fig. 10 were performed. Cinanserin, which is a specific 5HT antagonist, was included in each experiment so that the amount of high-affinity binding which remained in the presence of increasing concentrations of the uptake inhibitors could be calculated. To determine the potency of the uptake inhibitors against middle-affinity binding, experiments were performed in the presence of a cinanse-rin concentration (800 nM) which completely blocked [³H]5HT binding to the highest affinity site; the residual binding therefore represented only the middle-affinity site. Table 5 summarises the inhibitory potency of these agents against

TABLE 4
Effect of 5HT antagonists on the 5HT-induced platelet shape change and on the high-affinity binding of [³H]5HT to intact rat platelets

Compound	IC₅₀ (nM) against	
	5HT-Induced shape change	High-affinity [³H]5HT binding
Pizotifen	1.2	1.3
Cinanserin	2.8	1.4
Cyproheptadine	3.0	1.0
l-LSD	2.4	1.0
d-LSD	5.5	1.3
Methysergide	5.5	2.0
Xylamidine	16.0	11.0
Chlorpromazine	32.0	24.0
Atropine	1600.0	750.0

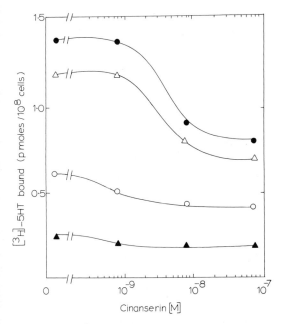

Fig. 10. Effect of Lilly 110140 on the specific binding of [³H]5HT to rat blood platelets at 4°C. (●—●), saline; (△–△), +Lilly 110140 (0.08 μM); (○–○), +Lilly 110140 (0.8 μM); (▲–▲), +Lilly 110140 (8.0 μM). Drugs and/or saline were preincubated with 0.1 ml PRP samples for 1 min at 4°C prior to the addition of 40 nM [³H]5HT.

high- and middle-affinity binding, 5HT uptake and the platelet shape-change induced by 5HT. There was high correlation between the inhibitory potency of these agents against high-affinity binding and the platelet shape-change, and a similar relationship was found when middle-affinity binding was compared with 5HT uptake.

There are certain accepted criteria which have to be fulfilled before the tissue binding of a ligand can be equated with an interaction of the ligand with its physiological receptor (Paton and Rang, 1965): binding should be reversible and

TABLE 5
Effect of 5HT uptake inhibitors on the uptake of [³H]5HT, the 5HT-induced platelet shape change and the high- and medium-affinity binding of [³H]5HT to intact rat blood platelets

| Compound | IC$_{50}$ (μM) against | | | |
	5HT-induced platelet shape change	High-affinity [³H]5HT binding	5HT uptake	Medium-affinity [³H]5HT binding
Chlorimipramine	0.40	0.50	0.20	0.43
Imipramine	0.25	0.10	0.70	0.61
Lilly 110140	4.00	0.40	0.50	0.40
Lilly 103947	0.82	—	0.25	0.52
Amitriptyline	—	—	1.20	1.15
Desipramine	0.40	—	7.50	4.50

saturable, with a rate of association similar to the rate of onset of the physiological response and with an affinity constant similar to that for the production of the response. Also, competitive inhibitors of this response should be equiactive against binding. The binding of 5HT to rat blood platelets was saturable, reversible and rapid in onset, reaching equilibrium within 60 sec. Because of the heterogeneous nature of the binding sites it was impossible to calculate accurate association and dissociation constants for the binding process, but there was significant binding within 10 sec even although the binding reaction was studied at 4°C. Using rat platelets, both the uptake process and the 5HT-induced shape-change are maximal within 10 sec at 37°C. The discrepancies between the rate of onset of binding and the rate of onset of the physiological response may be related to the lower temperature used in the study of the binding reaction.

The affinity constant $(2 \times 10^{-7} M)$ for the binding of [³H] 5HT to the middle-affinity site is comparable with the K_m for the uptake process in rat blood platelets $(8 \times 10^{-7} M)$ and in rat brain slices $(1.7 \times 10^{-7} M)$ (Shaskan and Snyder, 1970; Drummond and Gordon, 1976). Because the rate of 5HT uptake by rat platelets is extremely rapid (Buczko et al., 1975; Drummond and Gordon, 1976), accurate estimation of the initial rate (and hence the K_m) is difficult. Recently, Azzaro and Smith (1975) have shown that the methods currently available for the estimation of K_m values for amine transport processes do not necessarily measure solely the plasma membrane component of this system, and this is a further difficulty which must be considered when attempting to relate the receptor binding K_a^{-1} to the kinetic K_m value.

There is a large discrepancy between the K_a^{-1} for the high-affinity binding of 5HT $(6 \times 10^{-9} M)$ and the concentration of 5HT which causes a half-maximal shape change $(8 \times 10^{-7} M)$ (Drummond and Gordon, 1975a). Various other derivatives of 5HT which can also induce the platelet shape change by an action on 5HT receptors (e.g., 5-chloro-α-methyltryptamine, 3-(2-aminoethyl)-5-hydroxyindene and 3-(2-aminoethyl)-5-hydroxybenzofuran) were also at least 100 times more potent at inhibiting high-affinity [³H]5HT binding than in producing the shape-change (Drummond and Gordon, unpublished). These discrepancies may be largely due to the insensitivity of the optical system used to measure the shape-change, but it is also possible that we may be measuring the binding of 5HT to a desensitized receptor. Responses to 5HT in platelets are prone to tachyphylaxis (Baumgartner and Born, 1968; Hilton and Cumings, 1971; Evans and Gordon, 1974); this is rapid in onset, and it is entirely possible that, in our studies, desensitization of the high-affinity site could have occurred in the time required to separate the platelet-bound and free [³H]5HT. Cohen et al. (1974) have recently shown that the affinity of the nicotinic cholinergic receptor for agonists is increased after the receptor is desensitised, and this may also be true for other receptors. This possibility should be considered in all binding studies using radiolabelled agonists.

Gaddum and Picarelli (1957) originally classified 5HT receptors into two types; 'D' (sensitive to d-LSD and phenoxybenzamine) and 'M' (sensitive to morphine and atropine). The results presented above confirm the findings of Michal (1969) who showed that the platelet 5HT receptor has the general characteristics of a 'D'-type receptor. Various workers have, however, presented evidence that 5HT receptors on different tissues are more heterogeneous than is allowed by the classification of Gaddum and Picarelli (Wurzel, 1966; Saxena, Van Howelingen and Bonta, 1970; Vargaftig and Lefort, 1974) and this is especially true when one considers the known agonist action of d-LSD and methysergide on some tissues (Anden et al., 1968; Eyre, 1971; Haigler and Aghajanian, 1974). While neither d-LSD nor methysergide induced the rat platelet shape-change at concentrations up to 10^{-5} M (Drummond and Gordon, unpublished), both d- and l-LSD were potent antagonists at nanomolar concentrations. The non-hallucinogenic optical isomer, l-LSD, has been reported to be much less active than d-LSD as a 5HT antagonist (see Gyermek, 1961), and consequently our finding suggests either that 5HT receptors on different tissues are heterogeneous with regard to their sensitivity to inhibition by the optical isomers of LSD, or that the two batches of l-LSD made available to us were highly contaminated with the d-isomer.

Our observation that tricyclic antidepressants can inhibit high-affinity [^{3}H]5HT binding and the 5HT-induced shape-change confirms an earlier report that these drugs can also act as 5HT antagonists by a mechanism unrelated to their effects on uptake (Domenjoz and Theobald, 1959). The close correlation between the structure-activity relationships for inhibition of middle-affinity [^{3}H]5HT binding and inhibition of the active uptake of 5HT suggests that this binding site is related to the postulated 5HT transport carrier. Moreover, the fact that these drugs compete with 5HT for binding to this site supports the hypothesis that these drugs inhibit 5HT uptake by a direct action on the 5HT-binding carrier molecule.

Born and Bricknell (1959) studied the binding of [^{14}C]5HT to intact human blood platelets and concluded that there were approximately 10^4 5HT uptake receptors per cell. Because of the low specific activity of the radiolabelled 5HT available, these workers were unable to characterise these receptors fully. Our results enabled us to calculate that there are approximately 21,000 uptake receptors per cell, and are therefore in reasonable agreement with this early work. Since the maximum velocity of 5HT uptake by rat platelets is 63 pmoles/10 sec/10^8 cells (Drummond and Gordon, 1976), it is possible to estimate that a transport carrier moves one molecule of 5HT every 0.5 sec, assuming that each carrier binds one molecule of 5HT.

If we assume that the rat platelet is a flat disc with a diameter of 2.5 μm, then the receptor density for the high- and middle-affinity binding sites can be calculated to be 170 per μm^2 and 2500 per μm^2 respectively. However, the platelet membrane is contiguous with a surface-connected tubule system (Behnke, 1970) and if 5HT receptors are present within these invaginations the receptor density on the platelet surface could be much lower than our estimates.

Several groups have attempted to characterise the platelet membrane constituent involved in the active transport of 5HT. Sneddon and Williams (1974) showed that low concentrations of trypsin, which did not induce either the platelet release reaction or platelet damage, could specifically inhibit the uptake of 5HT by rat platelets. This suggests that the transport carrier for 5HT is protein in nature but it remains to be seen whether the inhibitory action of trypsin is an indirect effect resulting from the redistribution of membrane constituents or a direct effect on the carrier molecule itself. Other workers have been concerned with the role of platelet sialic acid in 5HT uptake: Glynn (1973) and Gielen and Viehöfer (1974) reported that prolonged incubation (30 min; 37°C) with unpurified neuraminidase reduced 5HT uptake by rabbit and human platelets, although the degree of inhibition recorded by the latter workers was slight. Glynn (1973) further showed that addition of a ganglioside preparation partially reversed the inhibition produced by the action of neuraminidase, and Szabados et al. (1975) found that by increasing the platelet sialic acid content they could enhance 5HT uptake. Although these studies apparently implicate platelet sialic acid-containing macromolecules in the uptake process, the specificity of the interaction has not been investigated.

5. Conclusions

The various reactions which human platelets undergo in response to biogenic amines are summarised in Fig. 11. Clearly, the blood platelet and the synaptic apparatus share many common features, but there are also several differences: the platelet uptake system for noradrenaline is unlike that in sympathetic nerves and hence the platelet should be considered as a model only for serotonergic and, perhaps, dopaminergic neurones. There is little information on dopamine-platelet interactions and therefore this discussion will only compare 5HT-platelet interactions with transmission at serotoninergic synapses.

Firstly, it is worth considering the possible functions of 5HT-related processes in blood platelets. If the role of the platelet is simply to transport 5HT from the enterochromaffin cells of the gut to the endothelial cells of the lung (White et al., 1975), it seems superfluous for the platelet to have a stimulatory site on its external membrane in addition to the uptake receptor. Although the stimulatory receptor may simply be an evolutionary legacy from amphibian and avian species in which 5HT has a primary role in haemostasis (see Belamarich et al., 1973) it clearly contributes to mammalian haemostasis also. Baumgartner and Born (1968), suggested that released platelet 5HT might initially potentiate haemostatic plug formation by combination with this stimulatory receptor, and then, since prolonged receptor occupation appeared to inhibit subsequent responses to aggregating agents in vitro, that this secondary inhibitory effect might help to restrict the intravascular growth of the plug. The platelet's active transport system for 5HT would be expected to limit the amine's effects on the stimulatory receptor, but it should be emphasized that ADP, which is released from platelets in parallel with 5HT, inhibits the active transport of 5HT (Drummond and Gordon, 1976). It would be interesting to determine whether the inhibitory effect of 5HT, observed after prolonged incubation, is mediated by inhibition of 5HT release in response to the haemostatic stimulus: if so, this could be similar to the feedback inhibition of neuronal firing which apparently occurs in 5HT-containing nerves (Haigler and

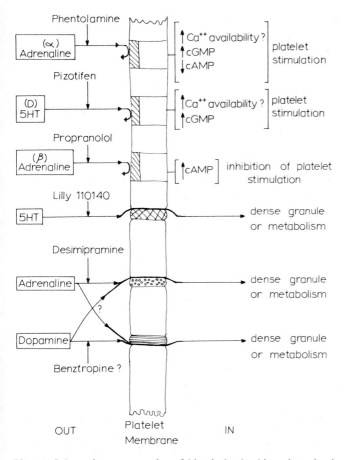

Fig. 11. Schematic representation of blood platelet–biogenic amine interactions.

Aghajanian, 1974; Hamon et al., 1974). A detailed comparison of these phenomena seems to be warranted.

There are several other features which are shared by the platelet and the serotonergic nerve terminal. The active transport and granular storage mechanisms appear to be almost identical, and platelets are useful models for the development of drugs directed against these processes. The innovatory work of Reimers, Allen, Feuerstein and Mustard (1975) on the compartmentalisation of 5HT in platelets and the estimation of intercompartmental 5HT fluxes could be applied to studies on the development of new antidepressant drugs (see Corrodi et al., 1975).

Schildkraut (1965) proposed that the anti-depressant action of the imipramine derivatives is related to their inhibitory effect on monoamine re-uptake into pre-synaptic nerve terminals. As a consequence of this, higher transmitter concentrations could be achieved at the post-synaptic stimulatory site, resulting in potentiation of transmitter activity. However, the potentiatory 'window' in the imipramine dose–response relationship is small because higher concentrations inhibit transmission–probably by blocking the post-synaptic 5HT- or catecholamine-stimulatory receptor (Domenjoz and Theobald, 1959; Sigg et al., 1963; Callingham, 1966; Bradshaw et al., 1974). If this spectrum of activity determines the anti-depressant action of these drugs (see Vetulani and Sulser, 1975), it would obviously be desirable to develop drugs that are potent monoamine uptake inhibitors but poor 5HT antagonists or α-blockers. The blood platelet is well suited for screening such agents, since it contains both stimulatory and uptake receptors on the same, easily obtainable, cell. Moreover, the effect of drugs on the two receptors can be measured under identical conditions by a simple and rapid assay (Barthel and Markwardt, 1975). The blood platelet could therefore be used as a cellular model not only for the presynaptic terminal, but for the entire serotoninergic synapse.

In the last four years, major advances have been made in the identification and characterisation of tissue receptors for various drugs and hormones using direct binding techniques (for reviews see Cuatrecasas, 1974; Birnbaumer et al., 1974), but despite its many advantages, the platelet has remained almost unexploited in this field. Most hormone–receptor binding studies have used plasma membrane-enriched cell fragments, and while these preparations contain receptor populations of increased specific activity, they also have a number of distinct disadvantages. Firstly, the degree of non-specific ligand binding (i.e., binding to non-receptor material) is relatively high, since the ligand has access to various physiologically inaccessible surfaces, notably the inner face of the plasma membrane. Secondly, because of the number of disruptive processes necessary to obtain these plasma membrane preparations, it is difficult to extrapolate quantitatively from one preparation to another. The blood platelet, however, is easily obtained as an intact, homogeneous cell suspension and problems related to ligand diffusion through a multicellular matrix, non-specific binding to unphysiological surfaces and heterogeneity of cell type are therefore minimal. By way of an example, the results reported in Section 4 indicate that greater than 90% of [^{3}H]5HT bound to intact rat platelets is associated with a pharmacologically-identifiable receptor.

The platelet contains specific receptors for a wide variety of hormones and drugs, and the ease with which human platelets can be obtained would allow the estimation of an individual's receptor status in a variety of physiological and pathological conditions.

Acknowledgements

I am grateful to Dr. J.L. Gordon for many helpful discussions and to Mrs. M. Drummond for typing this manuscript.

References

Abdulla, Y.H. (1969) J. Atheroscler. Res., *9*, 171.
Abrams, W.B. and Solomon, H.M. (1969) Clin. Pharmac. Ther., *10*, 702.
Ahtee, L. (1975) J. Pharm. Pharmacol., *27*, 177.
Ahtee, L. and Michal, F. (1972) Brit. J. Pharmac., *44*, 363.
Ahtee, L. and Saarnivaara, L. (1971) J. Pharm. Pharmac., *23*, 495.
Ahtee, L. and Saarnivaara, L. (1973) Brit. J. Pharmac., *47*, 808.
Ahtee, L., Tuomisto, J., Solatunturi, E. and Paasonen, M.K. (1968) Ann. Med. exp. Fenn., *46*, 429.
Anden, N.E., Corrodi, H., Fuxe, K. and Hokfelt, T. (1969) Brit. J. Pharmac., *34*, 1.
Ardlie, N.G., Glew, G. and Schwartz, C.J. (1966) Nature (London), *212*, 415.
Aurbach, G.D., Fedak, F.A., Woodward, C.J., Palmer, J.S., Hauser, D. and Troxler, F. (1974) Science, *186*, 1223.
Azzaro, A.J. and Smith, D.J. (1975) J. Neurochem., *24*, 811.
Barthel, W. and Markwardt, F. (1974) Biochem. Pharmac., *23*, 37.
Barthel, W. and Markwardt, F. (1975) Biochem. Pharmac., *24*, 1903.
Baumgartner, H.R. (1969) J. Physiol. (London), *201*, 409.
Baumgartner, H.R. and Born, G.V.R. (1968) Nature (London), *218*, 137.
Baumgartner, H.R. and Born, G.V.R. (1969) J. Physiol. (London), *201*, 397.
Baumgartner, H.R., Thoenen, H. and Tranzer, J.P. (1969) Experientia, *25*, 857.
Behnke, O. (1970) Ser. Haemat., *3*, 4, 3.
Belamarich, F.R. and Simoneit, L.W. (1973) Microvasc. Res., *6*, 229.
Belamarich, F.R., Stiller, R.A. and Shepro, D. (1973) Ser. Haemat., *6*, 3, 418.
Berneis, M.K., Da Prada, M. and Pletscher, A. (1969) Agents & Actions, *1*, 35.
Berneis, M.K., Da Prada, M. and Pletscher, A. (1974) Nature (London), *248*, 604.
Berry, D.G. and Miller, J.W. (1974) Eur. J. Pharmac., *28*, 164.
Berry, D.G. and Miller, J.W. (1975) Eur. J. Pharmac., *31*, 176.
Besterman, E.M.M. and Gillett, M.P.T. (1973) Nature New Biol., *241*, 223.
Birnbaumer, L., Pohl, S.L. and Kaumann, A.J. (1974) Adv. Cycl. Nucl. Res. (Greengard, P. and Robison, G.A., eds.), Vol. 4, p. 240, Raven Press, New York.
Booyse, F.M., Sternberger, L.A., Zschocke, D. and Rafelson, M.E. (1971) J. Histochem. Cytochem., *19*, 540.
Borga, O., Azarnoff, D., Forshall, G.P. and Sjoqvist, F. (1969) Biochem. Pharmac., *18*, 2135.
Born, G.V.R. (1962) Nature (London), *194*, 927.
Born, G.V.R. (1969) Proc. 4th Int. Cong. Pharmac. Schwabe, Basle.
Born, G.V.R. and Bricknell, J. (1959) J. Physiol. (London), *147*, 153.
Born, G.V.R. and Cross, M.J. (1963) J. Physiol. (London), *168*, 170.
Born, G.V.R. and Gillson, R.E. (1959) J. Physiol. (London), *146*, 472.
Born, G.V.R., Hornikiewicz, O. and Stafford, A. (1958) Brit. J. Pharmac., *13*, 411.
Born, G.V.R., Juengjaroen, K. and Michal, F. (1972) Brit. J. Pharmac., *44*, 117.
Born, G.V.R. and Smith, J.B. (1970) Brit. J. Pharmac., *39*, 765.
Boullin, D.J., Grahame-Smith, D.G., Grimes, R.P.J. and Woods, H.F. (1975a) Brit. J. Pharmac., *53*, 121.
Boullin, D.J., Grahame-Smith, D.G., Grimes, R.P.J. and Woods, H.F. (1975b) Brit. J. Pharmac., *2*, 37.
Boullin, D.J. and O'Brien, R.A. (1970) Brit. J. Pharmac., *39*, 779.
Boullin, D.J., Woods, H.F., Grimes, R.P.J., Grahame-Smith, D.G., Wiles, D., Gelder, M. and Kolakowska, T. (1975) Brit. J. Pharmac., *2*, 29.
Boullin, D.J., Woods, H.F., Youdim, M.B.H. and Callender, S. (1975) Fed. Proc., *34*, 220a.
Bradshaw, C.M., Roberts, M.H.T. and Szabadi, E. (1974) Brit. J. Pharmac., *52*, 349.
Brodie, B.B., Tomich, E.G., Kuntzman, R. and Shore, P.A. (1957) J. Pharmac. exp. Ther., *119*, 461.
Bruinvels, J. (1975) Nature (London), *257*, 606.
Buczko, W., de Gaetano, G. and Garattini, S. (1975) Brit. J. Pharmac., *53*, 563.
Bull, B.S., and Zucker, M.B. (1965) Proc. Soc. exp. Biol. Med., *120*, 296.
Buus Lassen, J., Squires, R.F., Christensen, J.A. and Molander, L. (1975) Psychopharmacologia (Berlin), *42*, 21.
Bygdeman, S. and Johnsen, O. (1969) Acta Physiol. Scand., *75*, 129.
Callingham, B.A. (1966) In Antidepressant Drugs, (Garattini, S. and Dukes, M.N.G., eds.), p. 35, Excerpta Medica, Amsterdam.
Campbell, I.C. and Todrick, A. (1973) Brit. J. Pharmac., *49*, 279.

Carlsson, A. (1970) J. Pharm. Pharmac., *22*, 729.
Carlsson, A., Corrodi, H., Fuxe, K. and Hokfelt, T. (1969a) Eur. J. Pharmac., *5*, 357.
Carlsson, A., Corrodi, H., Fuxe, K. and Hokfelt, T. (1969b) Eur. J. Pharmac., *5*, 367.
Clayton, S. and Cross, M.J. (1963) J. Physiol. (London), *169*, 82P.
Cohen, J.B., Weber, M. and Changeux, J.P. (1974) Mol. Pharmac., *10*, 904.
Constantine, J.W. (1966) Nature (London), *210*, 162.
Corrodi, H., Farnebo, L.O., Fuxe, K. and Hamberger, B. (1975) Eur. J. Pharmac., *30*, 172.
Crane, R.K. (1965) Fed. Proc., *24*, 1000.
Cuatrecasas, P. (1974) Ann. Rev. Biochem., *43*, 169.
Cumings, J.N. and Hilton, B.P. (1971) Brit. J. Pharmac., *42*, 611.
Da Prada, M., O'Brien, R.A., Tranzer, J.P. and Pletscher, A. (1973) J. Pharmac. exp. Ther., *186*, 213.
Da Prada, M., Obrist, R. and Pletscher, A. (1975a) Brit. J. Pharmac., *53*, 257.
Da Prada, M., Obrist, R. and Pletscher, A. (1975b) J. Pharm. Pharmac., *27*, 63.
Da Prada, M. and Pletscher, A. (1968) Brit. J. Pharmac., *34*, 591.
Da Prada, M. and Pletscher, A. (1969a) Life Sci., *8*, 65.
Da Prada, M. and Pletscher, A. (1969b) Experientia, *25*, 923.
Da Prada, M. and Pletscher, A. (1970) Life Sci., *9*, 1271.
Da Prada, M. and Pletscher, A. (1975) Eur. J. Pharmac., *32*, 179.
Da Prada, M., Pletscher, A., Tranzer, J.P. and Knuchel. H. (1967) Nature (London), *216*, 1315.
Da Prada, M., Von Berlepsch, K. and Pletscher, A. (1972) Naunyn Schmiedeberg's Arch. Pharmac., *275*, 315.
Davis, J.W., Yue, K.T.N. and Phillips, P.E. (1972) Thromb. Diath. haemorrh., *28*, 221.
De Clerck, F.F. and Reneman, R.S. (1973) Naunyn Schmiedeberg's Arch. Pharmac., *278*, 261.
Doery, J.C.G., Hirsh, J. and Mustard, J.F. (1973) Brit. J. Haemat., *25*, 657.
Domenjoz, R. and Theobald, W. (1959) Arch. Int. pharmacodyn. Ther., *120*, 450.
Drummond, A.H. and Gordon, J.L. (1974a) Thromb. Diath. haemorrh., *31*, 366.
Drummond, A.H. and Gordon, J.L. (1974b) J. Physiol. (London), *240*, 39P.
Drummond, A.H. and Gordon, J.L. (1975a) Biochem. J., *150*, 129.
Drummond, A.H. and Gordon, J.L. (1975b) Brit. J. Pharmac., *55*, 257.
Drummond, A.H. and Gordon, J.L. (1976) Brit. J. Pharmac. *56*, 417.
Enna, S.J., Da Prada, M. and Pletscher, A. (1974) J. Pharmac. exp. Ther., *191*, 164.
Erspamer, V. (1954) Pharmac. Rev., *6*, 425.
Estensen, R.D. and White, J.G. (1974) Amer. J. Path., *74*, 441.
Evans, R.J. and Gordon, J.L. (1974) Brit. J. Pharmac., *51*, 123P.
Eyre, P. (1971) Brit. J. Pharmac., *43*, 302.
Fuks, Z., Lanman, R.C. and Schanker, L.S. (1964) Int. J. Neuropharmac., *3*, 623.
Gaddum, J.H. and Picarelli, Z.P. (1957) Brit. J. Pharmac., *12*, 323.
Gielen, W. (1965) Hoppe Seyler's Z. Physiol. Chem., *342*, 170.
Gielen, W. and Viehöfer, B. (1974) Experientia, *30*, 1177.
Glynn, M.F.X. (1973) Amer. J. clin. Path., *60*, 636.
Goetz, U., Da Prada, M. and Pletscher, A. (1971) J. Pharmac. exp. Ther., *178*, 210.
Gordon, J.L. and Drummond, A.H. (1974) Biochem. J., *138*, 165.
Gordon, J.L. and Drummond, A.H. (1975) Biochem. Pharmac., *24*, 33.
Graham, J.D.P. (1964) Brit. J. Pharmac., *23*, 285.
Greenberg, J., Packham, M.A., Cazenave, J.P., Reimers, H.J. and Mustard, J.F. (1975) Lab. Invest., *32*, 476.
Grobecker, H. and Lemmer, B. (1971) Experientia, *27*, 299.
Gyermek, L. (1961) Pharmac. Rev., *13*, 399.
Haigler, H.J. and Aghajanian, G.K. (1974) J. Pharmac. exp. Ther., *188*, 688.
Hamon, M., Bourgoin, S., Jagger, J. and Glowinski, J. (1974) Brain. Res., *69*, 265.
Harbury, C.B. and Schrier, S.L. (1974) Thromb. Diath. haemorrh., *31*, 469.
Hardisty, R.M. and Stacey, R.S. (1955) J. Physiol. (London), *130*, 711.
Haslam, R.J. (1964) Nature (London), *202*, 765.
Haslam, R.J. (1967) in Physiology of Hemostasis and Thrombosis, (Johnson, S.A. and Seegers, W.H., eds.) p. 88, Charles C. Thomas, Springfield, Illinois.
Haslam, R.J. (1973) Ser. Haemat., *4*, 333.
Haslam, R.J. and Lynham, J.A. (1973) Life Sci., *11*, 1143.
Haslam, R.J. and Rosson, G.M. (1975) Mol. Pharmac. *11*, 528.
Heikkila, R.E., Orlansky, H. and Cohen, G. (1975) Biochem. Pharmac., *24*, 847.
Heinrich, P., Da Prada, M. and Pletscher, A. (1972) Biochem. Biophys. Res. Commun., *46*, 1769.

Hilton, B.P. and Cumings, J.N. (1971) J. clin. Path., *24*, 250.
Hilton, B.P. (1974) J. Neurol. Neurosurg. Psychiatr., *37*, 593.
Holmsen, H. (1972) Clin. Haemat., *1*, 235.
Holmsen, H. and Day, H.J. (1971) Ser. Haemat., *4*, 1, 28.
Holmsen, H., Day, H.J. and Stormorken, H. (1969) Scand. J. Haemat. Suppl., *8*, 1.
Holmsen, H., Setkowsky, C.A. and Day, H.J. (1974) Biochem. J., *144*, 385.
Hughes, F.B. and Brodie, B.B. (1959) J. Pharmac. exp. Ther., *127*, 96.
Humphrey, J.H. and Toh, C.C. (1954) J. Physiol. (London), *124*, 300.
Iversen, L.L. (1967) The Uptake and Storage of Noradrenaline in Sympathetic Nerves, Cambridge University Press.
Kikugawa, K., Suehiro, H. and Ichino, M. (1973) J. med. Chem., *16*, 1389.
Kinlough-Rathbone, R.L., Perry, D.W. and Mustard, J.F. (1974) Fed. Proc., *33*, 611a.
Kipnis, D.M. and Parrish, J.E. (1965) Fed. Proc., *24*, 1051.
Klein, T.W., Szentivanyi, A. and Fishel, C.W. (1974) Proc. Soc. exp. Biol. Med., *147*, 681.
Lages, B., Scrutton, M.C. and Holmsen, H. (1975) J. Lab. clin. Med., *85*, 811.
Lands, A.M., Arnold, A., McAuliff, J.P., Luduena, F.P. and Brown, T.G. (1967) Nature (London), *214*, 597.
Lefkowitz, R.J., Mukherjee, C., Coverstone, M. and Caron, M.G. (1974) Biochem. Biophys. Res. Commun., *60*, 703.
Lemmer, B. (1973) Eur. J. Pharmac., *21*, 183.
Lemmer, B., Wiethold, G., Hellenbrecht, D., Bak, I.J. and Grobecker, H. (1972) Naunyn Schmiedeberg's Arch. Pharmac., *275*, 299.
Lessin, A.W., Long, R.F. and Parkes, M.W. (1965) Brit. J. Pharmac., *24*, 68.
Levitzki, A., Atlas, D. and Steer, M.L. (1974) Proc. Natl. Acad. Sci. U.S.A., *71*, 2773.
Levy-Toledano, S. (1971) In Platelet Aggregation (Caen, J.P., ed.), p. 155, Masson, Paris.
Lingjaerde, O. (1969) Febs. Lett., *3*, 103.
Lingjaerde, O. (1970) Eur. J. Pharmac., *13*, 76.
Loeb, W.F. and Mackey, B. (1973) J. med. Primat., *2*, 195.
Lovenberg, W., Jequir, E. and Sjoerdsma, A. (1968) Adv. in Pharmac., *6A*, 21. Academic Press, New York.
McCoy, E.E., Segal, D.J., Bayer, S.M. and Strynadka, K.D. (1974) New Engl. J. Med., *291*, 950.
Macfarlane, D.E. (1974) Fed. Proc. *33*, 269a.
McLean, J.R. and Potoczak, D. (1969) Arch. Biochem. Biophys., *132*, 416.
Macmillan, D.C. (1966) Nature (London), *211*, 140.
Madoff, M.A., Ebbe, S. and Baldini, M. (1964) J. clin. Invest., *43*, 870.
Marcus, A., Safier, L. and Ullman, O. in Biochemistry and Pharmacology of Blood Platelets (CIBA Foundation) p. 309, Elsevier, Amsterdam.
Markwardt, F. (1968) Ann. Med. exp. Fenn., *46*, 407.
Marmaras, V.J. and Mimikos, N. (1971) Experientia, *27*, 196.
Marshall, E.F., Stirling, G.S., Tait, A.C. and Todrick, A. (1960) Brit. J. Pharmac., *15*, 35.
Mason, R.G., Read, M.S. and Shermer, R.W. (1974) Amer. J. Path., *76*, 323.
Mester, L., Szabados, L., Born, G.V.R. and Michal, F. (1972) Nature New Biol., *236*, 213.
Michal, F. (1969) Nature (London), *221*, 1253.
Michal, F. (1971) Acta Med. Scand. Suppl., *525*, 146.
Michal, F. and Born, G.V.R. (1971) Nature New Biol., *231*, 220.
Michal, F., Maguire, M.H. and Gough, G. (1969) Nature (London), *222*, 1073.
Michal, F. and Motamed, M. (1975) Brit. J. Pharmac., *54*, 221P.
Michal, F. and Penglis, F. (1969) J. Pharmac. exp. Ther., *166*, 276.
Mills, D.C.B. (1970) Symp. zool. Soc. Lond., *27*, 99.
Mills, D.C.B. (1973) Nature New Biol., *243*, 220.
Mills, D.C.B., Robb, I.A. and Roberts, G.C.K. (1968) J. Physiol. (London), *195*, 715.
Mills, D.C.B. and Roberts, G.C.K. (1967a) Nature (London), *213*, 35.
Mills, D.C.B. and Roberts, G.C.K. (1967b) J. Physiol. (London), *193*, 443.
Mills, D.C.B. and Smith, J.B. (1971) Biochem. J., *121*, 185.
Mitchell, J.R.A. and Sharp, A.A. (1964) Brit. J. Haemat., *10*, 78.
Mustard, J.F. (1975) Drugs, *9*, 19.
Mustard, J.F. and Packham, M.A. (1970) Pharmac. Rev., *22*, 97.
Mustard, J.F., Perry, D.W., Ardlie, N.G. and Packham, M.A. (1972) Brit. J. Haemat., *22*, 193.
Mustard, J.F., Perry, D.W., Kinlough-Rathbone, R.L. and Packham, M.A. (1975) Amer. J. Physiol., *228*, 1757.

Nachman, R.L. and Ferris, B. (1974) J. biol. Chem., *249*, 704.
O'Brien, J.R. (1962) J. clin. Path., *15*, 452.
O'Brien, J.R. (1963) Nature (London), *200*, 763.
O'Brien, J.R. (1964) J. clin. Path., *17*, 275.
O'Brien, J.R. (1965) Nature (London), *212*, 1057.
O'Brien, J.R. and Heywood, J.B. (1966) J. clin. Path., *19*, 148.
O'Brien, J.R., Shoobridge, S.M. and Finch, W.J. (1969) J. clin. Path., *22*, 28.
O'Brien, J.R. and Woodhouse, M.A. (1968) Exp. Biol. Med., *3*, 90.
Paasonen, M.K. (1965) J. Pharm. Pharmac., *17*, 681.
Paasonen, M.K. (1968) Ann. Med. exp. Biol. Fenn., *46*, 416.
Paton, W.D.M. and Rang, H.P. (1965) Proc. Roy. Soc. Lond., Ser. B., Biol. Sci., *163*, 1.
Phillips, J.H. (1974a) Biochem. J., *144*, 311.
Phillips, J.H. (1974b) Biochem. J., *144*, 319.
Pignatti, P.F. and Cavalli-Sforza, L.L. (1975) Neurobiology, *5*, 65.
Pletscher, A. (1968) Brit. J. Pharmac., *32*, 1.
Pletscher, A., Da Prada, M. and Bartholini, G. (1965) Biochem. Pharmac., *14*, 1135.
Pletscher, A., Da Prada, M. and Berneis, K.H. (1971) Mem. Soc. Endocr., *19*, 767.
Pletscher, A., Da Prada, M., Berneis, K.H. and Tranzer, J.P. (1971) Experientia, *27*, 993.
Portoghese, P.S., Riley, T.N. and Miller, J.W. (1971) J. med. Chem., *14*, 561.
Puszkin, E.G. and Zucker, M.B. (1973) Nature New Biol., *245*, 277.
Reimers, H.J., Allen, D.J., Feuerstein, I.A. and Mustard, J.F. (1975) J. cell. Biol., *65*, 359.
Reimers, H.J., Mustard, J.F. and Packham, M.A. (1975) J. cell. Biol., *67*, 61.
Richter, A. and Smith, S.E. (1974) J. Pharm. Pharmac., *26*, 763.
Roizen, M.F., Weise, V., Moss, J. and Kopin, I.J. (1975) Life Sci., *16*, 1133.
Rosner, F., Ong, B.H., Paine, R.S. and Mahanand, D. (1965) Lancet, *i*, 1191.
Rossi, E.C. and Levin, N.W. (1973) J. clin. Invest., *52*, 2457.
Rysanek, K., Svehla, C., Spankova, H. and Mlejnkova, M. (1968) J. Pharm. Pharmac., *20*, 154.
Sano, I., Kakimoto, Y. and Taniguchi, K. (1958) Amer. J. Physiol., *195*, 495.
Sano, I., Kakimoto, Y., Taniguchi, K. and Takesada, M. (1958) Amer. J. Physiol., *197*, 81.
Sarges, R., Koe, B.K., Weissman, A. and Schaefer, J.P. (1974) J. Pharmac. exp. Ther., *191*, 393.
Saxena, P.R., van Howelingen, P. and Bonta, I.L. (1970) Eur. J. Pharmac., *13*, 295.
Schildkraut, J.J. (1965) Amer. J. Psychiat., *122*, 509.
Seaman, G.V.F. and Brooks, D.E. (1969) Fed. Proc., *28*, 576a.
Shaskan, E.G. and Snyder, S.H. (1970) J. Pharmac. exp. Ther., *175*, 404.
Sigg, E.B., Soffer, L. and Gyermek, L. (1963) J. Pharmac. exp. Ther., *142*, 13.
Sinakos, Z. and Caen, J.P. (1967) Thromb. Diath. haemorrh., *17*, 99.
Skoza, L., Zucker, M.B., Jerushalmy, Z. and Grant, R. (1967) Thromb. Diath. haemorrh., *18*, 713.
Slotkin, T.A. (1973) Life Sci., *13*, 675–683.
Smith, A.D. (1968) in The interaction of drugs and subcellular components (Campbell, P.N., ed.), Churchill Press, London.
Smith, J.B. and Macfarlane, D.E. (1974) in Prostaglandins (Ramwell, P.W., ed.), Vol. 2, p. 293, Plenum Press, New York.
Sneddon, J.M. (1969) Brit. J. Pharmac., *37*, 680.
Sneddon, J.M. (1971) Brit. J. Pharmac., *43*, 834.
Sneddon, J.M. (1973) in Progress in Neurobiology (Kerkut, G.A. and Phillis, J.W., eds.), p. 151, Pergamon Press, Oxford.
Sneddon, J.M. and Williams, K.I. (1974) Brit. J. Pharmac., *52*, 237.
Snyder, S.H. (1975) Biochem. Pharmac., *24*, 1371.
Solomon, H.M., Spirt, N.M. and Abrams, W.B. (1970) Clin. Pharmac. Ther., *11*, 838.
Stacey, R.S. (1961) Brit. J. Pharmac., *16*, 284.
Szabados, L., Mester, L., Michal, F. and Born. G.V.R. (1975) Biochem. J., *148*, 335.
Tangen, O., Andrae, J.L. and Nilsson, B.E. (1973) Scand. J. Haemat., *11*, 241.
Tangen, O., Berman, H.J. and Marfey, P. (1971) Thromb. Diath. haemorrh., *25*, 268.
Thomas, D.P. (1968) Exp. Biol. Med., *3*, 129.
Tochino, Y. and Schanker, L.S. (1965) Biochem. Pharmac., *14*, 1557.
Todrick, A. and Tait, A.C. (1969) J. Pharm. Pharmac., *21*, 751.
Tranzer, J.P., Da Prada, M. and Pletscher, A. (1966) Nature (London), *212*, 1574.
Trenchard, A., Turner, P., PAre, C.M.B. and Hills, M. (1975) Psychopharmacologia, *43*, 89.
Tschopp, T.B. (1970) Thromb. Diath. haemorrh., *23*, 601.

Tu, J.B. and Zellweger, H. (1965) Lancet, *ii*, 715.
Tuomisto, J. (1973) Naunyn Schmiedeberg's Arch. Pharmac., *279*, 361.
Tuomisto, J. (1974) J. Pharm. Pharmac., *26*, 92.
Tuomisto, J. and Walaszek, E.J. (1974) Med. Biol., *52*, 255.
Tuomisto, J., Walaszek, E.J., Smissman, E.E. and Pazdernik, T.L. (1974) J. Pharm. Sci., *63*, 1714.
Vargaftig, B.B. and Lefort, J. (1974) Eur. J. Pharmac., *25*, 216.
Vetulani, J. and Sulser, F. (1975) Nature (London), *257*, 495.
Walsh, P.N. (1972) Brit. J. Haemat., *22*, 205.
Weiss, H.J. (1975a) New Engl. J. Med., *293*, 531.
Weiss, H.J. (1975b) New Engl. J. Med., *293*, 580.
Weissbach, H. and Redfield, B.G. (1960) J. Biol. Chem., *235*, 3287.
White, J.G. (1970) Scand. J. Haemat., *7*, 145.
White, J.G. (1974) Thromb. Diath. haemorrh. Suppl., *60*, 159.
White, M.K., Hechtman, H.B. and Shepro, D. (1975) Microvasc. Res., *9*, 230.
Wong, D.T., Bymaster, F.P., Horng, J.S. and Molloy, B.B. (1975) J. Pharmac. exp. Ther., *193*, 804.
Wong, D.T., Horng, J.S., Bymaster, F.P., Hauser, K.L. and Molloy, B.B. (1974) Life Sci., *15*, 471.
Woolley, D.W. (1958) Proc. Natl. Acad. Sci. U.S.A., *44*, 1202.
Wurzel, M. (1966) Amer. J. Physiol., *211*, 1424.
Yates, C.M., Todrick, A. and Tait, A.C. (1964) J. Pharm. Pharmac., *16*, 460.
Zucker, M.B. (1972) Thromb. Diath. haemorrh., *28*, 393.
Zucker, M.B. and Borelli, J. (1956) Amer. J. Physiol., *186*, 105.
Zucker, M.B. and Borelli, J. (1958) Ann. N.Y. Acad. Sci., *75*, 203.
Zucker, M.B., Troll, W. and Belman, S. (1974) J. cell. Biol., *60*, 325.
Zucker, W.H., Shermer, R.W. and Mason, R.G. (1974) Amer. J. Pathol. *77*, 255.

CHAPTER 9

The interaction of platelets
with thrombin

P.W. MAJERUS, D.M. TOLLEFSEN and M.A. SHUMAN

Washington University School of Medicine, Hematology Division, Box 8125, 600 South Euclid,
St Louis, Missouri 63110, U.S.A.

1. Introduction

The details of the mechanisms by which platelets function in hemostasis are essentially unknown. While a number of experimental observations suggest that collagen, cyclic prostaglandin endoperoxides and ADP play central roles in the processes of platelet aggregation and secretion, the precise role of these agents in in vivo hemostasis and their relationship to each other are not clear.

The first step in hemostasis that can be defined morphologically is the adhesion of platelets to collagen or other substances found in the tissues beneath the vascular endothelium. This interaction does not explain the major growth of the platelet plug, however, since most platelets do not come into contact with the vessel wall. Most investigators postulate that subsequent aggregation and release are mediated by ADP or by prostaglandin G_2 or thromboxane A_2 (Hamberg et al., 1975), released by the platelets initially interacting with the vessel wall. In this view platelet aggregation and secretion occur prior to and independent of the coagulation reactions leading to fibrin formation (for recent review, see Weiss, 1975). An alternative hypothesis suggests that early reactions of platelet function in hemostasis are triggered by minute amounts of thrombin which are formed prior to generation of a fibrin clot. Thus, a number of potentially important hemostatic reactions are catalyzed by concentrations of thrombin well below that required to clot fibrinogen. These include the activation of factors VIII and V as well as the initiation of platelet aggregation and the release reaction. This hypothesis has not been subject to test since assays which could detect minute amounts of thrombin which may be generated early in hemostasis are not available.

Regardless of the uncertainties concerning the precise roles of the various platelet-aggregating agents during hemostasis, a considerable amount of information about platelet function has been accumulated by studying the effects of these agents in vitro. Thrombin has certain advantages over ADP and collagen for such studies. For example, ADP will not aggregate platelets that have been washed free

Gordon (ed) Platelets in Biology and Pathology
© *Elsevier/North-Holland Biomedical Press, 1976*

from plasma (Ardlie and Han, 1974), and the secretory reaction observed with ADP is variable and partial, depending on conditions used (Ardlie and Han, 1974; Mills et al., 1968). Collagen-induced aggregation depends critically on the source of the collagen preparation as well as on the state of polymerization of collagen monomers (Kang et al., 1974; Brass and Bensusan, 1974), which has proven difficult to control experimentally. On the other hand, purified thrombin is readily available, and it will cause secretion and aggregation at low concentrations (< 1 nM) in suspensions of washed platelets.*

The mechanism by which thrombin induces platelet aggregation and secretion has been investigated intensively during recent years. Davey and Luscher have reported that thrombin inactivated with diisopropyl fluorophosphate is unable to induce secretion and aggregation, while certain other proteases are able to induce these reactions (Davey and Luscher, 1967). These experiments suggest that a proteolytic step is involved in triggering the reactions, but no direct evidence for proteolysis has been obtained. Thrombin catalyzes the hydrolysis of single arginylglycine peptide bonds in the $A\alpha$ and $B\beta$ chains of fibrinogen (Bettelheim, 1956). Studies with other proteases suggest that arginyl specificity is also required for induction of secretion in platelets (Davey and Luscher, 1967; Martin et al., 1975). Several proteins that have been identified in platelets, including fibrinogen (Ganguly, 1972), platelet factor XIII (Kisselbach and Wagner, 1966), and the contractile protein thrombosthenin M (Cohen et al., 1969), have peptide bonds susceptible to hydrolysis by thrombin, but none of these has been shown to be hydrolyzed in intact platelets during aggregation and release.

Recently, Phillips and Agin have reported that a platelet membrane glycoprotein (mol. wt 118,000), which is labeled by the lactoperoxidase iodination technique and is therefore presumably located on the outer surface of the platelet, is reduced in quantity by 10–50% when intact platelets are exposed to thrombin (Phillips and Agin, 1974). They concluded that this protein is a substrate for thrombin. Proof of this, however, would require identification of the products of hydrolysis. Furthermore, these workers have not correlated hydrolysis of glycoprotein with platelet physiology. In their experiments hydrolysis was shown only after 30 min at 10 U thrombin/ml. These conditions using 100-fold greater thrombin concentration and 10-fold longer time than required for maximal platelet release by thrombin do not establish that glycoprotein hydrolysis has any relationship to the physiological effect of thrombin on platelets. We have described another membrane protein (mol. wt 190,000) designated 'thrombin-sensitive protein' that disappears similarly from intact platelets treated with thrombin (Baenziger et al., 1971). However, we subsequently showed that this protein is released into the medium from platelets in a form that is indistinguishable from that present in the untreated platelet (Baenziger, et al., 1972), and that it is released by certain phytohemagglutinins that have no proteolytic activity (Majerus and Brodie, 1972). We concluded that this protein is not a substrate for thrombin.

---

* For purposes of this paper, pure thrombin is considered to have a specific activity of 3000 U/mg as measured in a fibrinogen clotting assay (Fasco and Fenton, 1973), and a molecular weight of 37,000. Thus, 1 nM thrombin ≅ 0.1 U/ml.

The above-mentioned studies have been directed at determining the *mechanism* by which thrombin triggers platelet reactions while numerous other studies have defined effects of thrombin on platelets including those on cAMP metabolism (Brodie et al., 1972; Salzman, 1972), protein phosphorylation (Lyons et al., 1975), lipid synthesis (Lewis and Majerus, 1969), prostaglandin synthesis (Hamberg et al., 1974), carbohydrate metabolism, and on secretion and aggregation (Weiss, 1975). These latter observations however only define the components and physiology of the platelet release reaction and do not explain the action of thrombin per se. Thus, release and aggregation are accompanied by the above metabolic effects when produced by a wide variety of agents working by mechanisms undoubtedly quite different from that of thrombin.

In this chapter we describe a series of experiments from our laboratory which study thrombin in another way. We have defined a cell surface receptor for thrombin, binding to which appears to be the first step in the action of thrombin on platelets. These experiments have demonstrated that the platelet surface contains highly specific receptors for thrombin and that the receptor–thrombin interaction has properties which strikingly resemble the hormone–receptor interactions defined in studies of a variety of endocrine tissues. In fact, many of the characteristics of the platelet–thrombin reaction are better described in terms of a hormone–hormone receptor interaction than by a catalytic or enzymatic reaction. Detweiler and Feinman (1973a,b), have come to a similar conclusion from a completely different type of experimental study. They have undertaken a detailed kinetic analysis of the secretion of Ca^{2+} and ATP from platelets and have concluded that thrombin does not turn over when it triggers platelet reactions, a result consistent with a hormone–receptor interaction but not with a typical enzymatic reaction.

2. Thrombin binding to platelets

We have utilized radioiodinated thrombin to demonstrate a platelet surface receptor (Tollefsen et al., 1974). In order to perform valid binding studies, two conditions must be met. First, the thrombin used must be free of contaminating proteins so that the specific radioactivity of the thrombin can be used to calculate the amount bound to the cell. If contaminating proteins were iodinated but did not bind or were iodinated to a different extent than thrombin, the specific radioactivity estimate would be in error. Secondly, it is essential that the radioactive thrombin not be denatured by the iodination process. This latter condition is shown most clearly by experiments where unlabeled thrombin is shown to compete for binding with labeled thrombin (see below). For our studies we have used both human thrombin and bovine thrombin. Both proteins were pure as judged by SDS polyacrylamide gel electrophoresis and by their high specific clotting activity ($> 2,000$ U/mg protein).

Thrombin binds to platelets as shown in Fig. 1. A correction for nonspecific binding to platelets and to Millipore filters was necessary and was made by adding

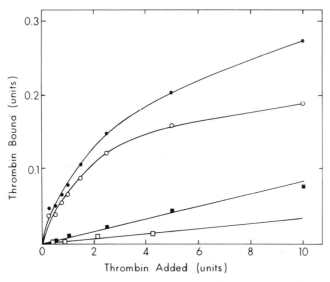

Fig. 1. Binding of ^{125}I-thrombin to platelets. Each incubation included 0.5×10^8 platelets and the specified amount of thrombin in 0.5 ml of Tris-buffered saline (pH 7.5), containing 5 mg/ml bovine serum albumin. Incubations were initiated by addition of platelets. After 30 min at room temperature, the platelets were collected by Millipore filtration: (●–●), total ^{125}I-thrombin; (■–■), non-specific binding of ^{125}I-thrombin in the presence of 200 units of unlabeled thrombin; (○–○), net ^{125}I-thrombin bound calculated by subtracting non-specific binding; (□–□), total ^{125}I-thrombin bound to 0.25×10^8 erythrocytes. (From Tollefsen, et al., 1974.)

excess unlabeled thrombin to duplicate reaction mixtures containing labeled thrombin. As shown in Fig. 1, the non-specific ^{125}I-thrombin bound was proportional to the total amount added and did not saturate with addition of excess unlabeled thrombin. We therefore corrected each value for ^{125}I-thrombin bound by subtracting the value obtained in the duplicate incubation containing excess unlabeled thrombin. The magnitude of the correction for nonspecific binding varied as shown in Fig. 1 from 7% to 30% of the total thrombin bound, the latter at the very high concentration of thrombin added. For all of the measurements, equilibrium binding occurred within 10 to 15 min. Figure 1 also shows that thrombin binds minimally to erythrocytes indicating that the thrombin receptor is specific for platelets. Additional experiments using human diploid skin fibroblasts indicate that human thrombin does not bind to these cells, further indicating the specificity of the thrombin receptor on platelets (N. Baenziger, unpublished observations).

To determine the number of thrombin receptor sites per platelet as well as their affinity, binding data were plotted (Figs. 2 and 3) according to the method of Steck and Wallach (1965). When plotted in this manner, the number of molecules bound at saturation can be calculated from the intercept on the ordinate and the apparent dissociation constant (K_{diss}) can be calculated from the intercept on the abscissa. From a number of different experiments similar to that shown in Fig. 2 using both human and bovine thrombin as well as different platelet preparations, we have

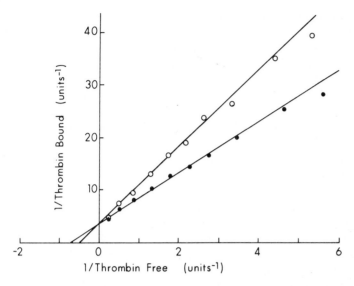

Fig. 2. Binding of ^{125}I-thrombin to platelets and competitive inhibition by DIP-thrombin. Incubations were conducted as in Fig. 1 with 0.213 to 4.25 units of ^{125}I-thrombin and 0.5×10^8 platelets in a total volume of 0.5 ml. Data are plotted according to the method of Steck and Wallach (1965). The intercept on the ordinate equals 1/thrombin bound at saturation per 0.5×10^8 platelets. The intercept on the abscissa equals -1/thrombin free per 0.5 ml (K_{diss}) at which level half-maximal binding occurs. (●–●), ^{125}I-thrombin; (○–○), ^{125}I-thrombin + 0.95 unit of unlabeled DIP-thrombin. (From Tollefsen, et al., 1974.)

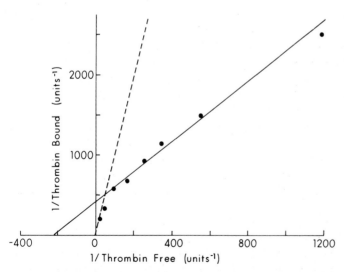

· Fig. 3. Binding of ^{125}I-thrombin to platelets. This experiment is analogous to that described in Fig. 2 except that lower levels of ^{125}I-thrombin (0.00125 to 0.050 U/0.5 ml) were used. (– – –), extrapolation of the data presented in Fig. 2 for ^{125}I-thrombin binding in the absence of DIP-thrombin. (From Tollefsen, et al., 1974.)

determined that platelets bind 30,000 to 50,000 thrombin molecules per cell with a dissociation constant which ranges from approximately 1 to 5 U/ml (10 to 50 nM thrombin). The range in the number of thrombin binding sites and the affinity is both due to differences in individual platelet preparations as well as to differences in various thrombin preparations. In general, it appears that human thrombin binds with slightly less affinity ($\cong$ 2-fold) than bovine thrombin to human platelets. Whether this small difference is due to an actual difference in the platelet binding site on human thrombin from that on bovine thrombin is not clear. The efficiency of the thrombin from the two species in inducing serotonin release is identical per amount of thrombin bound (Shuman and Majerus, 1976). When a small constant amount of unlabeled thrombin (0.2–2 U/ml in different experiments) is present during the measurement of binding of ^{125}I-thrombin, competitive inhibition of binding is observed. The inhibition constant (K_i) calculated for unlabeled thrombin is identical to the dissociation constant for ^{125}I-thrombin determined in the same experiment. Thus, we conclude that iodination does not alter the affinity of thrombin nor the number of platelet receptors to which it binds.

When thrombin binding to platelets is measured at very low thrombin levels (1 to 100 mU/ml), different binding characteristics are seen as shown in Fig. 3. At the lowest thrombin concentration an apparently linear relationship is observed when the results were plotted by the method of Steck and Wallach suggesting a small number of binding sites, approximately 300 to 600 per cell, having a very high thrombin binding affinity ranging from 0.005 to 0.02 U/ml using various preparations of human and bovine thrombin. At higher concentrations, the curve becomes distinctly non-linear and the points approach the line extrapolated from the data in Fig. 2. These results suggest that platelets possess at least two populations of thrombin binding sites. Depending on how data are plotted, other intermediate populations of receptor sites can be observed. The properties of the high affinity sites are similar to those for the other thrombin sites in that native unlabeled thrombin competes for these sites. From these experiments it is not clear whether the platelet contains more than one physically distinct class of thrombin binding sites or whether there is a single class of sites which showed negative cooperativity of binding, i.e., the affinity of receptor sites decreases as more thrombin is bound. Other experiments described below suggest that the latter hypothesis is more consistent with the data, i.e., that platelets contain a single class of thrombin receptor sites which show an interaction among sites leading to apparent negative cooperativity of binding.

3. Localization of bound thrombin

While the above-described binding experiments suggest a cell surface receptor for thrombin, it was necessary to establish that the thrombin bound was in fact located on the cell surface. We utilized electron microscopic autoradiography with highly radioiodinated thrombin to demonstrate that thrombin is localized on the cell surface (Fig. 4). Over one hundred cells were examined and total of 400

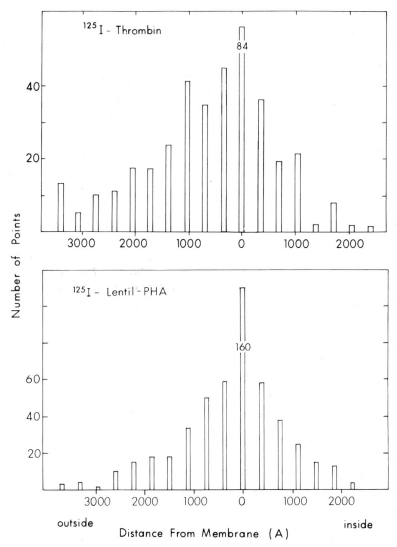

Fig. 4. Distribution of autoradiographic grains in relation to the platelet plasma membrane. The perpendicular distance was measured from the center of each grain to the plasma membrane. *Top*, 2.0 U/ml of ^{125}I-thrombin incubated with platelets for 10 min prior to fixation; *bottom*, 50 μg/ml of ^{125}I-lentil PHA, 10 min prior to fixation. (From Tollefsen, et al., 1974.)

thrombin grains were counted. For each grain on an autoradiograph, the perpendicular distance from the center of the grain to the nearest surface membrane was measured. For purposes of these measurements, the membranes of the platelet canalicular system were considered as surface membrane since these membranes are continuous with the platelet surface. Approximately 15% of the grains were judged to be associated with the channel system. The distribution of the grains is shown in Fig. 4. The mean position for ^{125}I-thrombin was 490 ± 90 Å S.E.M. outside the platelet membrane suggesting that the thrombin receptor is localized in the glycoprotein coat of the platelet surface. A similar localization was obtained using ^{125}I-lentil PHA (mean 240 ± 50 Å S.E.M. outside the platelet membrane). The latter protein is known to bind to a platelet surface oligosaccharide. As further support for surface localization of bound thrombin, we have also noted that ^{125}I-thrombin can be rapidly displaced from platelets by excess unlabeled thrombin as described below. Thrombin can be removed from both 'high- and low-affinity' sites in this manner.

4. Characteristics of the thrombin receptor

The binding of thrombin to human platelets apparently does not depend on an intact catalytic active site since thrombin inactivated with diisopropyl fluorophosphate (DIP) binds to platelets in a manner identical to native thrombin. There was equivalent binding of DIP-thrombin and native thrombin both at high- and low-affinity binding sites. Thus, native and DIP-thrombin compete for the same platelet receptor sites with equal affinity yet DIP-thrombin does not itself cause aggregation or release. In contrast, an acetylated thrombin derivative which retains esterase activity does not bind to human platelets at either high- or low-affinity sites, thus suggesting that some part of the thrombin molecule distinct from the catalytic site is required for the platelet receptor–thrombin interaction. A similar situation exists in regard to the clotting of fibrinogen where acetylated thrombin does not catalyze fibrinogen clotting. While the above experiments might suggest that proteolysis is required for the thrombin-induced release reaction, it is not necessary to postulate proteolysis to explain these results. Thus, inactivation of the active site of thrombin with DIP may result in some conformational change in the molecule, which though it does not interfere with binding to the platelet receptor does block some other functional property of the molecule required for triggering the release reaction. In the case of the interaction of insulin (or derivatives of insulin) with its receptor on fat cells or liver cells there is close correlation between binding affinity and biological activity (Cuatrecasas, 1974). Thus, there is no clear precedent for the dissociation of receptor binding and physiological activity seen with DIP-thrombin. Evidence that the DIP-thrombin–thrombin receptor interaction has some functional effect on the platelets is shown in the experiment depicted in Fig. 5. In this experiment, we show that DIP-thrombin is able to displace active thrombin from the platelets. In this manner one might expect DIP-thrombin to inhibit the release reaction induced by native thrombin. The dependence of [^{14}C]serotonin release on native thrombin concentration in the presence and absence of DIP-thrombin is shown in the figure. DIP-thrombin does not prevent thrombin-induced release of serotonin at concentrations which greatly inhibit the amount of native thrombin bound to the platelet, e.g., at 33 U/ml of DIP-thrombin plus 0.1 U/ml of native thrombin, binding is reduced by 90% to $0.2 \, \text{mU}/0.5 \times 10^8$ platelets, while the serotonin release of

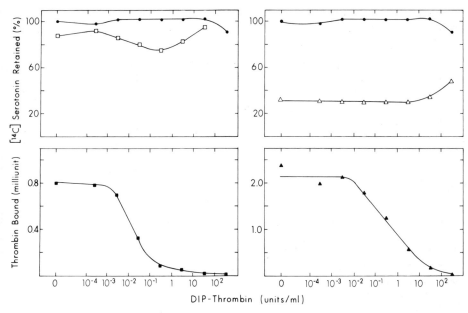

Fig. 5. Effect of DIP-thrombin on ^{125}I-thrombin binding and on [^{14}C]serotonin release. Two-minute incubations were performed at 0.01 U/ml (*left panels*) and 0.1 U/ml (*right panels*) of thrombin (total volume 0.5 ml). DIP-thrombin (unlabeled) was varied from 3.3×10^2 to 3.3×10^{-4} U/ml. Serotonin release is presented as serotonin retained in platelets collected on Millipore filters. (●–●), DIP-thrombin alone; (□–□), 0.01 U/ml of unlabeled thrombin; (△–△), 0.1 U/ml of unlabeled thrombin; (■–■), 0.01 U/ml of ^{125}I-thrombin; (▲–▲), 0.1 U/ml of ^{125}I-thrombin. (From Tollefsen, et al., 1974.)

approximately 70% is only slightly affected. By comparison 0.01 U/ml of native thrombin in the absence of DIP-thrombin resulted in 0.8 mU bound but only about 10% of maximum serotonin release occurred. Thus, it appears that DIP-thrombin has resulted in a marked increase in the efficiency of release per thrombin molecule bound. As outlined below, the release of serotonin correlates rather precisely with the number of thrombin molecules bound to the platelet. It is clear here that DIP-thrombin is not inert but, in fact, markedly potentiates the effect of native thrombin. The effects of DIP-thrombin are not explained by kinetic differences in binding or release since time course studies of the rate of thrombin binding and on serotonin release in presence and absence of DIP-thrombin show no difference. The basis for the difference between native and DIP-thrombin on platelet triggering remains unexplained. Other proteolytic enzymes including trypsin and papain are known to stimulate platelet aggregation and the release reaction (Davey and Luscher, 1967; Martin et al., 1975). We have studied whether these proteases interfere with thrombin interaction with the thrombin receptor. Neither trypsin nor papain had any effect on thrombin binding to human platelets. For these experiments it was necessary to use DIP-trypsin since native trypsin destroys thrombin itself. At concentrations of DIP-trypsin of 1 mg/ml, 100-fold greater than required to cause release by trypsin itself, there was no interference with thrombin binding indicating that the release reaction stimulated by trypsin does not proceed through the thrombin receptor mechanism.

In other experiments we studied the binding of prothrombin and the intermediates involved in the conversion of prothrombin to thrombin, including intermediate 1 and intermediate 2, on binding to platelets (Tollefsen et al., 1975). These experiments demonstrated that none of these three thrombin precursors binds to intact platelets, nor do they compete with thrombin for binding to the platelet receptor. It is particularly interesting that intermediate 2 does not bind since hydrolysis of a single peptide bond converts single chain intermediate 2 to the 2-chain disulfide bonded thrombin. Thus, intermediate 2 with the identical amino acid sequence of thrombin has essentially no affinity for the platelet receptor. The molecular conformation required for binding to platelets occurs only after the final step in prothrombin activation. The finding that the intermediates of prothrombin activation do not affect the thrombin-induced platelet reaction implies that these intermediates do not modulate platelet function mediated by thrombin. It is well established that phospholipid dispersions enhance the rate of prothrombin activation in vitro. Prothrombin and factor Xa bind to phospholipid vesicles in a process requiring calcium ions while thrombin does not bind. It is generally assumed that platelets provide the catalytic surface analogous to phospholipid vesicles for prothrombin activation in vivo. It is thus of interest that there was no detectable binding of prothrombin to platelets either before or after the thrombin-induced release reaction, regardless of the presence or absence of calcium ions. We do not conclude from this that prothrombin binding to platelets does not occur since further experiments are required to determine whether prothrombin binding can be detected under other conditions or by other techniques. Specifically, we would not have detected binding if the dissociation rate were very rapid such that a large fraction of the bound prothrombin dissociated within the time (5 sec) taken for dilution and filtration of platelet suspensions by the Millipore filtration binding technique used for these experiments.

5. *Further studies on the kinetics of thrombin binding*

When equilibrium binding data over the range 0.0002 to 10 U/ml of thrombin added are plotted according to the Hill equation (Levitski and Koshland, 1969), as shown in Fig. 6, a Hill coefficient of 0.775 is obtained. A value of less than 1.0 suggests, but does not prove, a negative cooperative interaction among a single population of platelet receptor sites for thrombin. From equilibrium binding measurements alone, it is not possible to distinguish negative cooperativity from heterogeneous receptor sites with different affinities for thrombin.

Many polypeptide hormones, including insulin (Hammond et al., 1972; Gavin et al., 1973), glucagon (Marinetti et al., 1972), adrenocorticotropic hormone (Lefkowitz et al., 1970), and oxytocin (Bockaert et al., 1972), exhibit equilibrium binding to their target tissues that is similar to that of thrombin. Recently,

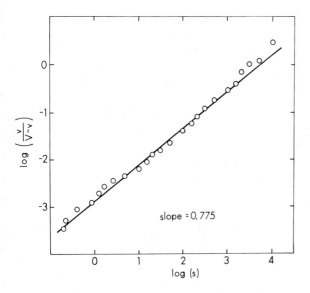

Fig. 6. Hill plot of thrombin binding to platelets. Incubations were conducted as in Fig. 1 with 0.2 mU/ml to 10 U/ml of labeled thrombin and a platelet concentration of 1×10^8/ml. Incubations were terminated by Millipore filtration after 30 min, and the amounts of bound and free thrombin were determined. The maximum number of thrombin molecules bound at a saturating thrombin concentration was calculated as in Fig. 2 by the method of Steck and Wallach (1965), using data from the six highest thrombin concentrations to construct the double reciprocal plot. s = free thrombin (mU/ml). v = thrombin bound (mU/10^8 platelets). V = maximum amount of thrombin bound at saturation (mU/10^8 platelets).

DeMeyts, et al. (1973), have devised a direct kinetic test of the negative cooperativity hypothesis of hormone binding. They studied the dissociation of ^{125}I-insulin from its receptor on human lymphocytes under two conditions: (a) by diluting the hormone-receptor complex to an extent sufficient to prevent rebinding of the dissociated hormone; and (b) by dilution to the same extent in a medium containing an excess of unlabeled hormone. They reasoned that if the receptor sites are independent, the dissociation rate should be the same in both cases. If the presence of unlabeled hormone increases the dissociation rate of the labeled hormone, a negative cooperative interaction must be occurring. The latter result was found in the case of insulin.

We have performed similar experiments with platelets and thrombin. Platelets were exposed to a relatively low level of ^{125}I-DIP-thrombin (0.04 U/ml) at which high affinity binding is observed, and after equilibrium had been reached the platelets were sedimented and resuspended in the original volume of buffer in the absence of thrombin or in the presence of 14 U/ml of unlabeled thrombin. The amount of ^{125}I-DIP-thrombin that remained bound to the platelets was measured at various times after resuspension (Fig. 7).

The total concentration of thrombin remaining in this experiment after resuspension is about 0.004 U/ml. This level of thrombin would reach a new equilibrium of binding, as determined in other experiments, at which the amount of thrombin

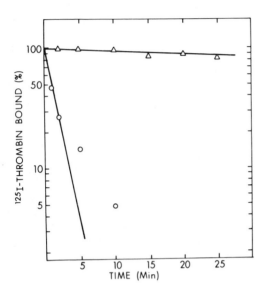

Fig. 7. Dissociation of thrombin from high-affinity binding sites. Platelets were incubated at a concentration of 1×10^8/ml with 0.04 U/ml of ^{125}I-DIP-thrombin. After 30 min the platelet suspension was centrifuged at $2250 \times g$ for 15 min at room temperature, and the supernate containing unbound thrombin was removed. The platelets were quickly resuspended in the original volume of isotonic Tris-buffered saline (10 ml) and divided into two portions, to one of which was added 14 U/ml of unlabeled thrombin. At various times after the addition of the unlabeled thrombin, 0.5 ml aliquots were removed and filtered to determine the thrombin bound. Data are plotted as the percentage of the thrombin originally bound (4.0 mU/10^8 platelets). (O–O), tube containing excess unlabeled thrombin. (△–△), tube without additional thrombin.

bound would be about 1/5 the amount bound at 0.04 U/ml. Thus, reassociation of labeled thrombin is negligible, at least at early time points.

As shown in Fig. 7, the dissociation rate is much greater in the presence than in the absence of excess unlabeled thrombin. This observation suggests that as the unlabeled thrombin itself binds to the platelets the association between platelet receptor sites and the ^{125}I-DIP-thrombin originally bound is weakened. This could be explained by a negative cooperative interaction among receptor sites for thrombin. If there were no site–site interaction, the dissociation rate of thrombin from high affinity sites would be independent of the binding of additional thrombin molecules to unoccupied sites.

The dissociation rate of low affinity thrombin binding (1.0 U/ml of ^{125}I-DIP-thrombin added) was also determined (Fig. 8). As one would predict, the initial rate of dissociation was similar to that obtained in the previous experiment (Fig. 7) in the presence of excess unlabeled thrombin. Association rates were also determined both at 0.04 U/ml and at 1.0 U/ml using the same preparation of ^{125}I-DIP-thrombin. These data are shown in Figs. 9 and 10.

Rate constants for thrombin binding were determined from the data above (see Table 1). First order rate constants for dissociation (k_2) were determined directly from the initial slopes of the semilogarithmic plots in Figs. 7 and 8. Rate constants

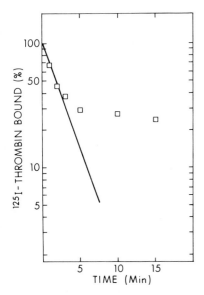

Fig. 8. Dissociation of thrombin from low-affinity binding sites. This experiment was carried out in the same manner as in Fig. 7, except that 1.0 U/ml of ^{125}I-DIP-thrombin was used. In addition, no unlabeled thrombin was added after resuspension of the platelets. The timer was started at the beginning of the resuspension, which took about 20 sec to complete. The amount of thrombin originally bound (100%) was 30 mU/10^8 platelets.

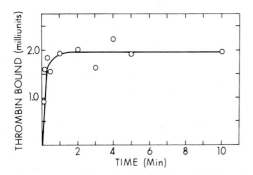

Fig. 9. Association of thrombin with platelets. Each time point represents a separate incubation containing 5×10^7 platelets in 0.5 ml of isotonic Tris-buffered saline with 0.04 U/ml of ^{125}I-DIP-thrombin. At the indicated times the incubations were terminated by Millipore filtration. The data are corrected for nonspecific binding as in Fig. 1.

for association (k_1) were calculated from the equation: initial association rate = $k_1[T][R]$, where $[T]$ is the initial free thrombin concentration and $[R]$ is the initial free concentration of platelet receptor sites for thrombin. In this calculation the number of receptor sites per platelet was assumed to be 40,000 for both low and high affinity binding. The apparent dissociation constants for thrombin binding at low and at high affinity were calculated from the equation: $K_{diss} = k_2/k_1$. The

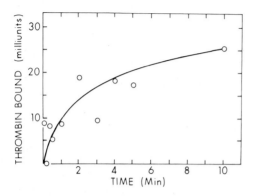

Fig. 10. Association of thrombin with platelets. This experiment was carried out as in Fig. 13, except that 1.0 U/ml of ^{125}I-DIP-thrombin was added.

TABLE 1
Rate constants for thrombin binding to human platelets

	High affinity	Low affinity
k_1	4.0×10^7 M^{-1} min^{-1}	4.2×10^6 M^{-1} min^{-1}
k_2	4.8×10^{-3} min^{-1}	4.0×10^{-1} min^{-1}
K_{diss} (calc)	1.2×10^{-10} M	9.5×10^{-8} M
	(= 0.011 U/ml)	(= 8.6 U/ml)

calculated dissociation constants agree rather closely with the dissociation constants determined from the direct binding studies described above. If the lower apparent number of thrombin binding sites at high affinity (500 per platelet) as determined by the method of Steck and Wallach (Fig. 3) is used in the calculation of k_1 rather than the total number of sites observed at high thrombin concentrations (40,000 per platelet), the K_{diss} calculated for high affinity binding is about two orders of magnitude less than the value actually observed. This provides a further suggestion that all 40,000 thrombin receptor sites are available for high affinity binding.

   In addition to thrombin and insulin, several other hormones exhibit dissociation rates in the presence of unlabeled ligand that suggest negative cooperativity. These include nerve growth factor binding to sympathetic neurons (Frazier et al., 1974), and catecholamine binding to erythrocyte membranes (Limbird et al., 1975). In contrast, the binding of human growth hormone to human leukocytes does not demonstrate negative cooperativity when tested in the same manner (DeMeyts et al., 1973).

6. Functional significance of the thrombin receptor

In the experiments described above, we have demonstrated that platelets contain a highly specific cell surface receptor for thrombin. It remained, however, to establish that the binding of thrombin to this receptor is associated with the physiological function of thrombin on platelets. While the high degree of specificity of the binding interaction would support the hypothesis, it is important to note that the amount of thrombin required to induce 50% of maximal serotonin release using washed platelets is at least an order of magnitude below the thrombin concentration required to saturate the thrombin receptor. The explanation for this discrepancy is unknown but a similar situation exists with respect to receptors for glucagon and insulin, where 5 to 10% of receptor saturation results in a maximal physiological response. Evidence for the functional significance of the thrombin receptor stems from two recent experiments. The first is indirect evidence which shows that human and bovine thrombin contained essentially identical platelet binding sites indicating preservation of this structure during evolution (Shuman and Majerus, 1976). We have prepared antibodies to homogeneous human and bovine thrombin and have shown significant immunological differences between these two thrombin molecules. Thus, the antibodies to human and bovine thrombin cross-react to a limited extent each precipitating approximately 10-fold more thrombin of its own species than the crossed species. The marked antigenic differences observed here are consistent with the known primary structural differences which have been observed from the sequence data available on human and bovine thrombin. Utilizing the data of Prager and Wilson (Prager and Wilson, 1971), which relate antigenic differences to amino acid sequence differences with proteins of known sequence, we estimate that human and bovine thrombin differ in amino acid sequence at between 10 to 25% of all amino acids. Despite these relatively large differences, functionally the two molecules appear to be nearly identical both with respect to the clotting of fibrinogen and with respect to the binding to platelets and induction of the release reaction. The finding that both species of thrombin, despite significant evolutionary differences in primary structure, retain essentially identical binding sites to platelets suggests that this part of the thrombin molecule is physiologically important and has been conserved phylogenetically. The second set of experiments provides direct evidence for the physiological role of the thrombin receptor (Shuman and Majerus, 1975).

In recent studies we observed that thrombin binding to platelets is markedly affected by the anion composition of the buffer solution in which the platelets and thrombin are suspended. This finding allowed us to correlate thrombin binding with the thrombin-induced release reaction. In our previous experiments we measured the binding of bovine and human thrombin to platelets in isotonic Tris-buffered saline solutions. When buffers containing anions other than chloride are used for binding experiments, marked changes in thrombin binding are observed. At low concentrations of thrombin (1 to 20 mU/ml), the amount of thrombin bound varies with the buffer used. From the initial linear portion of the binding curve shown in Fig. 11, there is 5-fold greater thrombin binding in Tris-buffered sodium acetate and 12-fold greater thrombin binding in Tris-buffered sodium cacodylate as compared to Tris-buffered sodium chloride. At higher concentration of thrombin (inset) the differences are less marked and at

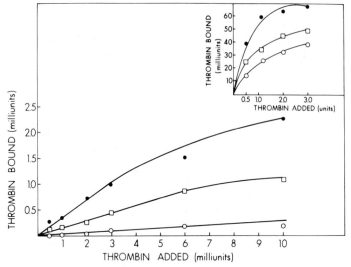

Fig. 11. Effect of anions on binding of ^{125}I-thrombin to platelets. (O–O), Tris-buffered saline; (●–●), Tris-buffered sodium cacodylate; (□–□), Tris-buffered sodium acetate. (From Shuman and Majerus, 1975.)

saturation (data not shown) approximately the same numbers of bindings sites are observed in all buffers.

We next measured whether the difference in thrombin binding is reflected in alterations in thrombin-induced serotonin release. As seen in Table 2 striking variation in response to thrombin is noted depending on the anion present. In this

TABLE 2
Effect of anions on thrombin-induced release of [^{14}C]serotonin from platelets

Buffer	Thrombin concentration required for half-maximal release of [^{14}C]serotonin*
	(U/ml)
Tris-buffered Na$_2$HPO$_4$/NaH$_2$PO$_4$	0.45
Tris-buffered sodium arsenate	0.3
Tris-buffered sodium chloride	0.056
Tris-buffered sodium acetate	0.012
Tris-buffered sodium cacodylate	0.006

Ten-minute incubations were conducted as described in Methods except that platelets were loaded with [^{14}C]serotonin.
* Release sensitivity was measured as the concentration of thrombin required for half-maximal serotonin release as determined by plotting the data obtained in each buffer as shown in Fig. 12 (from Shuman and Majerus, 1975).

experiment there is a 70-fold difference between the amount of thrombin required for half maximal serotonin release in phosphate buffer as compared to cacodylate buffer. While release sensitivity varied with anions, the maximum release obtainable was the same in all anions in any experiment. The full thrombin response curve from a different experiment is shown in Fig. 12 and illustrates that the total amount of release obtainable was the same in both buffers and the sensitivity varied by 33-fold in this experiment. When isotonic buffers were prepared by mixing various proportions of Tris–sodium cacodylate and Tris–sodium chloride, an increase in sensitivity to thrombin-induced serotonin release was seen as the proportion of cacodylate increased up to 0.14 M cacodylate. The requirement for high concentrations of cacodylate for this effect, plus the lack of any time dependence for the effect, suggests that the mechanism is related to the anion itself rather than to some metabolic effect which might be seen at lower concentrations of cacodylate. A number of control experiments were carried out which indicate that anions affect thrombin binding directly and are not toxic to the platelets. Thus, anions have no significant effect on the serotonin release reaction induced by either phytohemagglutinin or by collagen and additionally phyto-hemagglutinin binding to platelets is unaffected by anion composition of the buffer. It was impossible to determine whether or not the effect of anions is on the thrombin molecule or on the platelet cell surface receptor. We studied the effect of anion composition of buffers on the clotting of fibrinogen by thrombin and these experiments indicate that there is no effect of anions on the thrombin-fibrinogen interaction.

The ability to perturb binding without affecting platelet function allowed us to precisely correlate thrombin binding with [^{14}C]serotonin release. We compared the effects of cacodylate and chloride on thrombin binding to platelets with the

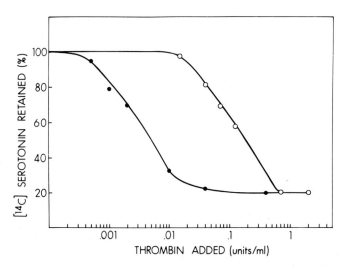

Fig. 12. Effect of anions on thrombin-induced [^{14}C]serotonin release. (O–O), Tris-buffered saline; (●–●), Tris-buffered sodium cacodylate. (From Shuman and Majerus, 1975.)

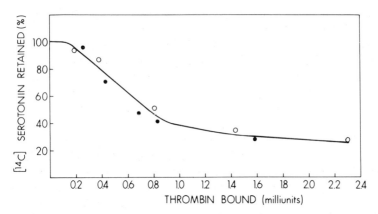

Fig. 13. Relationship of binding of ^{125}I-thrombin to platelets to [^{14}C]serotonin release. Platelets were loaded with [^{14}C]serotonin before incubation with ^{125}I-thrombin. [^{14}C]serotonin retained and ^{125}I-thrombin bound were determined after the platelets were collected on a Millipore filter by double-isotope counting. (●—●), Tris-buffered saline; (○—○), Tris-buffered sodium cacodylate. (From Shuman and Majerus, 1975.)

effects of these anions on [^{14}C]serotonin release in a double label experiment where ^{125}I-thrombin bound and [^{14}C]serotonin release were measured on the same platelets in the same reaction mixture as shown in Fig. 13. Although concentrations of thrombin necessary to induce an equivalent amount of serotonin release were much higher in sodium chloride than in sodium cacodylate (10-fold in this experiment) for a given amount of thrombin bound, the same degree of release was obtained in both anions. A similar correlation was seen in experiments using other anions in that the quantity of thrombin bound necessary to induce maximal release was constant in each experiment. Approximately 1 mU of thrombin bound per 5×10^7 platelets (equivalent to 100 molecules of thrombin per platelet) results in maximal serotonin release. These observations suggest that thrombin binding is a physiologically important first step in the thrombin-induced platelet release reaction.

7. Characterization of the thrombin receptor

The kinetic experiments suggest that there is a single class of thrombin receptors on platelets. Since all 40,000 receptors are likely of a single type, we postulate that the thrombin receptor on the platelet surface might be isolated and further characterized. Initial experiments have been directed at attempting to solubilize platelet membranes using a variety of ionic and non-ionic detergents and assay for thrombin-binding activity in the solubilized material. These experiments have met with little success. Ganguly (1974), has carried out similar experiments and has obtained a crude preparation of a Triton solubilized thrombin receptor, although it remains to be characterized. We have also carried out experiments using chemical cross-linking agents which can form covalent bonds between ^{125}I-thrombin and the platelet receptor in situ. In preliminary experiments we have shown that thrombin can be linked to platelets using very low concentrations of glutaraldehyde (0.01%) and that the platelets can then be dissolved and thereafter analyzed by SDS gel electrophoresis. Using ^{125}I-thrombin we have succeeded in cross-linking thrombin to its apparent receptor in this manner. These experiments suggest the molecular weight of the thrombin–thrombin receptor complex is approximately 200,000. It is impossible to know the true molecular weight of the receptor since we do not know whether the radioactive thrombin receptor complex contains one or more thrombin molecules per receptor or whether only one of the peptide chains of thrombin is included in the complex. Evidence that the cross-linked material does contain the thrombin receptor comes from experiments where the radioactivity in the cross-linked complex was measured by autoradiography of SDS gels. Thus, the cross-linked complex showed saturation characteristics ($K_{diss} \cong 3$ U/ml) similar to that determined from direct binding experiments. Further characterization of the cross-linked receptor awaits future experiments. We hope to use reversible cross-linking agents to facilitate regeneration of intact receptor. In other experiments using ^{131}I-lactoperoxidase-labeled platelets we find that cross-linking of thrombin to its receptor using intact platelets did not result in any change in mobility of any of the labeled glycoproteins suggesting that these proteins are not the thrombin receptor itself.

8. Summary

Our experiments indicate that human platelets contain approximately 40,000 cell-surface, highly specific receptor sites per platelet which bind thrombin with high affinity. Kinetic experiments suggest that there is interaction among the receptor sites such that the initial sites occupied bind thrombin with highest affinity altering the remaining sites with progressively decreasing affinity. This 'negative cooperativity' may explain the apparent 'threshold' observed in the thrombin–platelet reactions, i.e., a certain amount of thrombin added to platelets is required for sudden 'triggering of aggregation and release'. Both the kinetic and cross-linking experiments suggest that there is a single type of thrombin receptor on platelets. Perturbation of thrombin binding by anions indicates that binding of thrombin to the platelet receptor is a physiologically important first step in the thrombin-induced platelet reactions. These experiments suggest that the reaction of thrombin with platelets is analogous to a hormone-like reaction rather than a catalytic process.

Acknowledgments

We wish to acknowledge the assistance of Nancy Stanford in these experiments. Much of the work described in this report is contained in the Ph.D. thesis of D.M.

Tollefsen submitted to the Graduate School of Arts and Sciences of Washington University, May, 1975.

This work was supported by the National Institutes of Health grants HL-14147 (Specialized Center for Research in Thrombosis), and HL-16634.

References

Ardlie, N.G. and Han, P. (1974) Brit. J. Haematol., *26*, 331.
Baenziger, N.L., Brodie, G.N. and Majerus, P.W. (1971) Proc. Natl. Acad. Sci. U.S.A., *68*, 240.
Baenziger, N.L., Brodie, G.N. and Majerus, P.W. (1972) J. Biol. Chem., *247*, 2723.
Bettelheim, F.R. (1956) Biochim. Biophys. Acta, *19*, 121.
Bockaert, J., Imbert, M., Jard, S. and Morel, F. (1972) Mol. Pharmacol., *8*, 230.
Brass, L.F. and Bensusan, H.B. (1974) J. Clin. Invest., *54*, 1480.
Brodie, G.N., Baenziger, N.L., Chase, L.R. and Majerus, P.W. (1972) J. Clin. Invest., *51*, 81.
Cohen, I., Bohak, I., DeVries, A. and Katchalski, E. (1969) Eur. J. Biochem., *10*, 388.
Cuatrecasas, P. (1974) Ann. Rev. Biochem., *43*, 169.
Davey, M.G. and Luscher, E.F. (1967) Nature, *216*, 857.
DeMeyts, P., Roth, J., Neville, D.M. Jr., Gavin, J.R. III and Lesniak, M.A. (1973) Biochem. Biophys. Res. Commun., *55*, 154.
Detweiler, T.C. and Feinman, R.D. (1973a) Biochemistry, *12*, 2821.
Detweiler, T.C. and Feinman, R.D. (1973b) Biochemistry, *12*, 2462.
Fasco, M.J. and Fenton, J.W. II (1973) Arch. Biochem. Biophys., *159*, 802.
Frazier, W.A., Boyd, L.F. and Bradshaw, R.A. (1974) J. Biol. Chem., *249*, 5513.
Gavin, J.R. III, Gorden, P., Roth, J., Archer, J.A. and Buell, D.N. (1973) J. Biol. Chem., *248*, 2202.
Ganguly, P. (1972) J. Biol. Chem., *247*, 1809.
Ganguly, P. (1974) Nature, *247*, 306.
Hamberg, M., Svensson, J. and Samuelsson, B. (1975) Proc. Natl. Acad. Sci. U.S.A., *72*, 2994.
Hamberg, M., Svensson, J., Wakabayashi, T. and Samuelsson, B. (1974) Proc. Natl. Acad. Sci. U.S.A., *71*, 345.
Hammond, J.M., Jarett, L., Mariz, I.K. and Daughaday, W.H. (1972) Biochem. Biophys. Res. Commun., *49*, 1122.
Kang, A.H., Beachey, E.H. and Katzman, R.L. (1974) J. Biol. Chem., *249*, 1054.
Kisselbach, T.H. and Wagner, R.H. (1966) Am. J. Physiol., *211*, 1472.
Lefkowitz, R.J., Roth, J. and Pastan, I. (1970) Science, *170*, 633.
Levitski, A. and Koshland, D.E. Jr. (1969) Proc. Natl. Acad. Sci. U.S.A., *62*, 1121.
Lewis, N. and Majerus, P.W. (1969) J. Clin. Invest., *48*, 2114.
Limbird, L.E., DeMeyts, P. and Lefkowitz, R.J. (1975) Biochem. Biophys. Res. Commun., *64*, 1160.
Lyons, R.M., Stanford, N. and Majerus, P.W. (1975) J. Clin. Invest., *56*, 924.
Majerus, P.W. and Brodie, G.N. (1972) J. Biol. Chem., *247*, 4253.
Marinetti, G.V., Schlatz, L. and Reilly, K. (1972) in Insulin Action (Fritz, I., ed) p. 207, Academic Press, New York.
Martin, B.M., Feinman, R.D. and Detwiler, T.C. (1975) Biochemistry, *14*, 1308.
Mills, D.C.B., Robb, I.A. and Roberts, G.C.K. (1968) J. Physiol., *195*, 715.
Phillips, D.R. and Agin, P.P. (1974) Biochim. Biophys. Acta, *352*, 218.
Prager, E.M. and Wilson, A.C. (1971) J. Biol. Chem., *246*, 7010.
Salzman, E.W. (1972) N. Eng. J. Med., *286*, 358.
Shuman, M.A. and Majerus, P.W. (1975) J. Clin. Invest., *56*, 945.
Shuman, M.A. and Majerus, P.W. (1976) Blood, *47*, 43.
Steck, T.L. and Wallach, D.F.H. (1965) Biochim. Biophys. Acta, *97*, 510.
Tollefsen, D.M., Feagler, J.R. and Majerus, P.W. (1974) J. Biol. Chem., *249*, 2646.
Tollefsen, D.M., Jackson, C.M. and Majerus, P.W. (1975) J. Clin. Invest., *56*, 241.
Weiss, H.J. (1975) New Eng. J. Med., *293*, 531.

CHAPTER 10

Interaction of platelets with connective tissue

R.M. JAFFE

National Institutes of Health, Building 10, 4N309, Bethesda,
Maryland 20014, U.S.A.

1. Introduction

In 1842 two English physicians, George Gulliver and John Siddall, apparently made the first drawings identifying blood platelets (Robb-Smith, 1967). Gulliver called special attention to the role of 'white globules' (platelets) in hemostasis initiated by contact between blood and (connective) tissue, and recent reviewers of platelet function emphasize the importance of this same phenomenon (Packham and Mustard, 1971; Weiss, 1975). The details of hemostasis initiated by the platelet-connective tissue interaction phenomenon are, however, little clearer today than in Gulliver's time.

The role of platelets in thrombosis and hemostasis has been discussed extensively elsewhere (Spaet, 1972; Deykin, 1974; Sherry and Scriabine, 1974), and the molecular details of platelet-connective tissue interactions are a subject of considerable research interest (Michaeli and Orloff, 1976). Concurrently, connective tissue biophysical chemistry is progressing toward an understanding of the individual structural components and their interaction with each other. This discussion is a brief progress report emphasizing current work. In an effort to provide a coherent framework, many simplifications are made, and some of these may prove to obscure or mislead – especially in collagen chemistry where a sketchy presentation is made of a complex and evolving subject. I regret and am responsible for any inaccuracies occasioned by the brevity or structure of this discussion.

A topical review of connective tissue chemistry provides a useful background for a discussion of connective tissue:platelet interactions, and recent developments in collagen chemistry and nomenclature are therefore discussed in detail. Investigators of platelet:connective tissue interaction frequently apply descriptive terms to their connective tissue or collagen preparations which may imply characteristics of purity or physical chemistry which exceed the intent of the user; indeed, some of the apparently conflicting data recently reported may result from the choice of undefined descriptive terms and incomplete chemical or physical characterization of preparations employed.

Gordon (ed) Platelets in Biology and Pathology
© *Elsevier/North-Holland Biomedical Press, 1976*

2. Connective tissue chemistry and nomenclature

Connective tissue can be defined as an extracellular structural matrix (Balazs, 1970), and its major components are collagen (Piez, 1972; Gould, 1972), elastin (Franzblau, 1971), glycoprotein, and proteoglycan (Davison, 1973). Terms used to describe anatomic structures of connective tissue components include basement membrane, intima, and reticulin.

Basement membrane is an ultrastructurally amorphous complex of connective tissue components, including glycoprotein, collagen (or collagen-like) protein and, possibly, proteoglycan (Kefalides, 1973; Vracko, 1974).

Intima is a term applied to an ultrastructurally amorphous material normally seen in muscular blood vessels between the luminal side of the internal elastic lamina and the endothelial basement membrane. The intima contains proteoglycan (Davison, 1973), glycoprotein, collagen, and elastin (Ross and Bornstein, 1969; Vracko, 1974).

Reticulin, which is a descriptive term for the argyrophilic filamentous network of mesenchymal tissues, is apparently a complex of proteoglycan/glycoprotein and collagen (Vracko, 1974)–possibly the collagen subtype III recently described (see Table 1).

The structural and functional components of a typical muscular blood vessel are represented in Fig. 1. It is possible that the arrangement and/or composition of these components varies at different sites in the organism, and such differences may influence the properties of the connective tissue, including its reactivity toward platelets.

TABLE 1
Collagen subtypes and tissue distribution

Collagen type	Tissue of origin	Subunit chain composition
I	Bone, tendon, ligament, skin, dentin, fibrocartilage adventitia, lung	$[\alpha 1(I)]_2 \alpha 2$
II	hyaline cartilage	$[\alpha 1(II)]_3$
III	Fetal skin, Media of Muscular Arteries Lung ? Other (parenchyma)	$[\alpha 1(III)]_3$
IV	Basement Membrane ? Lense Capsule ? Other	$[\alpha 1(IV)]_3$

2.1. Collagen

This protein will now be discussed, with emphasis on the physical characteristics of collagen and its polymers. Nomenclature is specifically addressed because of the proliferation of similar terms referring to collagens of different physical and/or

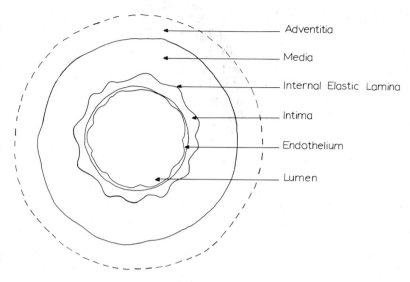

Morphologic structure	Composition
Adventitia	Adipose tissue
	Collagen (type I)
	Proteoglycan
	Glycoprotein
	Fibroblasts
Media	? Type III collagen ⎫
	Glycoprotein ⎬ Reticulin
	Proteoglycan ⎭
	? Type IV collagen
	Smooth muscle cells
Internal elastic lamina	Elastin
	Glycoprotein
	Collagen (? type)
	? Proteoglycan
Intima	Glycoprotein
	Collagen (? Types I + III)
	Elastin
	Proteoglycan
Endothelium	Glycoprotein
	Collagen (? Type IV)
	? Proteoglycan
	Endothelial cells

Fig. 1. Diagram of muscular blood vessel and its components.

chemical properties. Recent reviews have dealt with several aspects of collagen biosynthesis (Grant and Prockop, 1972; Bornstein, 1974), chemistry and structure (Traub and Piez, 1971; Piez, 1972).

Collagen is the major structural protein of mammals, and is the dominant protein in medium and large blood vessels, tendons, dentin, cartilage, and bone. In addition, it is present in appreciable quantities in lung, ligaments, cornea and the lense.

Collagen can be considered a repeating tripeptide (GLY-X-Y), and X and Y may be any aminoacid although imino and neutral aminoacids are most frequent (Fig. 2(A)). Collagen also contains unusual aminoacids (hydroxylated proline and lysine); lysine-derived aldehydes; galactosylhydroxylsine (GH) and glucosyl-galactosylhydroxylysine (GGH) (Fig. 2(B)); and crosslinks (Fig. 2(C)). The collagen helix is polyproline Type II (Gould, 1971; Ramachandran et al., 1973), which means that (unlike most other proteins) side chains of aminoacid residues are pointed regularly to the outside. Collagen is a 3000 Å × 15 Å rod-like mac-romolecule (mol. wt. about 295,000) composed of three subunit chains, and non-helical polypeptides exist at both the amino and the carboxytermini of the molecule. These 'telopeptides' usually comprise 16 to 25 residues (Fig. 2(D)), and can be cleaved with proteolytic enzymes other than collagenase (Piez, 1972).

Functional subtypes of collagen exist. Collagen in bone, mature skin, tendon, dentin, vascular adventitia, scar tissue, and ligament is primarily Type I (Traub and Piez, 1971; Miller and Matsuka, 1974), and fibrocartilage may also be of this type (Eyre and Muir, 1975). Two distinct subunit chains have been identified, and the chain composition of native type I collagen can be represented as $[\alpha 1(I)]_2 \alpha 2$. Type II collagen, which occurs in articular cartilage (Eyre and Muir, 1975), has three identical subunit chains and can be represented as $[\alpha 1(II)]_3$. Another species of collagen has been found in the media of muscular arteries (Trelstad, 1974) and

A. Primary sequence of collagen (1052 residues)

   Amino terminal telopeptide $-(Gly-X-Y)_{337}-$ Carboxy terminal telopeptide
     (16 residues)   (25 residues)

B. Unusual amino acid residues in collagen

   4-Hydroxyproline (and 3-Hydroxyproline in Types III and IV)
   Hydroxylysine
   Allysine (aminoadipicacid semialdehyde, from deamination of lysine)
   Hydroxyallysine (semialdehyde from deamination of hydroxylysine)
   Galactosylhydroxylysine (galactose linked to hydroxyl of hydroxylysine)
   Glucosylgalactosylhydroxylysine ($O-\beta-D$-glucose linked to galactose)

C. Crosslinks in collagen (°intermolecular; °°intramolecular)

   °Lysinonorleucine (adduct of lysine & allysine)
   °Hydroxylysinonorleucine (adduct of hydroxylysine & allysine)
   °Dihydroxylysinonorleucine (adduct of hydroxylysine & hydroxyallysine)
   °°Aldol (aldol condensation of two allysines)
   °Histidinylaldol (Michael addition of histidine & aldol)
   °Histidinylhydroxymerodesmosine (adduct of aldol, hydroxylysine & histidine)

D. Schematic view of collagen molecule

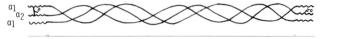

   aminoterminal telopeptide   2960 A   carboxyterminal telopeptide
   with aldol residue   polyproline type II helix   with allysine residue

Fig. 2.

skin, especially fetal skin (Epstein, 1974). This collagen, which may be widely distributed (Epstein and Munderloh, 1975), has been called Type III collagen, and can be represented as $[\alpha 1(\text{III})]_3$. Basement membrane is classified by some as Type IV collagen (Kefalides, 1973), and contains three identical subunits $[\alpha 1(\text{IV})]_3$ (Table 1). The characteristics of these collagen subtypes are presented below, with emphasis on those which influence physical or chemical reactivity toward platelets.

Type I collagen (Table 2(A)) has more proline than hydroxyproline, about one-fifth of lysines are hydroxylated, and about one-fifth of the hydroxylysines are glycosylated with galactose (which means less than 1 galactose per 1000 residues). About half the galactosyl residues contain a single glucose moiety. The aminoacid sequence near the galactose is unusual in its lack of imino acids (Traub and Piez, 1971; Miller and Matsuka, 1974; Gallop and Paz, 1975). Type I collagen usually forms ultrastructurally distinctive fibrils in vivo and in vitro with repeating 'D' periods (typically 670 Å) along the length of the polymers, each molecule spanning 4.4 'D' repeats. Other polymeric forms of Type I collagen also occur (Table 3).

Type II collagen (Table 2(B)) is more extensively hydroxylated at proline and lysine and contains 5–8-fold more carbohydrate than Type I collagen.

Type III collagen (Table 2(C)) is reported to contain less proline than hydroxy-proline, and one-third to one-seventh of the lysines are hydroxylated. Glycosylation appears limited, with roughly equal glucose and galactose content, and Type III collagen apparently contains cystine, unlike Types I and II (Trelstad, 1974; Epstein, 1974; Byers et al., 1974). Type III collagen forms reticular polymers of narrow diameter in vitro and, possibly, in vivo (Wiedemann et al., 1975).

The basement membrane protein that can be classified as Type IV collagen (Table 2(D)) is extensively hydroxylated at proline and contains 80% of its lysines as hydroxylysine. Consequently, it contains large amounts of glucose and galactose, and other sugars as well. Cystine is also reportedly present (Kefalides,

TABLE 2
Content of certain amino acids in different collagen types

| Collagen type | Residues per 1000 amino acids | | | | |
	OH-PRO/PRO	OH-LYS/LYS	GH/GGH	1/2 Cystine	GLY/VAL
(A) I	97/119	6/27	0.6/0.7	N.D.	324/20
(B) II	104/111	21/12	3.8/5.3	N.D.	327/15
(C) III (aorta)	120/95[a]	15/24	low/0.4	3	347/20
(D) IV (aorta)	122/86[b]	39/12	0.2/1.2	7	330/28
(E) IV (GBM[c])	141/61[b]	45/10	2/34	8	310/29

[a] May contain 3-hydroxyproline.
[b] Contains 3-hydroxyproline.
[c] GBM = glomerular (human) basement membrane.
    Studies which provided the data summarised above were: Piez et al. (1963); Miller and Lunde (1973); Kefalides (1973); Trelstad (1974).

TABLE 3
Some polymeric forms of Type I collagen (after Doyle et al., 1975)

Name	Description	Typical conditions of formation
Native	Fibril with repeating 670 Å period showing asymmetric banding ('D' period)	Usual 'in vivo' fibril or fiber Neutral pH, phosphate or acetate buffer 'in vitro'
DPS[a]	Fibril with repeating 670 Å period showing symmetric banding	Acid pH, high ionic strength or following pepsin digestion
FLS[b]	Fibril with repeating 900 (FLS III), 1700 (FLS IV), or 2600 Å (FLS I and FLS II) period showing symmetric banding	Low ionic strength and flexible polyanion (e.g., glycosaminoglycan or α 1-acid glycoprotein) in vitro or in pathologic conditions in vivo
SLS[c]	Fibril with repeating 2680 Å period showing asymmetric banding	Low ionic strength and cation (e.g., ATP)
Oblique Striated	Fibril with 'D' period polar subfibrils staggered with respect to nearest neighbor by about 90 Å	Usually seen in Type II collagen, neutral pH, 'in vitro'

[a] DPS = 'D' period symmetric banding.
[b] FLS = Fibrous long spacing.
[c] SLS = Segment long spacing.

1973). Tactoidal or reticular forms are observed in vitro, but basement membrane is ultrastructurally amorphous in vivo (Vracko, 1974).

The nomenclature of collagen components is complex and reflects the polymorphism of the protein (Hulmes et al., 1973). The protein is synthesized from common aminoacids, initially as a polypeptide sometimes called protocollagen (Table 4(A)). Once hydroxylated and glycosylated the protein is ready for secretion from the cell: it is then called procollagen and contains long amino- and carboxyl-terminal 'non-collagen' telopeptides (Table 4(B)) which are cleaved by neutral peptidases to yield the mature collagen molecule (Table 4(C)). The term collagen should refer only to the individual native molecule described above. Trivial or descriptive names for this molecule are tropocollagen, collagen monomer, and unit collagen. Purity of collagen preparations can be determined by aminoacid and carbohydrate analysis, and their physical state by viscometry, electron microscopy, and optical techniques using absorbance or reflectance.

Collagen solutions at 4°C and acid pH exist as individual molecules, and polymers form only at high ionic strength or after pepsin treatment. At 4°C and neutral pH, however, collagen tends to self polymerize to multimers; this accelerates at higher temperatures and is retarded by divalent cations (Gross and Kirk, 1958; Wood, 1960; Wood and Keech, 1960a,b; Bard and Chapman, 1973). The nature of the polymer depends on the pH, ionic strength, and presence or absence of other modifying agents such as ATP, glycosaminoglycan, or glycoprotein (Table 3).

TABLE 4
Nomenclature and characteristics of collagen assembly

Name	Other Names	Characteristics
(A) Protocollagen	–	Under- or pre-hydroxylated/non-glycosylated protein
(B) Procollagen	p-Collagen[a]	Hydroxylated, glycosylated protein contains long N-terminal and C-terminal 'non-collagen' telopeptides which are cleared separately
(C) Collagen[b]	Tropocollagen[b] Collagen monomer[b] Unit collagen[b]	Contains short N-terminal and C-terminal 'non-collagen' telopeptides (viscosity low)
(D) ?[c]	Multimeric collagen[d] Monomeric collagen[d] 'Protofibril'[e] 'Nuclei'[e]	Small collagen polymer (viscosity intermediate). Amorphous filaments by E/M
(E) Fibril	Fibrillar collagen	Large, ordered collagen polymer distributed in spectrophotometrically clear liquid (viscosity high). Banded filaments by E/M (see Table 3)
(F) Fiber	Fibrous collagen	Large, ordered polymeric precipitate forming opaque precipitate in liquid (viscosity can not be measured). Banded filaments by E/M

[a] Can be used to represent procollagen with a cleaved telopeptide.
[b] Equivalent terms.
[c] No term is in general use.
[d] Equivalent terms (not shown to be equivalent to "protofibril").
[e] Equivalent terms.

During the polymerization of collagen a latent period exists before light scattering is observed, known as the nucleation phase. Based on this and other data Smith (1958) and Petrushka and Hodge (1964) suggested that the macromolecular assembly of collagen proceeds through a small polymer of (perhaps) 4 or 5 molecules. This 'protofibril' may be the subunit from which larger ordered polymers (fibrils and fibers) assemble.

A preparation of collagen which is physically and functionally distinct from the single molecule has been reported, called monomeric or multimeric collagen (Jaffe and Deykin, 1972; 1974), but no relation to the 'protofibril' has yet been established (Table 4(D)).

Larger polymers of collagen, ultrastructurally and viscometrically identifiable, are known as fibrils (Table 4E)). The different subtypes of collagen have different fibrillar forms, and Type I collagen itself can form physically distinct polymers in the presence of other compounds: for instance, nucleotides (e.g., ATP) and glycoprotein (e.g., α1-acid glycoprotein) can influence the spacing of the fibrils. Fibrils thus formed are known as segment long spacing (SLS) or fibrous long spacing (FLS) collagen (Table 3). Polymers of collagen can also form which are amorphous and have no identifiable ultrastructural banding (Hulmes et al., 1973; Jaffe and Deykin, 1974). Collagen fibrils can polymerize into grossly visible, insoluble fibers, which have defined ultrastructural morphology (Table 4(F)).

Thus, collagen can assemble in vitro into multimers, fibrils, fibers or random polymers with different geometry, physical chemistry and functional properties. Each of the chemical and physical characteristics of the molecule may influence reactivity of platelets.

The subunit structure of collagen is now also being elucidated. Purified collagen can be dissociated (denatured) into subunit chains (Piez, 1972). Denatured collagen is known as gelatin. Subunits with molecular weight one-third native collagen (typically 95,000) are known as alpha (α) chains, and subunits with molecular weight two-thirds native collagen (typically 190,000) are known as beta (β) chains (Table 5). Beta chains form from alpha chains by lysine-derived crosslinks (Fig. 2(C)).

Collagen is susceptible to cleavage by cyanogen bromide at methionyl residues (Nordwig and Dick, 1965), and the peptides derived from this treatment can be isolated by molecular sieve chromatography; these are named by the order they elute from the columns. Figure 3 shows the alignment and some characteristics of

TABLE 5
Subunit chains of collagen (gelatin)

Designation	Approximate molecular weight (daltons)			
	Type I	Type II	Type III	Type IV
α = alpha = single chain	95,000	101,000	108,000	120,000
β = beta = dimer of αs	190,000	202,000	216,000	240,000

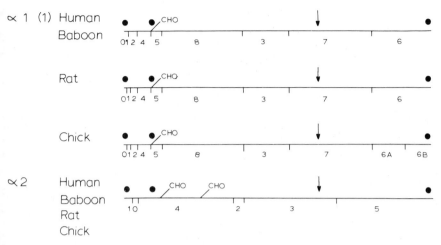

Fig. 3. Cyanogen bromide peptide order in Type I collagen, showing regions of crosslinking and glycosylation (carbohydration). After Piez.

$\alpha 1$ (I) and $\alpha 2$ refer to the subunit chains of Type I collagen.
  ●: Cross-linking region.
CHO: Carbohydrate (galactose, or glucose–galactose) attached to hydroxylysine residue.
  ↓ : Collagenase-sensitive region in native molecule.

cyanogen bromide peptides in the native molecule for certain Type I collagens. Cyanogen bromide peptides of cartilage (Type II) collagen have also been reported (Miller and Lunde, 1973). Platelet interaction with denatured collagen and cyanogen bromide peptides will be discussed below.

Collagen is usually purified by solubilization in 1 M sodium chloride ('neutral salt soluble collagen') or in 0.5 M citric acid or acetic acid ('acid soluble collagen'). Sometimes, enzymatic digestion is employed to increase the yield. In the platelet literature, the term 'acid soluble' collagen is sometimes applied to dispersions of polymeric, partially purified connective tissue without characterization of the product physically or biochemically (Cazenave et al., 1973). Unless criteria for purity (e.g., amino acid and carbohydrate analysis) are met, the term 'connective tissue suspension' should probably be applied to such preparations, even if the dominant protein is collagen. The source of the preparation (e.g., tendon collagen) should be given when chemical and physical characterization is not available. In this discussion, an effort will be made to distinguish studies employing such connective tissue dispersions from those employing characterized collagens.

2.2. Elastin

Elastin is a highly crosslinked, insoluble connective tissue protein composed primarily of neutral aminoacids (Franzblau, 1971), derived from a precursor protein which is partially characterized (Smith, 1973). Elastin appears ultrastructurally amorphous (Kadar, 1974) but has a distinct order to its assembly which permits stretching and relaxation with little applied force (Hoeve, 1974).

2.3. Glycoproteins and proteoglycans

Proteoglycans are hydrophilic matrices, and their substituent glycosaminoglycans are now being characterized in several tissues such as articular cartilage, lung and blood vessel (Rosenberg, 1973; Brandt, 1974; Horwitz and Crystal, 1975).

The biosynthesis and structure of proteoglycans are reviewed elsewhere (Roden, 1970; Roden et al., 1971) but, briefly, they are composed of low molecular weight proteins to which sugar polymers are attached, usually through serine hydroxyl groups. Chondroitin-4-sulfate, chondroitin-6-sulfate, heparin sulfate, heparan sulfate, dermatan sulfate and hyaluronic acid are most often encountered.

Connective tissue glycoproteins, which are an important component of blood vessels, may play a role in platelet: vascular interactions. Many studies of platelet reactivity have been made using connective tissue homogenates or partially purified connective tissue. Certain components of connective tissue can be purified and used either alone or in combination with other components to study platelet reactions. Most of this discussion will deal with platelet studies which employ connective tissue and its constituents.

2.4. Hemostatic disorders associated with defined defects in connective tissue

Ehlers-Danlos Syndrome (Table 6(A)) represents a group of (perhaps) seven diseases characterized by hyperextensibility of joints, 'cigarette-paper' scarring, tissue friability and easy bruising or bleeding (Beighton, 1970; McKusick, 1972a). One well-defined example, Type VI (the so-called ocular type), is characterized by hydroxylysine deficient collagen caused by a decrease in the enzyme lysyl hydroxylase (Krane et al., 1972), and these patients show unusual crosslinking in skin and bone collagen (Eyre and Glimcher, 1972). Type VII Ehlers-Danlos syndrome, which apparently is caused by a defect in the conversion of procollagen to collagen (Lichtenstein et al., 1973), is similar to dermatosparaxis, a condition of cattle characterized by abnormal and disarrayed collagen fibrils and fibers and increased procollagen content (Furthmayer et al., 1972).

Marfan's syndrome (Table 6(B)) is characterized by laxity in connective tissue structural elements (McKusick, 1972b), and the defect appears to reside in both elastin and collagen although no biochemical lesion has yet been defined. Morphologically, cystic medial necrosis and bruisability are evident. Homocystinemia (Table 6(C)) shares certain morphologic features with Marfan's syndrome (Kang and Trelstad, 1973).

Two other connective tissue syndromes have recnetly been elucidated in part: Menke's kinky hair syndrome (Menke et al., 1962), which is related to decreased copper absorption and, as a consequence, an increase in soluble (not cross-linked) elastin and collagen, may result from deficiency in the copper-dependent lysyl deaminase enzyme required in the first step of cross-linking (Table 6(D)). The

TABLE 6
Clinical disorders of connective tissue

Syndrome	Molecular defect	Morphologic defect	Hemostatic abnormality	Animal model
(A) Ehlers-Danlos: Type I–V	?	Decreased elasticity and hyperextensibility	Bruisability	Spaniel and Mink (Hegreberg et al., 1970)
Type VI	Lysyl hydroxylase deficiency	Decreased elasticity and hyperextensibility	Bruisability	?
Type VII	?Procollagen peptidase deficiency	Abnormal polymerization of collagen fibrils	Bleeding	Dermatosparaxic cattle (Furthmayer et al., 1972)
(B) Marfan's	?Elastin/collagen crosslinking	Decreased elasticity and hyperextensibility	Bruising or none	?
(C) Homocystinemia	?Elastin/collagen crosslinking	Decreased elasticity	Variable	Homocystinemic Baboon (Harker et al., 1974)
(D) Menke's	Decreased copper absorption	Increase in soluble elastin and collagen	?	Copper deficient swine and chicks (Carnes, 1971)
(E) Osteogenesis Imperfecta	?	Abnormal formation of collagen fibers in bone	Variable	?

other syndrome, osteogenesis imperfecta (Table 6(E)), may result from abnormal assembly of bone collagen fibers (Teitelbaum et al., 1974).

3. Platelet adhesion to connective tissue

The interaction between platelets and connective tissue or its components can be separated (for purposes of discussion) into two phases:
(1) adhesion (specific contact);
(2) aggregation and clumping.

Contact refers to any non-specific physical interaction between platelets and connective tissue; *adhesion* follows contact and means a specific interaction between platelets and connective tissue; *aggregation* means clusters of platelets adjacent to connective tissue.

In response to the stimulus of adhesion or aggregation, platelets may *release* certain organelle contents and transform their membrane to develop coagulant activity.

This discussion will address in turn contact and adhesion, clumping and aggregation, and release reactions.

3.1. Platelet–collagen adhesion

Most workers conclude that contact with subendothelial connective tissue is required to initiate platelet adhesion to the vascular wall (French, 1969; Baumgart-ner and Haudenschild, 1972; Spaet and Stemerman, 1972; Hovig, 1974). Although there are some ultrastructural studies which show platelet processes apparently adhering to endothelial cells at sites of minimal vascular injury (Marchesi, 1964; Ashford and Freiman, 1968) these observations remain unconvincing–mainly because it is difficult to exclude platelet pseudopod adhesion to subendothelium at sites distant from the sites illustrated (Spaet and Stemerman, 1972). However, one intriguing and unexplained observation is that of Johnson et al. (1969), who showed ATPase-staining material on the subendothelium in areas of platelet contact, and interpreted this as residual endothelial cell material interposed between platelets and subendothelium.

Bounameaux (1959) and Hugues (1962) were the first to call attention to a possible specific role of collagen in platelet adhesion to subendothelial or tendon fibers, and this observation was supported by Zucker and Borrelli (1962) and by Hovig (1963). Other workers, however, have emphasized that non-collagen components of connective tissue may also be involved in platelet adhesion (Stemerman et al., 1971).

Experimental design can influence results, and most studies of platelet adhesion to connective tissue or collagen are variations of four basic experimental designs:
(1) Platelet rich plasma or blood is exposed to a tissue component in the presence of some compound (e.g. EDTA or apyrase) which blocks platelet aggregation and/or release.

(2) Washed platelets are exposed to a tissue component in an environment free of divalent cations.

(3) Washed platelets are exposed to an artificial surface coated with the material under investigation.

(4) Platelets are allowed to bind radiolabeled collagen.

This discussion of adhesion will focus on particular experimental questions and indicate differences in experimental detail when such differences provide possible bases for understanding apparently conflicting results.

The influence of the following factors on platelet adhesion will be sequentially addressed: divalent cations; platelet sulfhydryl groups; plasma proteins; formaldehyde and glutaraldehyde fixation; antimetabolites; collagen structure and carbohydrate content; sugars and sugar nucleotides; non-steroidal anti-inflammatory drugs; tricyclic antidepressant drugs; and platelet sialic acid. Each factor is considered in terms of platelet adhesion to collagen or collagen-rich connective tissue. Platelet adhesion to elastin, glycoprotein, proteoglycan, and basement membrane will then be discussed.

3.1.1. Divalent cations

Human platelets adhere to suspensions of tendon in the absence of divalent cations (Hovig, 1964) and washed rat platelets bind radiolabeled collagen in the absence of divalent cations (MacIntyre and Gordon, 1975a) but Cazenave et al. (1973) showed that adherence of washed human or pig platelets to a surface coated with tendon collagen fibrils was greater in the presence of 2 mM calcium than when 9 mM EDTA was added to chelate the calcium. Also, rabbit platelets apparently do not adhere to subendothelial surface when 0.1% EDTA is present (Baumgartner, 1974).

3.1.2. Sulfhydryl groups

Reagents which block surface sulfhydryl groups (PCMBS, PHMB, and PHMBS) do not affect platelet adhesion to connective tissue, but platelet adhesion is reduced by incubation with 1 mM N-ethylmaleimide (NEM), a cell-penetrating sulfhydryl blocking reagent (Al-Mondhiry and Spaet, 1970). Zucker and Jerushalmy (1967), however, reported that 1 mM NEM caused loss of pre-labeled [^{14}C]serotonin and ^{51}Cr from platelets, which indicates that the cells had been damaged, and Behnke (1970) reported disappearance of platelet microtubules and ballooning of plasma membranes in response to 1 mM NEM. MacIntyre and Gordon (1975a) found that a lower concentration (0.1 mM) did not inhibit the binding of collagen to washed rat platelets.

3.1.3. Plasma proteins

Plasma proteins (particularly fibrinogen) may enhance platelet adhesion to connective tissue and collagen (Lyman et al., 1971) although platelet: collagen adhesion and aggregation in 'afibrinogenemic' patients is apparently normal (Gugler and Lüscher, 1965; Rodman et al., 1966). Lyman et al. (1971) showed that acylated or desialized fibrinogen supported platelet adhesion to collagen like native fibrinogen, but plasmin-digested fibrinogen did not. These workers also reported that purified bovine nasal and humeral cartilage proteoglycans (but not glycosaminoglycans) were more active than fibrinogen, on a molar basis, at enhancing collagen-platelet adhesion.

Bang et al. (1972) showed that gamma globulin, fibrinogen, and Hageman Factor preparations could enhance adhesion in washed platelet preparations. The ability of gamma globulins to support platelet adhesion was inhibited by acylation of amino groups with various anhydrides, and Bang et al. (1972) suggested that the cationic nature of the proteins was one of the factors responsible for their effect.

3.1.4. Aldehyde fixation

MacIntyre and Gordon (1975a) found that brief exposure of platelets to formaldehyde did not inhibit their ability to bind radiolabeled collagen whereas glutaraldehyde fixation did, and suggested that the difference might be due to glutaraldehyde crosslinking membrane proteins.

3.1.5. Antimetabolites

Incubation of platelets with the metabolic poisons 2-deoxyglucose (15 mM) and antimycin A (5 μg/ml) does not reduce collagen binding to platelets, and exposure to low temperatures or reducing platelet glycogen by 50% does not inhibit platelet adhesion to tendon fibers (Lyman et al., 1971).

3.1.6. Collagen structure and carbohydrate content

Gordon and Dingle (1974), using iodinated neutral salt soluble rat skin collagen and washed rat platelets resuspended in calcium-free Tyrodes solution (pH 7.3), concluded that the collagen had to be polymerized in order to bind to the platelets.

Kronick and Jimenez (1975) reported that small collagen fibrils ($s_w > 10$ sec) can bind to washed, resuspended human platelets at physiologic ionic strength, whereas individual collagen molecules do not bind to platelets under these conditions, although at low ionic strength (50 mM NaCl), both individual collagen molecules and collagen polymers can bind. Under these conditions, a nonhydroxylated procollagen ('protocollagen') containing no carbohydrate can also bind to platelets, but the specificity of collagen binding to platelets at low ionic strength remains to be demonstrated.

Brass and Bensusan (1975) coupled collagen and collagen fibrils to cyanogen bromide activated Sepharose 2B, and found that washed human platelets adhered to both columns, although those containing collagen fibrils were more active. The ionic strength at which these experiments were carried out was not stated, and no information was provided about the state of the collagen after coupling to sepharose. A more detailed account of the results obtained with collagen fibrils has, however, now been published (Brass et al., 1976).

Jaffe and Deykin (unpublished results) examined binding of chick bone (Type I) and cartilage (Type II) collagen to human platelets in plasma, having obtained the collagens by organ culture in media containing tritiated glycine, lysine, and proline. The collagen molecule ('unit collagen') did not bind to platelets after 30 minutes incubation at 30°C or 37°C, whereas collagen multimers exhibited a time-dependent increase in binding, and collagen fibrils bound rapidly to platelets (Table 7).

TABLE 7
Platelet interaction with Type I collagen

Collagen form	Binding of platelets	Aggregation of platelets	Platelet release
Collagen	Not observed	No	?
Multimeric collagen	With lag ($\sim$120s)	With lag ($\sim$180s)	?
Fibrillar collagen	Immediate	With lag ($\sim$60s)	Yes
Fibrous collagen	Immediate	With lag ($\sim$60s)	Yes
Connective tissue suspensions	Not known	With lag ($\sim$60s)	Yes

Cazenave et al. (1973) extracted collagen from bovine tail tendon with cold acetic acid and used this material to coat a glass tube under standard conditions at 22°C. The surface contained ultrastructurally banded collagen fibrils, and the term 'acid soluble collagen' was applied to the connective tissue extract used, but no criteria of protein purity or physical studies to show complete de-polymerization of the collagen were reported. The possibility that de-polymerization did not occur is strengthened by their observation that 10 mM glucosamine did not inhibit fibril deposition during the coating process, and yet glucosamine prevents fibril formation of soluble collagen (Legrand et al., 1968). This collagen preparation is therefore not equivalent to the acid soluble collagen referred to earlier in this discussion.

Jimenez et al. (1975) showed that cartilage procollagen did not bind to platelets, and this collagen does not form ordered polymers, although it has the same carbohydrate content as native cartilage collagen—which does form ordered polymers and does bind to platelets.

3.1.7. Sugars, aminosugars, and sugar-nucleotides

Cazenave and coworkers (1974b) found that glucosamine, uridine diphosphate (UDP), and UDP-Glucose (UDPG), at (1 mM), did not affect adherence of platelets to collagen-coated surfaces. These studies were stimulated by an earlier suggestion that a UDPG transferase might mediate collagen adhesion to platelets (Jamieson et al., 1971) and UDP (and ADP) inhibit the enzyme.

Jamieson, Smith, and Kosow (1975) later emphasized, however, that the ineffectiveness of these sugars on platelet adhesion to collagen is not incompatible with several possible mechanisms by which UDP-Glucose transferase could mediate platelet:collagen adhesion.

3.1.8. Drugs

Aspirin (ASA; acetyl salicylate) and prostaglandin E_1 (PGE$_1$) do not inhibit binding of radiolabeled collagen to washed rat platelets (MacIntyre and Gordon, 1975a) but Cazenave et al. (1974a) found that ASA, phenylbutazone, RA 233, and RA 433 all reduced the adhesion of washed platelets to collagen-coated surfaces. The ASA effect was 3-fold greater with human than pig platelets. Spaet and Lejnieks (1969) had previously found that aspirin did not inhibit adhesion of platelets to connective tissue fibers in EDTA plasma, and Baumgartner and Muggli (1974) and Weiss et al. (1975) recently reported that ASA treated rabbit and human platelets adhere normally to exposed rabbit subendothelium. Cazenave et al. (1975), however, reported that ASA does inhibit rabbit platelet adhesion to damaged rabbit subendothelium. The experimental designs are similar, inasmuch as platelets are exposed to mechanically damaged, everted rabbit aortae, but there are some differences in experimental approach which may relate to the divergent results: (1) Baumgartner and co-workers allowed citrated platelet-rich plasma to flow over everted rabbit aortic segments at physiologic rates, while Cazenave rotated everted rabbit aortic segments in washed platelets resuspended in Tyrodes buffer containing 0.35% albumin and calcium. (2) Cazenave et al. have apyrase present, while Baumgartner and his colleagues do not.

Tricyclic antidepressants such as imipramine inhibit amine (e.g., serotonin) uptake and release by platelets at therapeutic dosages (1 μM or less), but although these drugs can inhibit platelet adhesion to collagen fibrils (Mohammed and Mason, 1974; Cazenave et al., 1974a), concentrations of 100 μM or more are required. This effect is therefore of minimal pharmacological significance.

3.1.9. Platelet sialic acid

It might be argued that platelet surface charge could play an important role in platelet: collagen interaction, but Greenberg et al. (1975) reported that removing over 50% of platelet surface sialic acid residues with neuraminidase did not inhibit platelet adherence to collagen fibril coated surfaces, or to de-endothelialized, everted rabbit aorta segments. It therefore seems that the negative charge of sialic acid does not play a major role in platelet:collagen interaction.

3.2. Platelet:elastin adhesion

Some studies have suggested that platelets adhere to elastin (Jorgensen, 1971; Spaet and Stemerman, 1972), but the preparations tested probably contained collagen (Franzblau, 1971), even though no ultrastructurally identifiable collagen fibers were present. Digesting subendothelium with collagenase and trypsin leaves elastin intact, and such digests induce little platelet adhesion (Baumgartner, 1974). In vitro studies also suggest that purified elastin is a poor thrombogenic surface (Hoffman, 1975) and Ts'ao and Glagov (1970) reported that aortic elastic lamina and elastin fragments do not support platelet adhesion.

3.3. Platelet:glycoprotein adhesion

Extracellular non-collagenous filaments ('microfibrils') are characterized as glycoprotein and are distinct from collagen (Ross and Bornstein, 1969). Studies showing platelet adhesion to sub-endothelial 'microfibrils' (Stemerman et al., 1971) should perhaps be re-interpreted, as recent work has not confirmed that platelets adhere to non-collagenous glycoproteins in the subendothelium (Weiss et al., 1975).

3.4. Platelet:proteoglycan adhesion

Proteoglycans have not been systematically studied with regard to their reactivity toward platelets, but there is indirect evidence that they may reduce platelet interaction with adhesive subendothelial components (Carraway, 1975) either by forming a mechanical barrier or by directly inhibiting platelet adhesion. Sheppard and French (1971) showed platelets adhering to subendothelial mucopolysaccharide, but as they used ruthenium red staining to identify the mucopolysaccaride, and this technique is not specific, their conclusions remain to be confirmed.

3.5. Platelet:basement membrane adhesion

Basement membrane is a complex structure (Balazs, 1970), and when flowing blood is exposed to it platelets adhere (T'sao et al., 1970; Baumgartner, 1974; Carraway, 1975) although large platelet aggregates rarely occur. When compared to collagen fibrils on a weight basis, isolated glomerular basement membrane is much less active at inducing platelet adhesion and degranulation (T'sao, 1971) and collagenase digestion is associated with a 50 fold reduction in platelet adhesion to rabbit aorta basement membrane (Baumgartner, 1974). The collagenase used was not assayed for the presence of other enzymes, however, and it may be premature to conclude that collagen is the main active component of basement membrane.

Platelets adhere to human glomerular basement lamina devoid of morphologically identifiable collagen fibers (T'sao, 1971; Huang et al., 1974) but these adherent platelets do not release granule contents of the Huang et al. (1974) concluded that platelet aggregation reportedly induced by glomerular basal lamina (Hugues and Mahieu, 1970) was caused by associated collagen fibers. It will be of interest to learn whether purified basement membrane collagen (Type IV) is intrinsically less active than Type I collagen in inducing platelet adhesion, or whether non-collagen components associated with basement membrane collagen reduce platelet reactivity toward basement membrane collagen.

3.6. Summary

The available evidence about platelet : connective tissue adhesion can be summarized as follows:

(1) Platelets have variable affinity for subendothelial connective tissue, depending upon the molecular composition of the subendothelium.

(2) Divalent cations, and platelet membrane sulfhydryl groups, are not required for platelet binding to connective tissue or collagen.

(3) Plasma proteins enhance (but are not a prerequisite for) platelet : collagen binding.

(4) Treatment of platelets with metabolic poisons, or brief exposure to formaldehyde, does not inhibit platelet : collagen binding.

(5) Collagen polymers (?fibrils) have a high avidity for platelets.

(6) Collagen telopeptides and cross-links are not required for platelet : collagen adhesion, and the role of collagen carbohydrate is unresolved.

(7) High concentrations of tricyclic antidepressants reduce platelet : collagen adhesion, but there are conflicting reports about aspirin's effectiveness.

(8) Platelet sialic acid is not required for platelet : collagen adhesion.

(9) Purified elastin and non-collagen glycoproteins do not support platelet adhesion, and basement membrane appears to be less active than collagen fibrils in inducing platelet adhesion.

4. Platelet aggregation induced by connective tissue

Platelets aggregate when exposed to collagen-rich connective tissue suspensions (Zucker and Borrelli, 1962), and preparations of connective tissue used in platelet aggregation studies are usually minced or acid-swollen collagen-rich tendon, although purified polymeric collagen is sometimes used by some workers (Jaffe and Deykin, 1974; Brass and Bensusan, 1974; Katzman et al., 1973).

4.1. Divalent cations, sulfhydryl groups and plasma proteins

Divalent cations are required for aggregation and chelating agents such as EDTA are inhibitory (Hovig, 1964), as are reagents which block platelet sulfhydryl groups. Plasma proteins enhance aggregation, although their presence is apparently not essential (Lyman et al., 1971; Wilner et al., 1968). The role of complement is obscure: Jobin and Tremblay (1969) emphasized that compounds which inhibit complement activation also block collagen-induced platelet aggregation, and Salicylaldoxime which antagonises the C3a component of complement is reported to block 'collagen'- and thrombin-induced platelet aggregation, though not thrombin digestion of fibrinogen. Late components of complement, however, are not required for collagen-induced platelet aggregation–at least in the rabbit (Christian and Gordon, 1975).

4.2. Collagen structure

Purified collagen, reconstituted as fibrils, induces platelet aggregation. No property of the collagen fibril is reported which distinguish it from connective tissue suspensions in this respect, and the structural details of the collagen molecule essential for platelet aggregation have been most extensively investigated.

4.2.1. Collagen helix and telopeptides

As mentioned above, the collagen molecule contains a helical portion, and amino and carboxy terminal telopeptides which do not display the 'collagen' helix. These telopeptides can be digested away from the collagen molecule with pepsin or pronase without affecting platelet aggregation (Wilner et al., 1968; Jaffe and Deykin, 1974). It should be noted that this modified collagen can form fibrils.

4.2.2. ε-Amino groups of lysine

Wilner and co-workers (1968) treated acid-dispersible collagen with reagents (nitrous acid, acetic anhydride, 2,4-dinitrofluorobenzene, and 2,4,6-trinitrobenzenesulfonic acid) which blocked the free amino groups of lysine, and found that the treated collagen lost its ability to aggregate platelets. They concluded that free amino groups in general, and specifically the ε-amino groups of lysine, were essential for the platelet-aggregating activity of collagen. However, Rauterberg and Kuhn (1968) showed that such treatment may lead to random orientation of the collagen chains, as may succinylation of collagen (Gustavson, 1961), which was also employed by Wilner and coworkers. Brass and Bensusan (1974) reported that guanidinylation of ε-amino groups (which converts the lysines to homoarginine) enhances fibril formation and produces a collagen fibril which induces platelet aggregation, and Jaffe and Deykin (1974) permethylated collagen ε-amino groups without loss of fibril formation or loss of aggregating activity. Permethylated lysine retains a positive charge, although it is chemically and sterically converted to a secondary, rather than primary, amine, and so, the role of positively charged amines in collagen-induced platelet aggregation remains unresolved (Nossel et al., 1969).

4.2.3. Carboxyl groups

Wilner and co-workers (1971) showed that esterification of carboxyl residues in collagen does not inhibit platelet aggregation by collagen; we confirmed this observation, and also noted that esterification did not affect collagen's fibril structure (Jaffe and Deykin, unpublished observation).

4.2.4. Collagen-associated carbohydrate

Following the hypothesis advanced by Roseman (1970) that membrane-bound glycosyltransferases could mediate cell adhesion, two laboratories reported

UDP-Glucose transferases in platelets (Bosmann, 1971; Barber and Jamieson, 1971). The platelet transferase apparently accepts collagen as a substrate (Jamieson et al., 1971) although the transfer of glucose to collagen under physiological conditions has not been confirmed. The hypothesis does not require covalent transfer of glucose to collagen from the enzyme to act as a collagen receptor (Jamieson et al., 1975), but the affinity (K_m) and saturability of the platelet transferase by collagen need to be reported before collagen could be considered a specific substrate for the enzyme. Spiro and Spiro (1971) have reviewed the difficulties in documenting the specificity of a collagen glucosyltransferase.

Chesney and co-workers (1972) lent support to the transferase theory by demonstrating that treatment of acid-soluble collagen with galactose oxidase impaired its ability to aggregate platelets. They concluded that galactose was essential for platelet aggregation, serving as a receptor for platelet glucosyltransferase. However, Muggli and Baumgartner (1973) showed that galactose oxidase treatment of soluble collagen monomers impairs their ability to polymerize, and Simons et al. (1975) supported these conclusions. These data agree with the suggestion of Morgan et al. (1970) that collagen carbohydrate influences fibril formation. Galactose oxidase treatment of preformed rat skin collagen fibrils does not inhibit human platelet aggregation, (Puett et al., 1973), and similar results have been reported for rabbit subendothelium treated with galactose oxidase (Muggli and Baumgartner, 1973).

Galactose oxidase or periodate oxidation of collagen carbohydrate leads to perturbed melting curves, inhibition of collagen multimer formation, and loss of platelet aggregating ability (Simons et al., 1975). Puett et al. (1973) reported that periodate oxidation of more than 90% of collagen carbohydrate in preformed rat skin collagen fibrils had no effect on human platelet aggregation, but Kang et al. (1974) found that periodate oxidation of chick skin collagen fibrils reduced platelet aggregating activity. However, there was no characterization of the oxidized product to distinguish effects on the structure of the collagen fibril from specific effects on the carbohydrate.

Jaffe and Deykin (1974) found no difference in platelet-aggregating activity between Type I and Type II collagen (of similar fibril size) although there is a 6-fold difference in GH content (see Table IIA and B). An invertebrate collagen from ascaris cuticle, when polymerized into a fibril, induces platelet aggregation although it contains no detectable GH (Josse and Harrington, 1964; Jaffe and Deykin, 1974). As pointed out by Jamieson (1974), however, the role of GH may be expressed in adhesion and not in aggregation, and Kang et al. (1974) have emphasized that there may be carbohydrate-dependent and independent mechanisms by which collagen can deduce platelet aggregation.

4.2.5. Collagen polymers

There is considerable evidence showing that platelet aggregation requires a quaternary structural (architectural) arrangement of the collagen. The collagen molecule alone does not induce platelet aggregation, whereas an intermediate collagen polymer (multimeric collagen) induces platelet aggregation after a lag of about 3 min, and collagen fibrils or connective tissue particles induce aggregation after a lag of about 1 minute (Muggli and Baumgartner, 1973; Deykin, 1974; Brass and Bensusan, 1974).

Chemicals which retard the formation of fibrils (0.1 M arginine, 0.1 M urea 0.1 M penicillamine, N-protonated sugars such as glucosamine) prolong the lag phase of platelet aggregation induced by multimeric collagen, although they have no effect on platelet aggregation induced by preformed collagen fibrils (Brass and Bensusan, 1974; Jaffe and Deykin, 1974). Similarly, galactose oxidase treatment (which retards collagen fibril formation) does not affect platelet aggregation induced by preformed collagen fibrils (Muggli and Baumgartner, 1973). Collagen fibril formation may be enhanced or stabilized by carbohydrate (Morgan et al., 1970), hydroxyproline (Ramachandran et al., 1975), and by the sequence regularity of the molecule (Salem and Traub, 1975).

Some of the physical properties and functional features of different collagen preparations are summarized in Table 8.

TABLE 8
Characteristics of physical forms of Type I collagen

Name	pH	Temperature	Viscosity (dl/g)	Ultra structure (E/M)
Collagen ('tropocollagen', 'collagen monomer', 'unit collagen')	4	4°C	13.8	No structure seen (up to 50,000 magnification)
Multimeric collagen ('monomeric collagen')	7–8	4°C	16.7	Amorphous filaments, e.g., 75 Å × 6000 Å
Fibrillar collagen	7–8	15°C–30°C	24.3	Banded filaments, e.g., 700 Å × μ
Fibrous collagen	7–8	> 30°C	*	Banded fibers, e.g., μ × μ

* Not homogeneously in medium so viscosity can not be approximated.

4.2.6. Collagen cross-links

Collagen contains unusual aminoacids, derived from lysine, which serve as intra- and intermolecular cross-links (Traub and Piez, 1971; Grant and Prockop, 1972; Veis and Brownell, 1975), and the possibility that these cross-links play a role in collagen-induced platelet aggregation has been assessed in two ways. Cross-links can be reduced by treatment with sodium borohydride which selectively converts the aldehydes to alcohols and the Schiff bases to covalent secondary amines. Such treatment does not affect platelet aggregation by collagen. Also, the aminothiol penicillamine (which binds collagen aldehydes and displaces Schiff bases) does not affect platelet aggregation by collagen fibrils (Jaffe and Deykin, 1974; Simons et al., 1975).

4.2.7. Glycosides, sugar-nucleotides, and aminosugars

Glucosyl galactosyl hydroxylysine (GGH) and galactosyl hydroxylysine (GH) at concentrations of 18 μM and 29 μM respectively did not inhibit platelet aggregation induced by human or rat skin collagen, although GH (but not GGH) apparently bound to platelets (Puett et al., 1973). Similarly, the nucleotide UDP and sugar-nucleotide UDP-glucose did not inhibit platelet aggregation by collagen polymers. The amino sugar glucosamine retards collagen polymerization (Hayashi and Nagai, 1972), but does not affect platelet aggregation by collagen preparations which are already polymerized (Brass and Bensusan, 1974).

Katzman et al. (1973) observed that platelet aggregation induced by the α1 chain of chick skin collagen could be inhibited by high concentrations ($\geqslant$ 15 mM) of glucosamine, GH and GGH. This could be because aggregation induced by the chick skin collagen alpha chain involves an unusual mechanism, or it may be due to physical effects of these agents on the alpha chain structure in solution.

4.2.8. Denatured collagen (gelatin) and subunits

Denaturing collagen by heating, or digesting it with collagenase, abolishes its ability to induce platelet aggregation at normal concentrations (Wilner et al., 1968). The products of digestion do not inhibit platelet aggregation induced by native collagen fibrils (Puett et al., 1973; Jaffe and Deykin, 1974; Simons et al., 1975). However, very high concentrations of denatured collagen (gelatin) from chick or rat skin can induce platelet aggregation (Puett et al., 1973; Kang et al., 1974), although these preparations are inactive if heated to 56°C for 30 min just prior to use (Jaffe and Deykin, unpublished).

Similarly, subunit chains of chick and rat skin collagen can induce platelet aggregation at high concentration (Puett et al., 1973; Kang et al., 1974). After heating to 56°C for 30 min the rat skin α-chains are inactive (Puett et al., 1973), but a recent report suggests that chick skin α-chains heated to 45°C can induce platelet release (Chiang et al., 1975).

Houck and Chang (1971) found that several collagen peptides produced by collagenase digestion and isolated by chromatography on Dowex resin could induce aggregation of rat platelets; however, the conditions employed workers favoured association of the peptides, and the platelet aggregation pattern obtained was unusual in showing no initial lag period.

4.2.9. Cyanogen bromide peptides

Kang and co-workers (1974) tested the collagen peptides derived from purified chick skin α-chains by cyanogen bromide digestion and found that the 34 residue α1 CB5 peptide (see Table 9) could induce platelet aggregation. Periodate oxidation or chymotrypsin digestion of this peptide abolished its activity. The carboxy terminal peptide (α1 CB5-C2), containing residues 7 through 34 and no carbohydrate, inhibited platelet aggregation induced by native collagen, whereas the amino terminal peptide (α1 CB5-C1), containing residues 1–6, had no effect.

TABLE 9
Sequence of α1-CB5 peptide

GlC-Gal-0
|
1

                      ↓

RAT   Hyl-Gly-His-Arg-Gly-Phe-Ser-Gly-Leu-Asp-Gly-Ala-Lys-Gly-ASN-THR-Gly-Pro-Ala-Gly-Pro-Lys-Gly-Glu-
CHICK Hyl-Gly-His-Arg-Gly-Phe-Ser-Gly-Leu-Asp-Gly-Ala-Lys-Gly-GLN-HYP-Gly-Pro-Ala-Gly-Pro-Lys-Gly-Glu-

RAT   Hyp-Gly-Ser-Hyp-Gly-Glx-ASX-Gly-Ala-HYP-Gly-Gln-Hse[a]
CHICK Hyp-Gly-Ser-Hyp-Gly-Glx-HYP-Gly-Ala-ASX-Gly-Gln-Hse[a]

Arrow (↓) represents chymotrypsin sensitive bond.
[a] Homoserine results from the cyanogen bromide cleavage of methionine residues.

The homologous peptide (α 1 CB5) from rat skin collagen neither induced platelet aggregation, nor inhibited aggregation induced by collagen (Puett et al., 1973) and the α 1 CB5 peptide from human skin collagen is also inactive (Michaeli and Swanson, unpublished).

The chick skin α 1 CB5 peptide differs from the homologous rat and human peptides at several residues (Table 9), which might explain the difference in activity, but it may be significant that the chick skin α 1 CB5 peptide was isolated at 45°C whereas the rat and human skin peptides were heated to 56°C immediately prior to use.

Gallop and Paz (1975) commented that chick α 1(I)CB5 is more likely to renature than rat α 1(I)CB5, because there is hydroxyproline at residues 118 and 133 in the chick peptide where the rat peptide has threonine and asparagyl residues; hydroxyproline contributes to fibril formation and stability (Ramachandran et al., 1975).

4.3. Inhibition by drugs

Platelet aggregation induced by collagen can be inhibited by many non-steroidal anti-inflammatory drugs including aspirin, phenylbutazone, amidopyrine, fenoprofen, mefenamic acid and indomethacin (O'Brien, 1968; Zucker and Peterson, 1970; Herrmann et al., 1972). Aspirin's effect ex vivo lasts for several days (Stuart et al., 1972), and there has been considerable controversy about its mechanism of action. It has been suggested that this involves acetylation of a plasma protein (Okonkwo and Sise, 1971; Scharrer et al., 1973), but the intensity and duration of aspirin's effect ex vivo are comparable in washed platelet suspensions and in platelet-rich plasma (MacIntyre and Gordon, 1975b) which indicates that its main effect is on the platelets themselves. Al-Mondhiry et al. (1970) suggested that aspirin could acetylate a protein on the platelet membrane, and recent elegant work from Majerus's laboratory has established that the protein in question is the cyclo-oxygenase involved in prostaglandin synthesis (Roth and Majerus, 1975). The significance of this is discussed in Chapter 13.

Thilo and Von Kaulla (1970) commented that salicylic acid derivatives which induced fibrinolysis could also inhibit collagen-induced platelet aggregation, and lipophilic, serine protease inhibitors could often inhibit collagen-induced platelet aggregation at levels 10–100 times lower than those required to increase fibrinolysis.

Several pyrimido–pyrimidine compounds inhibit collagen-induced aggregation of rabbit platelets ex vivo at doses of 15 mg/kg. Dipyridamole (persantin) was more active than its congeners RA433 and RA233 in both rabbit and rat (Didisheim and Owen, 1970; Cucuianu et al., 1971).

Benzazepine derivatives (particularly nortriptyline and amitriptyline) at concentrations of 10–50 μM inhibit collagen-induced platelet aggregation in vitro, and chlorophenoxyisobutyrate (Atromid-S) or its ester have a slight inhibitory effect both in vitro and ex vivo (Mills and Roberts, 1967; O'Brien and Heywood, 1966).

Phentolamine and dihydroergotamine (alpha adrenergic blocking drugs) can inhibit collagen-induced platelet aggregation, whereas propranolol (a beta ad-renergic blocker) is a much weaker inhibitor, but ADP-induced platelet aggrega-tion is similarly inhibited by phentolamine and propranolol (Nordoy, 1963; Hampton et al., 1967; Thomas, 1968).

4.4. Effects of changes in platelet or plasma constituents

Carvalho et al. (1974) reported a 5-fold increase in platelet sensitivity to collagen in a group of hypercholesterolemic patients, and Shattil et al. (1975) showed that incubating washed human platelets with cholesterol-rich liposomes increased the sensitivity of the platelets to collagen. Collagen-induced platelet aggregation is reduced in uremic patients (Baele et al., 1971) and lactacidemia may increase platelet adhesiveness (Broersma et al., 1970) although collagen-induced aggrega-tion is apparently not affected by 0.8% lactic acid (Goldschmidt, 1973). The pathological significance of these results, which may be considerable, awaits further evaluation.

4.5. Platelet aggregation induced by other connective tissue components

The only connective tissue component (other than purified collagen) which induces platelet aggregation in vitro is basement membrane, and, as discussed above (Section 3.5), it may be a collagen component which is responsible for this activity. Recent experiments indicate that purified elastin, and non-collagen fibrillar glycoprotein, do not induce platelet aggregation (Hoffman, 1975). It has, however, been suggested that platelet aggregation is enhanced by glycosaminogly-cans (Muir and Mustard, 1968).

Insoluble vitreous collagen, which has the same biochemical characteristics as basement membrane collagen and shows no ultrastructural banding (perhaps because of associated glycoprotein), reacts avidly with platelets (Swann et al., 1974).

4.6. Summary

The available evidence about connective tissue induced platelet aggregation can be summarized as follows:

(1) Suspensions of connective tissue or collagen fibrils aggregate platelets in microgram (nanomolar) amounts.

(2) Divalent cations and platelet sulfhydryl groups are required for platelet aggregation.

(3) Washed platelets aggregate in response to collagen fibrils in the presence of added albumin, and plasma proteins (especially fibrinogen) enhance aggregation.

(4) Collagen ε-amino groups of lysine, carboxylates of glutamic and aspartic acid, carbohydrate, and cross-links are not required for platelet aggregation, but collagen polymers (possibly fibrils) are necessary.

(5) The activity of different collagen types differs on a weight basis: Type IV collagen is least active. It is not known whether this reflects intrinsic differences in the collagen molecules or in their ability to form polymers.

(6) High concentrations of denatured collagen, certain subunit chains of collagen, and one chick skin collagen peptide induce platelet aggregation in milligram amounts.

(7) High concentrations of sugar-nucleotides and amino sugars apparently inhibit collagen-induced platelet aggregation, but it is not clear whether their effect is on collagen polymerization or on platelet-collagen interaction. Similarly, high concentrations of glucosamine, GH and GGH inhibit platelet aggregation induced by α 1(I) chains, but it is not known whether this is merely because they alter the structure of the α 1(I) chains in solution.

(8) Elastin, glycoproteins and proteoglycans do not induce platelet aggregation, and although basement membrane is a weak inducer of platelet aggregation, a collagen component may be responsible.

(9) Various drugs can inhibit platelet aggregation. Their exact sites of action are often not known (but see Chapter 13, for aspirin), and some may primarily affect the platelet release reaction (see the following section, and Chapter 3).

5. Platelet release reaction induced by collagen

Grette (1962) applied the term 'release reaction' to the thrombin-induced liberation of platelet components into the surrounding medium, but other agents (including collagen) can also stimulate platelets to release some of their constituents (Holmsen, 1965). The biology of the platelet release is discussed in Chapter 3.

5.1. Collagen structure

Chesney et al. (1974) reported that gel-filtered platelets did not release hydrolases in response to polymers of acid soluble collagen, but Holmsen (1975), also using gel-filtered platelets, reported that polymeric acid-soluble collagen released more hydrolases than thrombin. The polymeric form of the collagen employed was not characterized in these studies and may account for the differences in results.

Michaeli and Swanson (unpublished) found that the activity of the different types of collagen as release inducers was: Type I > Type II > Type III > Type IV, but they did not determine the polymeric structure of the collagens. In contrast, recent results from Kuhn's laboratory showed the rank order of activity to be Type III > Type I > Type II; the difference between III and I was, however, small when both were tested as preformed fibrils (Balleisen et al., 1975).

5.2. Collagen subunits

Chiang and co-workers (1975) reported that 200 μg chick skin α 1-chains, 100 μg chick skin α 1-CB5, and 50 μg chick skin collagen polymers all released serotonin from human platelets. The α 1-chain and α 1-CB5 peptide were apparently effective even when heated to 45°C prior to use, in contrast to similar preparations of rat skin collagen.

Michaeli and Swanson (unpublished) found that a 200 residue, noncarbohydrate containing peptide (α 1-CB6) derived from human skin collagen subunit chains by cyanogen bromide digestion, could inhibit the collagen-induced release of serotonin.

5.3. Inhibition by drugs

Aspirin inhibits collagen-induced release of platelet amines and nucleotides, by inhibiting prostaglandin formation (see Chapter 13). This inhibition can be overcome by increasing the concentration of collagen (Zucker and Peterson, 1970), but the collagen-induced release reaction in aspirin-treated platelets is presumably mediated by a prostaglandin-independent pathway. Both indomethacin and aspirin are potent inhibitors of the platelet release reaction, but mefenamic acid, phenylbutazone and salicylic acid are progressively less active inhibitors (Zucker and Peterson, 1970).

5.4. Summary

The available evidence about connective tissue induced platelet release can be summarized:

(1) Collagen fibrils can induce both release I and release II (see Chapter 3).

(2) On a weight basis, Type II and Type IV collagen are less potent than Type I and Type III at inducing release.

(3) Of the cyanogen bromide peptides tested, chick skin α 1-CB5 is uniquely able to induce the platelet release reaction.

(4) Drugs which inhibit the collagen-induced release reaction also inhibit collagen-induced platelet aggregation (see Section 4.3).

6. Stimulation of platelet coagulant activity by collagen

Platelet factor 3 (PF-3) catalyzes the activation of Factor X in the presence of calcium and Factors IXa and VIIIa (Spaet and Cintron, 1965) and the conversion of prothrombin to thrombin in the presence of Factor Xa (Papahadjopoulos and Hanahan, 1964). Collagen treatment increases the PF-3 activity in the reaction supernatant of washed rabbit, pig, and human platelets, whereas ADP increases PF-3 only in the supernatant of human platelets (Joist et al., 1974). However, since this PF-3 availability was associated with the loss of ^{51}Cr and the cytoplasmic enzyme lactic dehydrogenase it is possible that collagen-stimulated PF-3 availability is a consequence of platelet lysis.

Walsh and Biggs (1972) found a platelet coagulant activity induced by collagen which was independent of PF-3: this activity did not require Factor XII, was associated with the platelet membrane surface, and may be Factor XI (Walsh, 1972a,b).

7. *Effect of anti-platelet antibodies on platelet-collagen interaction*

Kaplan and Nachman (1974) raised antibodies to rabbit platelet membranes and platelet-associated membrane glycoproteins, and found that Fab fragments of the anti-membrane antibodies inhibited collagen-induced aggregation in an 'all-or-none' fashion, although the dose-response relationship for inhibition of aggregation induced by ADP and thrombin was nearly linear. These authors suggested that this might indicate a limited and saturable number of binding sites for collagen, all of similar affinity. They also found that the antibodies to platelet-associated glycoprotein did not block collagen-induced platelet aggregation.

Acknowledgements

This report was aided substantially by the generous availability of manuscripts in press and in preparation, especially from Drs. Dov Michaeli and Marian Packham. Florence Ross provided enthusiastic and enduring support, especially during the preparation of the manuscript. Lynn Huffman and Marcy Jaffe contributed graciously of their time and skill to this manuscript.

References

Al-Mondhiry, H. and Spaet, T.H. (1970) Proc. Soc. Exp. Biol. Med., *135*, 878.
Al-Mondhiry, H., Marcus, A.J. and Spaet, T.H. (1970) Proc. Soc. Exp. Biol. Med., *133*, 632.
Ashford, T.P. and Freiman, D.G. (1968) Am. J. Path., *53*, 599.
Baele, G., Vanden-Bogaert, P. and Barbier, F. (1971) Acta Med. Scand. Suppl., *525*, 131.
Balazs, E.A. (ed.) (1970) The chemistry and molecular biology of the Intercellular matrix. N.Y. Academic Press.
Balleisen, L., Gay, S., Marx, R. and Kühn, K. (1975) Klin. Wschr., *53*, 903.
Bang, N.U., Heidenreich, R.O. and Trygstad, C.W. (1972) Ann. N.Y. Acad. Sci., *201*, 280.
Barber, A.J. and Jamieson, G.A. (1971) Fed. Proc., *30*, 540.
Bard, J.B.L. and Chapman, J.A. (1973) Nature New Biol., *246*, 83.
Baumgartner, H.R. (1974) Thrombos. Diathes. Haemorrh. Suppl., *59*, 91.
Baumgartner, H.R. and Haudenschild, C. (1972) Ann. N.Y. Acad. Sci., *201*, 22.
Baumgartner, H. and Muggli, R. (1974) Thrombos. Diathes. Haemorrh. Suppl., *60*, 345.
Behnke, O. (1970) Scand. J. Haematol., *7*, 123.
Beighton, P. (1970) The Ehlers-Danlos Syndrome, p. 194, Heinemann, London.
Bornstein, P. (1974) Ann. Rev. Biochem., *43*, 567.
Bosmann, H.B. (1971) Biochem. Biophys. Res. Commun., *43*, 1118.
Bounameaux, Y. (1959) Compt. Rend. Soc. Biol. (Paris), *153*, 685.

Brandt, K.D. (1974) Adv. Exp. Med. Biol., *43*, 161.
Brass, L. and Bensusan, H.B. (1974) J. Clin. Invest., *54*, 1480.
Brass, L. and Bensusan, H. (1975) Fed. Proc., *34*, 241.
Brass, L.F., Faile, D. and Bensusan, H.B. (1976) J. Lab. Clin. Med., *87*, 525.
Broersma, R.J., Bullemer, D.G. and Mammen, E.F. (1970) Throm. Diath. Haemorrh., *24*, 55.
Butler, W.T. (1970) Biochemistry, *9*, 44.
Byers, P.H., McKenney, K.H., Lichtenstein, J.R. and Martin, G.R. (1974) Biochemistry, *13*, 5243.
Carnes, W.H. (1971) Proc., *30*, 995.
Carraway, K.L. (1975) Interaction of basement membranes with platelets. Annual Report NIH-
    NHLI-HB-4-2983, Biopolymers Program, Division of Blood Disease and Resources (available
    from N.T.I.S., Springfield, Va.).
Carvalho, A.C.A., Colman, R.W. and Lees, R.S. (1974) New Eng. J. Med., *290*, 434.
Cazenave, J.P., Packham, M.A. and Mustard, J.F. (1973) J. Lab. Clin. Med., *82*, 978.
Cazenave, J.P., Packham, M.A., Guccione, M.A. and Mustard, J.F. (1974a) J. Lab. Clin. Med., *83*,
    797.
Cazenave, J.P., Guccione, M.A., Mustard, J.F. and Packham, M.A. (1974b) Thrombos. Diathes.
    Haemorrh., *31*, 521.
Cazenave, J.P., Packham, M.A., Guccione, M.A. and Mustard, J.F. (1975) J. Lab. Clin. Med., *86*,
    551.
Chesney, C.McI., Harper, E. and Colman, R.W. (1972) J. Clin. Invest., *51*, 2693.
Chesney, C.McI., Harper, E. and Colman, R.W. (1974) J. Clin. Invest., *53*, 1647.
Chiang, T.M., Beachey, E.M. and Kang, A.H. (1975) J. Biol. Chem., *250*, 6916.
Christian, F.A. and Gordon, J.L. (1975) Immunology, *29*, 131.
Click, E.M. and Bornstein, P. (1970) Biochemistry, *9*, 4699.
Cucuianu, M.P., Nishizawa, E.E. and Mustard, J.F. (1971) J. Lab. Clin. Med., *77*, 958.
Davison, P.F. (1973) Crit. Rev. Biochem., *1*, 201.
Deykin, D. (1974) New Eng. J. Med., *290*, 144.
Didisheim, P. and Owen, C.A. (1970) Thrombos. Diathes. Haemorrh. Suppl., *42*, 267.
Doyle, B.B., Hukins, D.W.L., Hulmes, D.J.S., Miller, A. and Woodhead-Galloway, J. (1975) J. Mol.
    Biol., *91*, 79.
Epstein, E.H. (1974) J. Clin. Invest., *53*, 3225.
Epstein, E.H. and Munderloh, N.H. (1975) J. Biol. Chem., *250*, 9304.
Epstein, E.H., Scott, R.D., Miller, E.J. and Piez, K.A. (1971) J. Biol. Chem., *246*, 171.
Eyre, D.R. and Glimcher, M.J. (1972) Proc. Natl. Acad. Sci. U.S.A., *69*, 2594.
Eyre, D. and Muir, H. (1975) Biochem. J., *151*, 595.
Franzblau, C. (1971) in Comparative Biochemistry (Florkin and Stotz, eds), Vol. 26C, p. 659, Elsevier,
    Amsterdam.
French, J.E. (1969) in Thrombosis (Sherry, S., Brinkhous, K.M., Genton, E. and Stengle, J.M., eds), p.
    300, National Academy of Sciences, Washington.
Furthmayr, H., Timpl, R., Stark, M., Lapiere, C.M. and Kuhn, K. (1972) FEBS Lett., *28*, 247.
Gallop, P.M. and Paz, M.A. (1975) Physiol. Rev., *55*, 418.
Goldschmidt, B. (1973) Experientia *29*, 1399.
Gordon, J.L. and Dingle, J.T. (1974) J. Cell. Sci., *16*, 157.
Gould, B.S. (ed.) (1972) Treatise on collagen, Vol. 2, Academic Press, London and New York.
Grant, M.E. and Prockop, D.J. (1972) New Eng. J. Med., *286*, 194, 242, 291.
Greenberg, J., Packham, M.A., Cazenave, J.P., Reimers, H.J. and Mustard, J.F. (1975) Lab. Invest., *32*,
    476.
Grette, K. (1962) Acta Physiol. Scand. Suppl., *93*, 56.
Gross, J. and Kirk, D. (1958) J. Biol. Chem., *233*, 355.
Gugler, E. and Lüscher, E.F. (1965) Thrombos. Diathes. Haemorrh., *14*, 361.
Gustavson, K.H. (1961) Arkiv. Kemi., *17*, 541.
Hampton, J.R., Harrison, M.J.G., Honour, A.J. and Mitchell, J.R.A. (1967) Cardiovasc. Res., *1*, 101.
Harker, L.A., Slichter, S.J., Scott, C.R. and Ross, R. (1974) New Eng. J. Med., *291*, 537.
Hayashi, T. and Nagai, Y. (1972) J. Biochem., *72*, 749.
Hegreberg, G.A., Padgett, G.A. and Henson, J.B. (1970) Arch. Pathol., *90*, 159.
Herrmann, R.G., Marshall, W.S., Crowe, V.G. and Frank, J.D. (1972) Proc. Soc. Exp. Biol. Med., *139*,
    548.
Hoeve, C.A. (1974) Biopolymers., *13*, 677.
Hoffman, A.S. (1975) Report of NHLI Biopolymers Division Contract NO1-HB-2970-1. (Available
    through NTIS, Springfield, Va.)

290 | *R.M. Jaffe*

Holmsen, H. (1965) Scand. J. Lab. Clin. Invest., *17*, 239.
Holmsen, H. (1975) Ciba Fdn. Symp., *35*, 175.
Horwitz, A. and Crystal, R.G. (1975) J. Clin. Invest., *56*, 1312.
Houck, J. and Chang, C. (1971) Proc. Soc. Exp. Biol. Med., *138*, 342.
Hovig, T. (1963) Thrombos. Diathes. Haemorrh., *9*, 264.
Hovig, T. (1964) Thrombos. Diathes. Haemorrh., *12*, 179.
Hovig, T. (1974) in Platelets: Production, Function, Transfusion, and Storage (Baldini, M.G. and Ebbe, S., ed), p. 221, Grune and Straton, New York.
Huang, T.W., Lagunoff, D. and Benditt, E.P. (1974) Lab. Invest., *31*, 156.
Hugues, J. (1962) Thrombos. Diathes. Haemorrh., *8*, 241.
Hugues, J. and Mahieu, P. (1970) Thrombos. Diathes. Haemorrh., *24*, 395.
Hulmes, D.J.S., Miller, A., Parry, D.A.D., Piez, K.A. and Woodhead-Galloway, J. (1973) J. Mol. Biol., *79*, 137.
Jaffe, R. and Deykin, D. (1972) Fed. Proc., *31*, 241.
Jaffe, R. and Deykin, D. (1974) J. Clin. Invest., *53*, 875.
Jamieson, G.A. (1974) in Platelets and Thrombosis (Sherry, S. and Scriabine, A. ed), p. 139, University Park Press, Baltimore.
Jamieson, G.A., Urban, C.L. and Barber, A.J. (1971) Nature New Biol., *234*, 5.
Jamieson, G.A., Smith, D.F. and Kosow, D.P. (1975) Thrombos. Diathes. Haemorrh., *33*, 668.
Jimenez, S., Kronick, P., Lau, R. and Kefalides, N. (1975) Report of contract NO1-HB-2982 Biopolymers Program, Division of Blood Diseases and Resources, NHLI. Available through National Technical Information Services, Springfield, Va.
Jobin, F. and Tremblay, F. (1969) Thrombos. Diathes. Haemorrh., *22*, 466.
Johnson, S.A., Wojich, J.D., Webber, A.J. and Yun, J. (1969) in Dynamics of Thrombus Formation and Dissolution (Johnson and Guest, eds), Lippincott, Philadelphia.
Joist, H.J., Dolezel, G., Lloyd, J.V., Kinlough-Rathbone, R.L. and Mustard, J.F. (1974) J. Lab. Clin. Med., *84*, 474.
Jorgensen, L. (1971) Pathbiol. Ann., *1*, 139.
Josse, J. and Harrington, W.F. (1964) J. Mol. Biol., *9*, 269.
Kadar, A. (1974) Pathol. Eur., *9*, 133.
Kang, A.M., Igarashi, S. and Gross, J. (1972) Biochemistry, *8*, 3200.
Kang, A.H., Beachey, E.H. and Katzman, R.L. (1974) Biol. Chem., *249*, 1054.
Kang, A.H. and Trelstad, R.L. (1973) J. Clin. Invest., *52*, 2571.
Kaplan, K.L. and Nachman, R.L. (1974) Brit. J. Haemat., *28*, 551.
Katzman, R.L., Kang, A.H. and Beachey, E.H. (1973) Science, *181*, 670.
Kefalides, N.A. (1973) Int. Rev. Conn. Tis. Res., *6*, 63.
Krane, S.M., Pinell, S.R. and Erbe, R.W. (1972) Proc. Natl. Acad. Sci. U.S.A., *69*, 2899.
Kronick, P. and Jimenez, S. (1975) Fed. Proc., *33*, 1536.
Lichtenstein, J.R., Martin, G.R., Kohn, L.D., Byers, P.H. and McKusick, V.A. (1973) Science, *182*, 298.
Lyman, B., Rosenberg, L. and Karpatkin, S. (1971) J. Clin. Invest.
MacIntyre, D.E. and Gordon, J.L. (1975a) Thrombos. Diathes. Haemorrh., *34*, 332.
MacIntyre, D.E. and Gordon, J.L. (1975b) J. Pharm. Pharmacol., *27*, 19.
Marchesi, V.T. (1964) Ann. N.Y. Acad. Sci., *116*, 774.
McKusick, V.A. (1972a) in Heritable Disorders of Connective Tissue (4th ed), p. 292, Mosby, St. Louis, Mo.
McKusick, V.A. (1972b) in Heritable Disorders of Connective Tissue (4th ed.), p. 184, Mosby, St. Louis, Mo.
Menke, J.H., Alter, M., Steigleder, G.K., Weakley, D.R. and Sung, J.H. (1962) Pediatrics, *29*, 764.
Michaeli, D. and Orloff, K.G. (in press) in Progress in Thrombosis and Hemostasis (Spaet, T.H., ed), Vol. 3, Grune and Stratton, New York.
Miller, E.J. and Lunde, L.G. (1973) Biochemistry, *12*, 3153.
Miller, E.J. and Matsuka, V.T. (1974) Fed. Proc., *33*, 1197.
Mills, D.C.B. and Roberts, G.C.K. (1967) Nature (London), *213*, 35.
Mohammed, S.F. and Mason, R.G. (1974) Proc. Soc. Exp. Biol. Med., *148*, 1106.
Morgan, P.H., Jacobs, H.G., Segrest, J.P. and Cunningham, L.W. (1970) J. Biol. Chem., *245*, 5042.
Muggli, R. and Baumgartner, H.R. (1973) Thrombos. Res., *3*, 715.
Muir, H.M. and Mustard, J.F. (1968) in 'Le Role de la Paroi Arterielle dans l'Atherogenese', Centre national de la recherche scientifique, *169*, 589.
Nordoy, A. (1963) Nature, *200*, 763.

Nordwig, A. and Dick, P. (1965) Biochim. Biophys. Acta, *97*, 179.
Nossel, H.L., Wilner, G.D. and LeRoy, E.C. (1969) Nature, *221*, 75.
O'Brien, J.R. (1968) Lancet, *1*, 894.
O'Brien, J.R. and Heywood, J. (1966) Thrombos. Diathes. Haemorrh., *16*, 768.
Okonkwo, P. and Sise, H. (1971) Thrombos. Diathes. Haemorrh., *25*, 279.
Packham, M.A. and Mustard, J.F. (1971) Sem. Hematol., *8*, 30.
Papahadjopoulos, D. and Hanahan, D.J. (1964) Biochim. Biophys. Acta, *90*, 436.
Petruska, J.A. and Hodge, A.J. (1964) Proc. Natl. Acad. Sci. U.S.A., *51*, 871.
Piez, K. (1972) Curr. Top. Biochem., *21*, 102.
Piez, K.A., Eigner, E.A. and Lewis, M.S. (1963) Biochemistry, *2*, 58.
Piez, K.A., Miller, E.J., Lane, J.M. and Butler, W.T. (1969) Biochem. Biophys. Res. Commun., *37*, 801.
Puett, D., Wasserman, B.K., Ford, J.D. and Cunningham, L.W. (1973) J. Clin. Invest., *52*, 2495.
Ramachandran, G.N., Bansal, M. and Bhatnagar, R.S. (1973) Biochim. Biophys. Acta, *322*, 166.
Ramachandran, G.N., Bansal, M. and Ramakrishnan, C. (1975) Curr. Sci., *44*, 1.
Rauterberg, J. and Kuhn, K. (1968) Hoppe-Seyler's Z. Physiol. Chem., *349*, 611.
Robb-Smith, A.H.T. (1967) Brit. J. Haemat., *13*, 618.
Roden, L. (1970) in Metabolic Conjugation and Metabolic Hydrolysis (Fishman, ed), Vol. 2, Academic Press, New York.
Roden, L., Baker, J.R., Cifonelli, J.A. and Mathews, M.B. (1972) Meth. Enzymol., *28*, 73.
Rodman, N.F. Jr., Mason, R.G., Painter, J.G. and Brinkhous, K.M. (1966) Lab. Invest., *15*, 641.
Roseman, S. (1970) Chem. Phys. Lipids., *5*, 270.
Rosenberg, L. (1973) Fed. Proc., *32*, 1467.
Ross, R. and Bornstein, P. (1969) J. Cell Biol., *40*, 366.
Roth, G.J. and Majerus, P.W. (1975) J. Clin. Invest., *56*, 624.
Salem, G. and Traub, W. (1975) FEBS Lett., *51*, 94.
Scharrer, L., Gundlach, E., Schultze, U., Schaudinn, L. and Breddin, K. (1973) Int. Soc. Thrombos. Haemostas., IV Congress, Vienna. 360. (Abstract).
Sheppard, B.L. and French, J.E. (1971) Proc. Roy. Soc. (L) Ser B., *176*, 427.
Shattil, S.J., Anaya-Glindo, R., Bennett, T., Colman, R.W. and Cooper, R.A. (1975) J. Clin. Invest., *55*, 636.
Sherry, S. and Scriabine, A. (1974) Platelets and Thrombosis. Balt. Univ. Park Press.
Simons, E.R., Chesney, C.McI., Colman, R.W., Harper, E. and Samberg, E. (1975) Thrombos. Res., *7*, 123.
Smith, D.W. (1973) J. Biol. Chem., *248*, 8157.
Smith, J.W. (1958) Nature *219*, 157.
Spaet, T.H. (ed.) (1972) Progress in Hemostasis and Thrombosis, Vol. 1, Grune and Stratton, New York.
Spaet, T.H. and Cintron, J. (1965) Br. J. Haemat., *11*, 269.
Spaet, T.H. and Lejnieks, I. (1969) Proc. Soc. Exp. Biol. Med., *132*, 1038.
Spaet, T.H. and Stemerman, M.B. (1972) Ann. N.Y. Acad. Sci., *201*, 13.
Spiro, R.G. and Spiro, M.J. (1971) J. Biol. Chem., *246*, 4899.
Stemerman, M.B., Baumgartner, H.R. and Spaet, T.H. (1971) Lab. Invest., *24*, 179.
Stuart, M.J., Murphy, S., Oski, F.A., Evans, A.E., Donaldson, M.H. and Gardner, F.H. (1972) New Eng. J. Med., *287*, 1105.
Swann, D.A., Chesney, C.M., Constable, L.J., Colman, R.W., Caulfield, J.B. and Harper, E. (1974) J. Lab. Clin. Med., *84*, 264.
Teitelbaum, S.L., Kraft, W.J., Lang, R. and Avioli, L.V. (1974) Calc. Tissue Res., *17*, 75.
Thilo, D. and Von Kaulla, K.N. (1970) J. Med. Chem., *13*, 503.
Thomas, D.P. (1968) Exp. Biol. Med., *3*, 129.
Traub, W. and Piez, K. (1971) Adv. Protein Chem., *25*, 243.
Trelstad, R. (1974) Biochem. Biophys. Res. Comm., *57*, 717.
Ts'ao, Chung-hsin (1971) Thrombos. Diathes. Haemorrh., *25*, 507.
Ts'ao, Chung-hsin and Glagov, S. (1970) Brit. J. Exp. Path., *51*, 423.
Veis, A. and Brownell, A.G. (1975) Crit. Rev. Biochem., *2*, 417.
Vracko, R. (1974) Am. J. Path., *77*, 314.
Walsh, P.N. (1972a) Br. J. Haemat., *22*, 393.
Walsh, P.N. (1972b) Br. J. Haemat., *22*, 237.
Walsh, P.N., and Biggs, R. (1972) Br. J. Haemat., *22*, 743.
Weiss, H.J. (1975) New Eng. J. Med., *293*, 531.
Weiss, H.J., Tschopp, T.B. and Baumgartner, H.R. (1975) New Eng. J. Med., *293*, 619.

Wiedemann, H., Chung, E., Fujii, T., Miller, E.J. and Kuhn, K. (1975) Europ. J. Biochem., *51*, 363.
Wilner, G.D., Nossel, H.L. and LeRoy, E.C. (1968) J. Clin. Invest., *47*, 2616.
Wilner, G.D., Nossel, H.L. and Procupez, T.L. (1971) Am. J. Physiol., *220*, 1074.
Wood, G.C. (1960) Biochem. J., *75*, 605.
Wood, G.C. and Keech, M.K. (1960a) Biochem. J., *75*, 588.
Wood, G.C. and Keech, M.K. (1960b) Biochem. J., *75*, 598.
Zucker, M.B. and Borrelli, J. (1962) Proc. Soc. Exp. Biol. Med., *109*, 779.
Zucker, M.B. and Jerushalmy, Z. (1967) in Physiology of Hemostasis and Thrombosis (Johnson and Seegers, eds), p. 249, Chas. C. Thomas, Springfield, Ill.
Zucker, M.B. and Peterson, J. (1970) J. Lab. Clin. Med., *76*, 66.

CHAPTER 11

Identification and characterisation of a platelet specific release product: β-thromboglobulin

S. MOORE and D.S. PEPPER

Blood Transfusion Service, Royal Infirmary, Edinburgh, EH3 9HB, Scotland

1. Introduction

The role of platelets in haemostasis is well documented, but no reliable method as yet exists for quantitating platelet function in vivo. We approached this basic problem in our laboratory by developing a highly sensitive immunological assay for a platelet-specific protein which is secreted during the platelet release reaction.

Platelet aggregation, accompanied by the secretion of platelet granule contents into the surrounding medium (the 'release reaction') is accepted as the most important biological reaction of platelets in vivo, and one of the main physiological stimuli for platelets is thrombin (see Chapter 9). We therefore decided to study the release reaction during thrombin-induced aggregation of washed human platelets in vitro as a model system for investigating the secretion of a platelet-specific protein.

The earliest recorded evidence of a platelet specific β-globulin comes from the work of Salmon and Bounameaux (1958), on bovine platelets and Sokal (1962), on human platelets, but neither of these workers could determine whether the protein was located in the platelet cytoplasm (and would therefore not be secreted) or in the granules (and therefore might be secreted) because they used whole platelet lysates. Subsequently, Nachman (1965), Davey and Luscher (1968), and Dzoga et al. (1972), all showed that a platelet-specific β-globulin could be detected in serum from clotted whole blood, but not in plasma or serum from clotted platelet poor plasma. No other data were presented concerning the nature and localisation of this protein. The existence of a platelet-specific protein with antiheparin activity (platelet factor 4) has also been reported (Van Creveld and Paulsson, 1951, 1952; Niewiarowski et al., 1968; Barber et al., 1972), and recent work from this and other laboratories has been concerned with the characterisation of PF4 (Moore et al., 1975a).

The work described below is an account of the investigations performed in this laboratory which enabled us to identify, purify and characterise the platelet specific β-globulin, which is the most abundant component of the material

Gordon (ed) Platelets in Biology and Pathology
© *Elsevier/North-Holland Biomedical Press, 1976*

secreted during the release reaction (Moore et al., 1975b). This protein we designated 'β-thromboglobulin'.

2. Preparation of platelet release products

Human platelets were obtained within 24 h of venepuncture in the form of platelet-rich plasma prepared by conventional techniques for therapeutic use. The platelet rich plasma was centrifuged at $4000 \times g$ for 10 min, and the supernatant platelet poor plasma discarded. To remove the plasma proteins remaining the platelets were washed with a solution composed of Ringers lactate, 5% glucose, and 10% trisodium citrate (7:2:1 by vol.) followed by centrifugation at $4000 \times g$ for 10 min. The platelet button was resuspended in the same solution, pre-equilibrated to 37°C, and $CaCl_2$ was added to a final concentration of 10 mM. The platelet release reaction was induced by the addition of bovine thrombin at a final concentration of 1 IU/ml to the stirred suspension. Visible aggregation occurred within 15 sec. After 2 min the aggregated platelets were removed by centrifugation at $12,000 \times g$ for 10 min and the supernatant, which contained all the soluble material released from the aggregated platelets was carefully removed and stored at $-40°C$ until required for further investigation.

Note The platelet rich plasma from approximately 1 litre of whole blood yielded 1 mg of purified β-thromboglobulin.

3. Identification and preliminary purification of β-thromboglobulin

3.1. Preliminary fractionation

A preliminary investigation of the molecular size distribution of the released proteins indicated approximately 60% with a molecular weight < 100,000 ('low molecular weight') and approximately 40% of molecular weight > 200,000 ('high molecular weight'). The quantity of protein of molecular weight 100–200,000 was very small. This suggested that a useful first step in the investigation would be to separate the 'high'- and 'low'-molecular weight fractions by gel filtration. The maximum resolution in gel filtration technique is obtained at a K_d^* value of 0.5. In

*
$$K_d = \frac{V_e - V_o}{V_s - V_o}$$

where V_o is the void volume determined from the elution position of a totally excluded molecule, e.g., Blue Dextran 2000, V_s the solvent volume determined from the elution position of a totally included molecule, e.g., glucose and V_e the elution position of the compound under investigation. The Ackers equation is expressed as $r_s = a_o + b_o \operatorname{erfc}^{-1}(1 - K_d)$ where a_o and b_o are constants relating to the particular gel type in use. (Values of the inverse error function were obtained from: Tables of the error function and its derivatives (1954) N.B.S. Applied Mathematics Series 41, United States Government Printing Office, Washington, D.C.)

this case a gel matrix was required to give a K_d of 0.5 for a protein of 150,000 molecular weight. Agarose 4% (Biogel A15m or Sepharose 4B) has the required property.

The release products were concentrated by pressure ultrafiltration using an Amicon PM10 membrane and fractionated on Biogel A15m (see Fig. 1). It was evident from the elution profile that the 'low'-molecular weight proteins were partially resolved into two peaks, fractions 60 to 68 and 69 to 76 respectively. The possibility that either of these peaks contained a platelet specific protein was initially investigated by the immunoelectrophoresis of fractions 65 and 71 against anti-whole human serum in which case only precipitin lines corresponding to albumin were noted. For fraction 65 this reaction was very strong but in the case of fraction 71 only a very weak reaction was observed suggesting that the majority of proteins present in fractions 69 to 76 was not present in human serum. The optimum conditions for the resolution of these two fractions required the use of a lower porosity gel. To aid the choice of the correct gel type and also to enable the measurement of diffusion coefficients by the method of Siegel and Monty (1966) all gel filtration columns were calibrated (see footnote, page 294), by the method of Ackers (1967) in terms of Stokes radius (r_s) and the inverse error function of the distribution coefficient, $\text{erfc}^{-1}(1 - K_d)$, by using proteins of known r_s (see Table 1). Values of r_s are readily calculated from diffusion coefficients (D) and vice versa using the Stokes–Einstein equation.

Fractions 69 to 76 from the Biogel A15m fractionation were fractionated on Sephadex G-200 (see Fig. 2). Three peaks I, II, and III were resolved and r_s values of 5.05 nm, 3.65 nm and 2.85 nm calculated for I, II and III respectively. Peak I was thought to be an IgG from the correspondence of the measured r_s to the reported value of 5.3 nm (Smith, 1968). Peak II was identified by immunological techniques to be albumin. The measured r_s of 2.85 nm for peak III did not correspond to reported values for any known plasma or serum protein.

The possible platelet specificity was further investigated using 48-h-old platelets. These platelets were prepared for therapeutic procedures but discarded as unfit for use 48 h after venepuncture. The procedure described above for the preparation of release products from fresh platelets was followed, but addition of thrombin failed to produce any significant visible aggregation. Subsequent fractionation of the supernatant of these thrombin treated platelets on Biogel A15m (see Fig. 3) showed that the component of r_s 2.85 nm was absent. In addition the chart record from the UV monitor attached to the column outlet did not show the peak of material eluting at V_t which was found for fresh platelets. The presence of this UV absorbing material is characteristic of the presence of nucleotides and 5-hydroxytryptamine which are released during platelet aggregation (Grette, 1962). This, together with the lack of visible aggregation, indicated that the release reaction had not occurred probably because of ageing effects in the platelets during storage. Subsequent work described below confirmed this view since it was found that non-specific leakage of β-thromboglobulin had occurred into the supernatant plasma of the platelet concentrates during storage.

This evidence suggested that the 2.85 nm component was specifically released

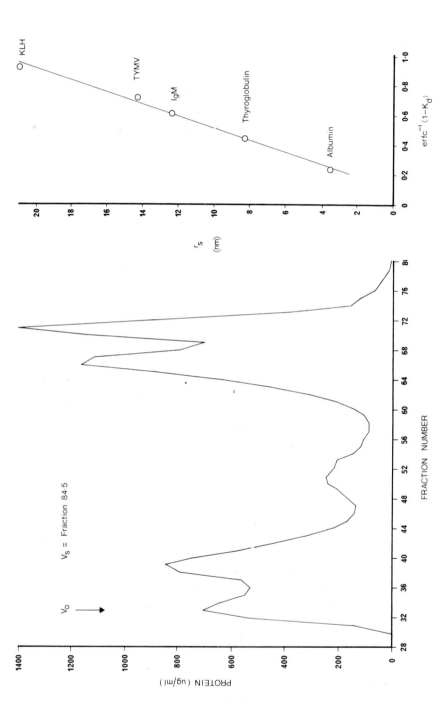

Fig. 1. (*Left*): Chromatography of the soluble material remaining after thrombin induced platelet aggregation. The soluble material was concentrated by ultrafiltration on an Amicon PM10 membrane (Amicon corp) at 25 lb/in² to a protein concentration of 17.5 mg/ml and 6 ml applied to a column containing Biogel A15m of bed dimensions 1070 × 22 mm, equilibrated and eluted with 25 mM Tris, 1 mM EDTA, 3.8 mM borate, 0.15 M NaCl, pH 8.8 at 22 ml/h. Fractions of 4.75 ml were collected and analysed for protein. (*Right*): Calibration of Biogel A15m (Bio-Rad Labs) 200–400 mesh. A 2 ml sample of each protein (5 mg/ml) was applied and eluted as in *Left*. Erfc⁻¹(1 − K_d) values were calculated from the elution volumes and plotted against r_s

TABLE 1
Protein standards used in the determination of S,D and molecular weight

	r_s (nm)	$s_{20,w}$	Subunit mol. wt.
Key-hole limpet haemocyanin (KLH)	21	—	—
Turnip yellow mosaic virus (TYMV)	15	—	—
IgM	12.4	—	—
Fibrinogen	—	7.63	—
Thyroglobulin	8.5	—	—
Transferrin	—	5.09	—
IgG	5.4	—	—
Albumin	3.55	4.63	—
Haemoglobulin	—	4.2	—
Ovalbumin	2.9	3.55	43,000
Chymotrypsinogen	2.24	2.58	25,700
Myoglobin	2.07	2.04	—
β-Lactoglobulin	—	—	18,000
Cytochrome c	1.64	1.71	12,300
Kallikrein inactivator	1.47	—	6,513
Bacitracin	0.89	—	—

during aggregation. To investigate the platelet specificity of this component, fractions 66 to 73 (peak III) from the Sephadex G-200 fractionation were pooled and used to induce antibody formation in rabbits (Moore et al., 1975b). Ouchterlony double immunodiffusion (Fig. 4) was used to characterise the antibodies. Figure 4 shows that peak III contained a platelet specific protein as the major component. In addition albumin antibodies were detected which indicated the presence of albumin in peak III though this must have been at a very low concentration since a precipitin reaction was not observed with peak III. This was confirmed by cellulose acetate electrophoresis (Fig. 5). At least three other components (minor antigens) which were apparently platelet specific were observed in peak III though these were present in low concentration since a less concentrated sample of peak III did not produce these lines. No reaction was noted with fibrinogen, red cell haemolysate or bovine thrombin. A systematic study of the major organs of the body and the various classes of leukocyte in the blood have shown no evidence of the platelet specific antigen other than at very low concentrations which were consistent with the inherent platelet residues in the samples. The major antigenic component was, however, detected in the supernatant of 48-h-old platelet concentrates (a consequence of leakage from the platelets during storage) and in serum prepared by clotting whole blood (due to platelet aggregation and the release reaction which occur during coagulation). At this stage a name was sought for this platelet-specific protein, and since electrophoresis on cellulose acetate (Fig. 5) showed a mobility equivalent to serum β-globulins, β-thromboglobulin was chosen as a suitable name: 'thrombo' is descriptive of the source (platelets, or 'thrombocytes') and β-globulin of its electrophoretic mobility.

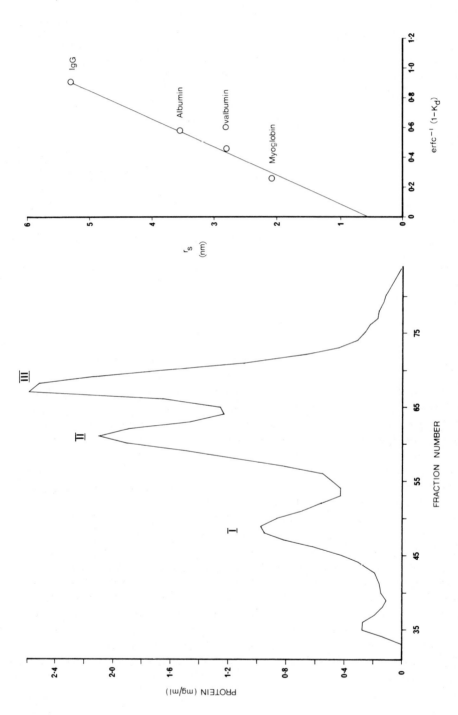

Fig. 2. (*Left*): Sephadex G-200 chromatography of 'low molecular weight' released proteins. The column of bed dimensions 1050×24.5 mm, was equilibrated and eluted with 25 mM Tris, 1 mM EDTA, 3.8 mM borate, 0.15 M NaCl, pH 8.8 at 22 ml/h. Fractions of 4.75 ml were collected. Pooled concentrated fractions 63–75 (190 mg protein) from the Biogel A15m fractionation of release products (see Fig. 1 (*Left*)) were chromatographed and the fractions analysed for protein. (*Right*): Calibration of Sephadex G-200. Procedure as in Fig. 1 (*Left*).

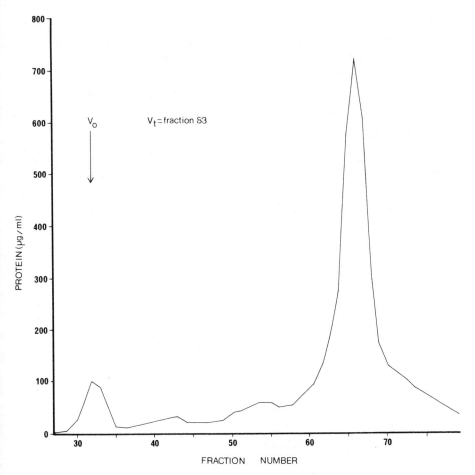

Fig. 3. As for Fig. 1 (*Left*) except that the sample consisted of the soluble material remaining after thrombin treatment of 48 h old washed platelets.

3.2. Preliminary characterisation

β-thromboglobulin was sedimented on a sucrose density gradient which was subsequently fractionated and analysed for protein (see Fig. 6). Proteins of known $s_{20,w}$ (see Table 1) were run in parallel. An s-value of 3.0 was determined, from which we calculated the molecular weight to be 36,000, using a value of 7.54 for the diffusion coefficient (determined by gel filtration) and assuming a value of 0.733 for $\bar{v}$. The value of $\bar{v}$ was subsequently substantiated by calculation from the amino acid analysis data (see below).

3.3. Further purification

As noted above the β-thromboglobulin preparation was contaminated with albumin and unidentified platelet specific antigens, and therefore we sought to

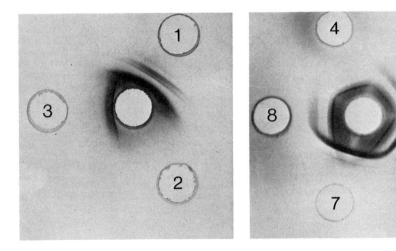

Fig. 4. Ouchterlony immunodiffusion. Agarose (1%) in 25 mM Tris, 1 mM EDTA, 3.8 mM borate, 0.15 M NaCl, pH 8.8. Centre well–rabbit antiserum to peak III protein. Peripheral wells–1. Lyophilised peak III (2 mg/ml); 2. Washed red cell haemolysate; 3. Human serum albumin (3 mg/ml); 4. Platelet poor plasma; 5. Supernatant from 2-day-old platelet rich plasma; 6. Supernatant from 2-day-old, three times freeze thawed platelet rich plasma; 7. Lyophilised peak III (500 μg/ml); 8. Serum from non anticoagulated whole blood allowed to clot at 37°C.

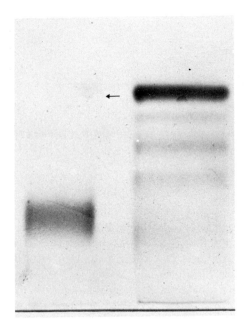

Fig. 5. Cellulose acetate electrophoresis. Sodium barbitone, 0.04 M, pH 9.9. 18 V/cm for 25 min. Samples were applied as follows: 1. Lyophilised peak III (3 μl, 3 mg/ml); 2. Undiluted human serum (3 μl). The arrow indicates the position of albumin present in trace amounts in peak III which does not show in the photograph.

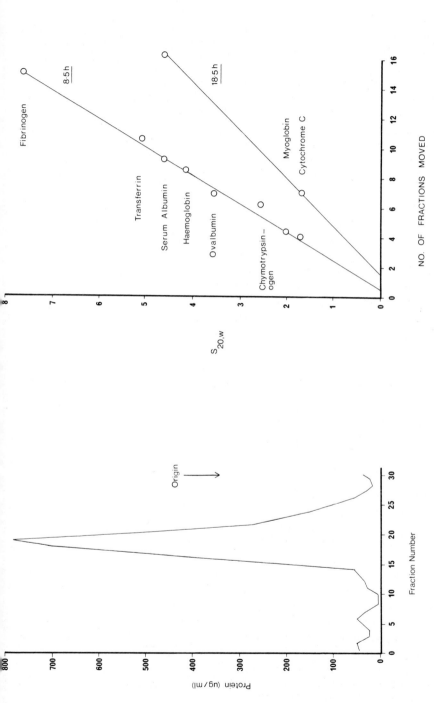

Fig. 6 (*Left*): Sucrose density gradient ultracentrifugation. 0.15 ml of peak III protein (9.8 mg/ml) was applied to a 6 to 30% (w/w) linear sucrose density gradient buffered by 25 mM Tris, 1 mM EDTA, 3.8 mM borate, 0.15 M NaCl, pH 8.8. The gradient was centrifuged at 420,000 × g (max) and 4°C for 18.5 h then fractionated into 0.2 ml aliquots and analysed for protein. (*Right*): Calibration of sucrose density gradients. Conditions as Fig. 6 (*Left*) except that proteins of known $s_{20,w}$ (5 mg/ml) were applied. The sedimentation distances were expressed as the number of fractions moved and plotted against $s_{20,w}$.

remove these contaminants. We noted that β-thromboglobulin and β-lactoglobulin were similar in molecular weight, S,D, and acid dissociation, although when we isolated human β-lactoglobulin there was no immunological cross reaction with β-thromboglobulin. Since albumin is a single chain polypeptide, we reasoned that if β-thromboglobulin dissociates in acid like β-lactoglobulin this might help in separating β-thromboglobulin from albumin by gel filtration–particularly since albumin undergoes a conformational change at low pH to give a more unfolded structure. To investigate this possibility fractions 66 to 73 from a Sephadex G-200 fractionation of 'low molecular weight' release products were pooled and dialysed overnight against 0.5% pyridine, 10% acetic acid (pH 3.2). The pooled fractions were deliberately chosen to contain a significant proportion of albumin to aid its subsequent identification. The dialysis precipitated some material which was removed by centrifugation and subsequently shown to redissolve in Tris–EDTA–borate (pH 8.8), and to be immunologically identical to the minor antigens seen in Fig. 4. The dialysis supernatant was fractionated on Sephadex G-75 and the fractions were analysed for protein (see Fig. 7). Subsequently, each fraction was individually dialysed against Tris–EDTA–borate (pH 8.8), and Ouchterlony immunodiffusion performed against the β-thromboglobulin (peak III) antiserum (see Fig. 8). The protein peak eluting at V_o was immunologically identical to albumin and that eluting in fractions 48 to 60 to β-thromboglobulin. An r_s value of 1.92 nm was calculated for this peak which indicated that dissociation had occurred. No 'Minor antigens' were detected in any of the fractions, thus confirming the identity of the precipitate. Of interest were the double precipitin lines to the β-thromboglobulin peak, all immunologically identical to the β-thromboglobulin preparation which had not been subjected to low pH dissociation. The nature of these lines was not known but polymorphism is suggested as a possible explanation.

3.4. Further characterisation

Since β-thromboglobulin dissociated at low pH a sedimentation at pH 3.2 was performed (see Fig. 9). This gave a value of 0.8 S, from which we calculated the molecular weight to be 6500 using the determined S and D values. This indicated that 'native' β-thromboglobulin was probably composed of six subunits. We then used SDS polyacrylamide gel electrophoresis as an independent method of determining subunit molecular weight. Proteins of known subunit molecular weight (see Table 1), were run in parallel and their migration distances plotted against log molecular weight (see Fig. 10). The migration distances of reduced and unreduced β-thromboglobulin (Fig. 10), were not identical and corresponded to apparent molecular weights of 5,800 and 10,700 respectively. We attributed this difference to conformational changes and consequent change in frictional ratio following reduction of intra chain disulphide bonds: we deduced that there were no inter chain bonds because the molecular weight in pyridine–acetic acid buffer pH 3.2 (a medium which does not reduce S–S bonds), corresponded to that of reduced β-thromboglobulin. The removal of albumin was apparently complete: no components of 68,000 molecular weight were present in the gels.

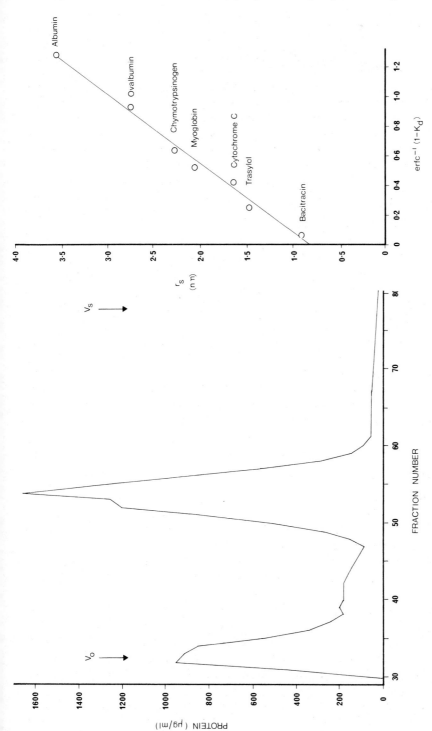

Fig. 7 (*Left*): Sephadex G-75 fractionation of crude β-thromboglobulin (peak III) at low pH. A 6 ml sample of pH 3.2 dialysate supernatant containing 13 mg/ml of protein was applied to a Sephadex G-75 column of bed dimensions 835 × 25 mm equilibrated and eluted with 0.5% pyridine, 10% acetic acid, pH 3.2 at 24 ml/h. 5.2 ml fractions were collected and analysed for protein. (*Right*): Calibration of Sephadex G-75. The column was equilibrated and eluted with 25 mM Tris, 1 mM EDTA, 3.8 mM borate, 0.15 M NaCl, pH 8.8. Procedure as for Fig. 1 (*Left*). V_0 and V_s were found to be independent of pH.

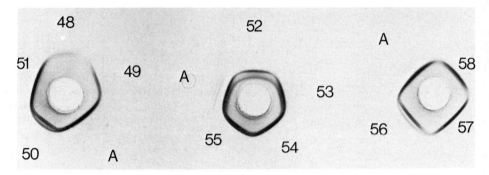

Fig. 8. Ouchterlony immunodiffusion. 1% agarose in 25 mM Tris, 1 mM EDTA, 3.8 mM borate, 0.15 M NaCl, pH 8.8. Samples were dialysed fractions (see text) from fractionation of crude β-thromboglobulin (peak III) on Sephadex G-75 at pH 3.2 (Fig. 7 *Left*). A = starting antigen (peak III). Numbers refer to the fraction numbers. Gels were washed in 0.15 M NaCl and then three times in distilled water, dried and stained in 0.2% amido black 12B in 45% methanol, 45% water, 10% acetic acid and destained in the same solvent.

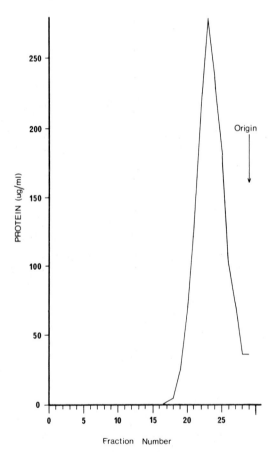

Fig. 9. Sucrose density gradient ultracentrifugation. Conditions as for Fig. 6 (*Left*) except the gradients were buffered with 0.5% pyridine, 10% acetic acid, pH 3.2. Standards were run in parallel on gradients buffered by 25 mM Tris, 1 mM EDTA, 3.8 mM borate, 0.15 M NaCl, pH 8.8.

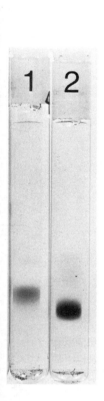

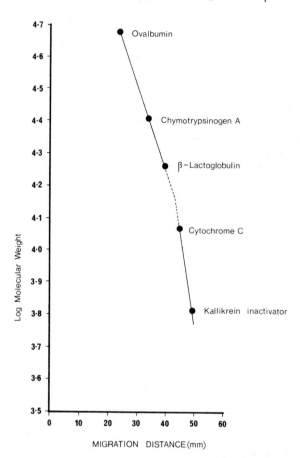

Fig. 10 (*Left*): Polyacrylamide gel electrophoresis in sodium dodecyl sulphate (SDS). Gel buffer: 0.3 M phosphate, pH 7.3; 0.3% SDS; 1.5 M urea. Electrode buffer: 0.1 M phosphate, pH 7.3; 0.1% SDS. Gel concentration: 7% (100:2.7 ratio of acrylamide to bis). Gel dimensions: 70 × 4.5 mm. Voltage: 12 V for 10 h. Gels were stained with amido black 12B in 45% methanol, 45% water, 10% acetic acid and destained in the same solvent. Sample No. 2 was diluted 1:1 with 2% SDS, 8 M urea, 10 mM dithiothreitol and No. 1 with 2% SDS, 8 M urea and heated for 10 min at 90°C. (*Right*): Plot of log molecular weight versus migration distance. Samples were proteins of known subunit molecular weight (see Table 1). Conditions as for Fig. 10 (*Left*).

An amino acid analysis of β-thromboglobulin was performed (see Table 2) and a $\bar{v}$ of 0.733 calculated by the method of Cohn and Edsall (1943). Of interest was the relatively high content of the hydrophobic residues leucine and isoleucine and the low content of the ultra violet absorbing residues phenylalanine and tyrosine: this explains the observed low ultra violet absorption of β-thromboglobulin. These findings are also characteristic of platelet factor 4 (Moore et al., 1975a). Also of interest was the finding that the most abundant single residue was lysine (usually glutamic acid in plasma proteins), which probably explains the basic nature of β-thromboglobulin (see below).

TABLE 2
The amino acid analysis of β-thromboglobulin

	g%	Residues/Mole*	Residues/100,000g*
Lysine	16.28	46	128
Histidine	2.94	8	22
Arginine	5.28	12	34
Aspartic acid	13.12	41	115
Threonine	4.93	17	47
Serine	4.98	20	56
Glutamic acid	14.12	39	109
Proline	3.34	12	34
Glycine	4.03	25	70
Alanine	4.80	24	67
Cysteine	3.16	11	31
Valine	2.83	10	28
Methionine	1.26	3	8
Isoleucine	7.08	22	61
Leucine	9.76	31	87
Tyrosine	1.79	4	11
Phenylalanine	0.29	1	3

* To nearest whole number.

At present one of the 'ultimate' techniques for the detection of protein heterogeneity is that of isoelectric focussing in polyacrylamide gel. Knowledge of antigen purity is important when developing quantitative immunological assay systems since it is essential to know exactly what is being measured. Figure 11 shows the result of focussing β-thromboglobulin purified by acid dissociation and fractionation on Sephadex G-75. It is obvious that the preparation is not completely homogeneous though it should be noted that a large quantity of protein was applied (150 μg). Focussing also showed that the pI of β-thromboglobulin was approximately 8. There was some evidence of polymorphism since two closely spaced bands were observed. More evidence for this is included in the next section. It should be noted that SDS polyacrylamide gel electrophoresis of the preparation did not detect any contaminants.

4. Heparin-agarose affinity chromatography

Affinity chromatography makes one-step purification feasible due to the highly specific reversible interactions which are employed in this technique. During the investigation of the antiheparin activity of platelet release products a heparin-agarose column was prepared in an attempt to isolate a soluble antiheparin thought to be distinct from the platelet factor 4 complex (Moore et al., 1975a). The sample applied to the column consisted of 'low molecular weight' proteins obtained from a Biogel A15m fractionation (see above) and contained albumin, minor antigens, β-thromboglobulin, 'IgG' and the 'antiheparin'. The column was eluted with a gradient of increasing ionic strength at constant pH. Subsequent analysis of the fractions for protein and antiheparin activity (see Fig. 12)

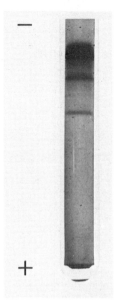

Fig. 11. Isoelectric focusing in polyacrylamide gels. Gel concentration: 7% (100:2.7 ratio of acrylamide to bis). Gels contained: 1% ampholine, pH 3–10; 0.1% ampholine pH 6–8; 10% sucrose. The gels were overlayered with 1% ampholine (pH 3–10) and samples layered under the 1% ampholine. The density of the samples and 1% ampholine were adjusted with sucrose such that the anode solution (see below) was of a lesser density. Anode solution: 1 M H_3PO_4 (lower). Cathode solution: 1 M NaOH (upper). Initial voltage: 30 V for 1 h. The voltage was subsequently raised while maintaining the current below 1 mA/gel to a final voltage of 320 V which was maintained for 3.5 h. The gels were fixed in 10% TCA, 5% $HgCl_2$ at 4°C for 12 h. and subsequently washed 6 times in 10% TCA, 5% $HgCl_2$, 2 h per wash, to remove 'ampholines'. Staining was performed as in Fig. 10 (*Left*). Sample 150 μg of β-thromboglobulin in 1% ampholine, pH 3–10.

confirmed the existence of the antiheparin which eluted with 1.5 M NaCl, completely separated from all other material. Of greater relevance to the work presented here was the observation of two peaks (fractions 50 to 70 and 71 to 95 respectively) which were both subsequently shown to be immunologically identical to β-thromboglobulin. SDS polyacrylamide gel electrophoresis (see Fig. 13) of these two peaks, the starting material, whole release products, β-thromboglobulin and the unadsorbed material confirmed this observation. This finding indicated that a charge difference must exist between the component protein of each peak and this was confirmed by isoelectric focussing which demonstrated a higher pI for the more strongly bound component. The origin of the apparent polymorphism of β-thromboglobulin is unknown and may be due to true polymorphism such as occurs for β-lactoglobulin and lactate dehydrogenase.

5. Radioimmunoassay of β-thromboglobulin

The technique of radioimmunoassay is well documented (Greenwood et al., 1963), and is capable of extremely high sensitivity and specificity. A radioimmunoassay

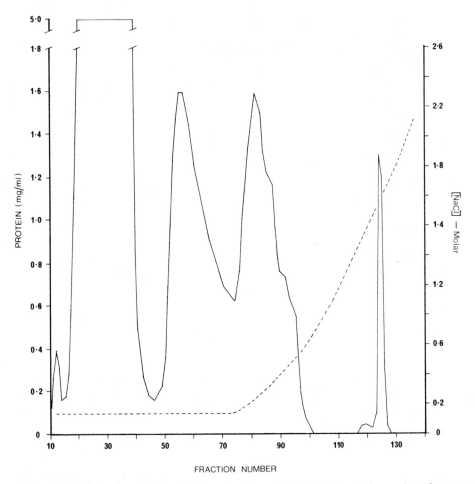

Fig. 12. Affinity chromatography of 'low molecular weight' released proteins on heparin-agarose. Heparin-agarose was prepared by a combination of the methods of Porath et al. (1973), and Andersson et al. (1974). Bed dimensions 250 × 15 mm. The column was equilibrated with 0.1 M phosphate (pH 8.0), 0.15 M NaCl. Sample: 34 ml of 'low molecular weight' released proteins (4.4 mg/ml) pre-dialysed against starting buffer. Column was eluted at 8 ml/h with an increasing ionic strength gradient at constant pH. 2 ml fractions were collected and analysed for protein (———) and NaCl concentration (------). Flow rate was 8 ml/h.

for β-thromboglobulin has been developed (Ludlam et al., 1975a,b), primarily for clinical investigations of platelet consumption in vivo which are outside the scope of this chapter. The assay is mentioned here because it has a much wider application in the field of platelet physiology, and an observation made during the early stages of developing the assay provides example of its potential use. It can be readily appreciated that when attempting to measure circulating levels of plasma β-thromboglobulin the techniques of blood sampling and processing should not induce platelet release, since this would lead to an overestimate of the

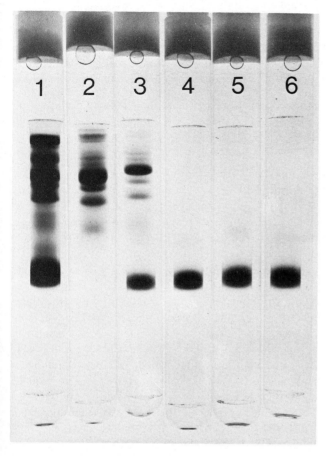

Fig. 13. SDS Polyacrylamide gel electrophoresis. Conditions as in Fig. 10. Samples: 1. Whole release products. 2. Pooled fraction 15 to 44 from Fig. 12. 3. Low mol. wt. released proteins (fractions 58–76) from Fig. 1 (*Left*). 4. Fraction 55, Fig. 12. 5. Fraction 81, Fig. 12. 6. β-Thromboglobulin purified by dialysis at pH 3.2 and fractionation on Sephadex G-75.

plasma β-thromboglobulin concentration. Initial measurements of the circulating levels of β-thromboglobulin gave erratic results for this very reason. By using the radioimmunoassay it was possible to compare the effects of various inhibitors of platelet aggregation including aspirin, prostaglandin E₁, theophylline, chloroadenosine, EDTA and cyclic AMP. These investigations led to the final choice of an anticoagulant/antiaggregant mixture for blood collection which contained EDTA, theophylline and prostaglandin E₁. This gave the lowest concentration of β-thromboglobulin in platelet poor plasma collected from 'normal' subjects. The assay was also used to investigate other aspects of the collection technique–for example, the storage temperature of samples prior to centrifugation, and the effect of using siliconised glass sample collection tubes. After all the conditions had been optimised the circulating level of β-thromboglobulin was in the range 20 to 50 ng/ml. By comparison, the level in clotted whole blood serum was 10 to 20 μg/ml. Since the ultimate sensitivity of the assay is approximately 50 pg/ml, the potential application of the radioimmunoassay to studies of platelet function in vitro and in vivo can be readily appreciated – particularly since β-thromboglobulin is the most abundant protein secreted during the release reaction.

6. Conclusion

The function of β-thromboglobulin remains obscure, partly because its detection and characterisation in our laboratories has been based only on its antigenicity and physical properties. No biological activity has yet been associated with it, and we have been unable to equate it with any known platelet enzyme or other protein. At the present time, the most striking feature of βTG is its relative inertness – it does not readily denature or aggregate, is freely soluble, does not precipitate at extremes of pH, and reassociates to a constant molecular weight even after acid dissociation.

It is tempting therefore to look for a 'physical' role for βTG, and its subcellular localization and concentration are compatible with this concept. We believe, from the published work of others, that the release products of platelets can be clearly demarcated into two groups: low molecular weight substances (ADP, ATP, 5HT, Ca^{2+}) in the very dense bodies, and high molecular weight products (fibrinogen, PF_4-complex, lysosomal enzymes, βTG) in the alpha granules. The release mechanisms for these two types of granules may or may not be different, but even if the mechanisms are the same, the contents of the very dense granules will diffuse out much more rapidly than those of the α granules because of the difference in molecular weight. Since the available evidence indicates that granules are more centrally located immediately before release, their constituents must diffuse through the entire platelet canalicular system to reach the exterior. Therefore, the relative differences in the rates of release of platelet constituents may depend more on their molecular size than on any other single factor.

Estimates of the βTG content in platelets vary, but from the yield of protein in large scale processes we can estimate a lower limit of 1 mg βTG protein per platelet unit (i.e., βTG represents at least 0.5% of the total platelet dry weight). Since we found that only about 5% of platelet protein is released by thrombin, we estimate that βTG is at least 10% by weight of the granule content. The βTG content in the supernatant plasma of outdated platelet concentrates suggests a somewhat higher figure – about 5 mg βTG per unit (i.e., 2.5% of the total platelet dry weight or 50% by weight of the granule contents). A third estimate can be obtained by triangulation of the various peaks observed in the first chromatograph of the total release products on Biogel A15m: over several successive runs, we observed that βTG peaks averaged 33% of the total protein released. Thus, three different sets of data indicate that βTG is a major component (and possibly the largest single contribution) of the proteins in platelet α granules, and that it is probably not present in the very dense granules. In view of the 'bland' nature of βTG and its presence in high concentration in the α granules, we are inclined to view it as a possible matrix or packing protein, which helps to stabilize the active constituents and is readily released by biological stimuli.

References

Ackers, G.K. (1967) J. Biol. Chem., *242*, 3237.
Anderson, M.M., Borg, H. and Andersson, L.-O. (1974) Thromb. Res., *5*, 439.
Barber, A.J., Kaser-Glanzmann, R., Jakabova, M. and Luscher, E.F. (1972) Biochim. Biophys. Acta, *286*, 312.
Cohn, E.J. and Edsall, J.T. (1943) Proteins, Amino Acids and Peptides as Dipolar Ions, p. 370, Reinhold, New York.
Davey, M.G. and Luscher, E.F. (1968) Biochim. Biophys. Acta, *165*, 490.
Dzoga, K., Stoltzner, G. and Wissler, R.W. (1972) Lab. Invest., *27*, 351.
Greenwood, F.C., Hunter, W.M. and Glover, J.S. (1963) Biochem. J., *89*, 114.
Grette, K. (1962) Acta Physiol. Scand., *56*, Suppl. 195.
Ludlam, C.A., Moore, S., Bolton, A.E., Pepper, D.S. and Cash, J.D. (1975a) Thrombosis. Res., *6*, 543.
Ludlam, C.A., Bolton, A.E., Moore, S. and Cash, J.D. (1975b) The Lancet, 259.
Moore, S., Pepper, D.S. and Cash, J.D. (1975a) Biochim. Biophys. Acta, *379*, 370.
Moore, S., Pepper, D.S. and Cash, J.D. (1975b) Biochim. Biophys. Acta, *379*, 360.
Niewiarowski, S., Poplawski, A., Lipinski, B. and Farbizewski, R. (1968) Exp. Biol. Med., *3*, 121.
Nachman, R.L. (1965) Blood, *25*, 703.
Porath, J., Aspberg, K., Drevin, H. and Axen, R. (1973) J. Chromatog., *86*, 53.
Salmon, J. and Bounameaux, Y. (1958) Thromb. Diath. Haemorrh., *2*, 93.
Siegel, L.M. and Monty, K.J. (1966) Biochim. Biophys. Acta, *112*, 346.
Smith, M.H. (1968) In Handbook of Biochemistry, Selected Data for Molecular Biology (Sober, H.A., ed), The Chemical Rubber Co., Cleveland.
Sokal, G. (1962) Acta Haematol. (Basel), *28*, 313.
Tables of the error function and its derivatives (1954) N.B.S. Applied Mathematics Series 41, United States Government Printing Office, Washington D.C.
Van Creveld, S. and Paulssen, M.M.P. (1951) The Lancet, 242.
Van Creveld, S. and Paulssen, M.M.P. (1952) The Lancet, 23.

CHAPTER 12

Platelets in immunological reactions

D.L. BROWN

Department of Immunology, Addenbrooke's Hospital, Hills Road, Cambridge CB2 2QQ, England

1. Introduction

Platelets are damaged by several immunological (allergic) or complement-mediated reactions in which the reactants are unrelated to the platelets themselves, but the reactions which cause 'bystander' platelet damage can be separated into two main classes depending on whether or not the platelets of the species examined are immune adherence positive, i.e., attracted to sites of fixation of the third component of complement, C3b. A commonly observed end point to many of these reactions is the clumping of platelets in masses – called *agglutination*, *adherence*, *aggregation* or *conglutination* depending on what the initial reaction was considered to be. This clumping may trigger the platelet release reaction (Grette, 1962; Stormorken, 1969; Weiss, 1975) simply by close juxtaposition of adjacent platelet membranes, thus reinforcing platelet aggregation. This aggregation response, the common end point of several different reactions, may be complicated by complement fixation, if the experimental conditions allow this, and platelet lysis may then result, making it difficult to determine which is the dominant event in the final path to platelet damage.

However, many details of the mechanism of platelet damage by complement have been worked out by the separate manipulation of the alternative and classical complement pathways, making use of the observation that they have different divalent cation requirements (Fine et al., 1972) and by the use of plasmas from animals or man congenitally deficient in single complement components (Alper and Rosen, 1974).

Several recent reviews have examined different aspects of platelet immune damage (Mustard and Packham, 1970; Osler and Siraganian, 1972; Becker and Henson, 1973; Pfueller and Lüscher, 1972c).

Gordon (ed) Platelets in Biology and Pathology
© *Elsevier/North-Holland Biomedical Press, 1976*

2. Historical review

Credit for first recognising that platelets can be directly involved in immunological phenomena should probably be given to Levaditi (1901) who observed adherence between platelets and *Vibrio cholerae* in the circulation of rabbits immunized against the microorganism, but not in normal unimmunized rabbits. *Vibrio cholerae* pretreated in vitro with immune serum, heated or unheated, also adhered to normal rabbit platelets in vivo. This phenomenon of immune adherence was extended to reactions with other bacteria, e.g., *E. coli*, *B. anthracis* and staphylococci by Aynaud (1911) and further shown to be applicable to the platelets of rats, mice and guinea pigs by Rieckenberg (1917).

Up to this point the phenomenon was thought to be primarily dependent on antibody and it was only in 1923 that Govaerts recognised the additional requirement for a heat-labile component, in experiments with dog and rabbit plasma in vitro. This part of the story was completed by a group working with Kritschewsky (1927) who studied the immune adherence of platelets with trypanosomes, leishmanias and the spirochaetes of relapsing fever and leptospirosis. They were aware that the heat-labile component was complement and that the platelets of man were unable to take part in the immune adherence reaction, unlike the platelets of laboratory species so far examined (Kritschewsky and Tscherikower, 1928). Much of the literature from this period has been reviewed in some detail by Lamanna (1957).

The term immune adherence was coined by Nelson (1956) to describe the reaction of complement-coated particles with primate red cells rather than with the platelets of certain nonprimate species and although there are minor differences between the two reactions, there is clear analogy (Nelson, 1963) in as much as both reactions follow fixation of the third component of complement (C3b). It therefore seems justified to use the term in the context of platelet reactions. Immune adherence was first recognised as occurring after the fixation of immune antibody and complement, though this view had to be broadened when it was found that the same immune adherence sites could be generated by naturally occurring antibodies (Swisher, 1956) and by particulate substances which apparently did not require conventional antibody at all. Starch granules and zymosan were particularly active in this respect (Nelson, 1956) and earlier workers had noted similar effects with colloidal particles such as indian ink, silver and quartz (quoted by Nelson, 1963). More recently Jobin and Tremblay (1969) have shown that a wide variety of nonorganic particles fix complement when coated with IgG and that this property coincides with a capacity to activate platelets.

Other aspects of the immunological reactivity of platelets were actively pursued at this time. In particular, it was recognised that intravenous challenge of sensitised animals with the appropriate antigen resulted in profound temporary thrombocytopenia and mixed aggregation between platelets and neutrophils. This effect was noted not only in nonprimates (Rocha e Silva, 1950) but also in primates (Kopeloff and Kopeloff, 1941; Kinsell et al., 1941); therefore, these effects could not be accounted for purely on the basis of an immune adherence reaction in vivo.

Stetson (1951a) found that platelets were involved at an early stage in the generalized Shwartzman reaction and went on to draw analogies between the local Shwartzman reaction and the Arthus reaction (Stetson, 1951b) in that platelet aggregates were a prominent feature of the necrotic and haemorrhagic skin lesions, though in the Arthus reaction, unlike the Shwartzman reaction, it was clear that the development of the lesions depended on combination between antibody and antigen close to a vessel wall. Another key observation at this time which helped to elucidate some of the mechanisms involved in the platelet release reaction was made by Humphrey and Jacques (1955). They showed that antigen-antibody complexes released vasoactive amines from rabbit platelets in a reaction which required normal plasma and Ca^{2+} ions. Heat inactivated plasma was only a quarter as effective and they concluded (1) that complement was required for the release and (2) since the reaction could take place in heparinized plasma that it was independent of the clotting system. A further significant observation was that AgAb complexes caused some vasoactive amine release from human platelets in the absence of plasma. This can be linked to the earlier finding of Ackroyd (1951) that certain unrelated immune complexes cause aggregation of human platelets in the absence of complement.

The role of complement components in the immune adherence reaction of rabbit and guinea pig platelets was more clearly defined by Siquiera and Nelson (1961) and by Gocke (1965). It can be concluded from a modern interpretation of their work that fixation of complement up to the C3 step is essential to generate immune adherence sites and the reaction is best performed with immune complexes in considerable antibody excess. Henson (1969) provided unequivocal proof that the complement component required for immune adherence is C3 since immune adherence reactivity could be generated in C6-deficient rabbit serum (i.e., fixing complement components C1, C4, C2, C3), but not in serum depleted of C3 by purified cobra venom factor (CVF).

Differences between rabbit and human platelets were further emphasized when Movat et al. (1965) found that aggregation and release of vasoactive amines and ADP from human platelets and pig platelets (both immune adherence negative species) by preformed immune complexes were best demonstrated with washed platelets rather than with platelet-rich plasma (PRP). Similar studies were carried out by Mueller-Eckhardt and Lüscher (1968a) who found that nucleotide release from human platelets by aggregated gammaglobulin and by preformed complexes could not by fully inhibited by EDTA (i.e., the reaction seemed to be partially independent of the divalent cation concentration), though aggregation and contraction of human platelets did not occur in EDTA. They also came to the conclusion (Mueller-Eckhardt and Lüscher, 1968b) that the aggregation reaction of human platelets with IgG-coated latex particles did not require complement and noted that the reaction was inhibited by serum or gammaglobulin.

The development of an understanding of the reactivity of platelets with antibody and complement up to the period 1958–68 can be summarized as follows:

(a) Platelets of many nonprimate species – e.g., dog, rabbit, guinea pig, rat and mouse – were known to be immune adherence positive and attracted to unrelated particles and surfaces which had fixed C3. Adherence was followed by a release reaction requiring divalent cations during which ADP and vasoactive amines were released.

(b) Platelets of primates (including man) and most ungulates–e.g., pig, sheep, horse, goat–were recognised to be immune adherence negative and were aggregated by preformed complexes, aggregated gammaglobulin or surfaces coated with IgG in a reaction for which the optimum conditions were to use washed platelets in a medium free of serum or plasma. A role for complement was not disproved though it did not appear to be an essential requirement.

In view of the fundamental differences between immune adherence positive and negative platelets it is convenient to consider recent studies of the two reactions separately.

3. Immunological reactivity of immune adherence positive platelets

3.1. Reaction with large particles coated with C_3

When zymosan is incubated in serum or in heparinized or citrated plasma, at 37°C it acquires a surface coating of several plasma proteins of which the dominant one antigenically and quantitatively is C3 (Mardiney and Müller-Eberhard, 1965). This acquisition of a C3-coating by zymosan arises principally from complement fixation via the alternative pathway (Brade et al., 1974; Nicholson et al., 1975) though, since fixation is less efficient in C2 deficient human serum and C4 deficient guinea pig serum (Martin, 1976) there appears to be at least a contribution from the classical pathway–possibly via IgG adsorbed to zymosan. The mechanism of complement activation and fixation may involve both pathways in a manner analogous to that described by Philips et al. (1972) for membrane-bound endotoxin. As incubation of zymosan in plasma or serum is continued at 37°C, C3 is first bound as C3b (the form of C3 which supports immune adherence) and is then progressively decayed by C3b inactivator (C3b-INA) to C3d (Lachmann and Müller-Eberhard, 1968; Ruddy and Austen, 1971; Gitlin et al., 1975). C3 in this form is negative for immune adherence. For this reason experiments in which complement coated zymosan (ZC) is generated in 10–15 min may not be entirely comparable with experiments in which the zymosan is in contact with serum or plasma for longer periods during which time considerable uncontrolled C3b decay may have taken place. In no experiments with platelets to date, however, have the relative amounts of C3b and C3d been measured.

Incubation at 37°C followed by vigorous washing at the same temperature is likely to destroy the classical or alternative pathway C3 convertases, respectively $\overline{C42}$ and $C3b\overline{B}$. At least one of these is required in intact membrane bound form in addition to sufficient C3b to generate the lytic phase of the complement system, C5-9 in the 'fluid' phase. In most experiments the washed C3b-coated particles, i.e., zymosan or red cells do not appear to have preserved the potential to trigger the lytic sequence on resuspension in fresh serum or plasma (Henson, 1970a; Brown et al., 1970; Marney et al., 1975).

When rabbit platelets are mixed with ZC either in the presence or the absence of plasma, aggregation develops immediately without a lag phase (Marney et al., 1975; Christian and Gordon, 1975). A similar mixed aggregation occurs when EC43b (complement coated red cells) are added to rabbit PRP (Brown et al., 1970). The aggregation is due to immune adherence and is independent of divalent cation concentration. However, the aggregation reaction remains strictly monophasic unless (1) Ca^{2+} ions are provided (Marney et al., 1975) or (2) heparinized normal plasma is present (Christian and Gordon, 1975). One interpretation of these observations is that the second wave of aggregation represents the Ca^{2+} dependent platelet release reaction. This view is supported by the finding that it can be inhibited by 10 mM AMP (Marney et al., 1975), though AMP and ADP at 1 mM concentration had no inhibitory effect according to Siraganian (1968b). The experiments of Christian and Gordon (1975) offer a slightly different interpretation in that the biphasic response of washed platelets to ZC can be generated only by normal plasma and not by C6-deficient plasma, suggesting that the lytic phase of the complement sequence is required. Platelet degranulation accompanied by rapid release of large amounts of ADP and vasoactive amines (40–70%) is associated with the second wave response. Since the ZC complex is preformed, the first phase of aggregation is normal in plasma decomplemented by treatment with CVF and the second phase can be triggered if sufficient Ca^{2+} ions are supplied (Marney et al., 1975).

The results of studies in vivo with preformed EC43 cells (i.e., red cells lacking both antibody and C42 complex) support the view (Brown et al., 1970), that the first wave of aggregation is principally immune adherence in that: (1) rabbit platelets form rosettes around EC43 cells injected intravenously, (2) the mixed rosettes are cleared from the circulation into the reticuloendothelial system without lysis of the red cells, resulting in severe temporary thrombocytopenia. (3) within 30–90 minutes the majority of the temporarily sequestered platelets return, unlysed, to the circulation.

3.2. Reaction with AgAb complexes formed in the reaction mixture

Two types of antigen–antibody (AgAb) complexes have been used and must be considered separately since they appear to damage platelets in different ways. Many experiments have been performed where the complexes are generated in the reaction mixture in considerable *antibody excess*. The advantages of complexes formed in this manner have been discussed at length by Gocke and Osler (1965). Henson and Cochrane (1969), and Osler and Siraganian (1972), and it seems that they fix complement efficiently because the complex slowly builds up in size. In contrast, complexes formed at equivalence flocculate very rapidly at

37°C and it is conceivable that complement fixation or release of active products is sterically hindered in the centre of the immune complex lattice.

Activation of the procoagulant, platelet factor 3 (PF3) in rabbit PRP by ovalbumin–antiovalbumin complexes occurs over a wide range of antigen concentration from X8 antigen excess to X512 antibody excess, but with marked reduction in activation around equivalence (Fig. 1).

The aggregation pattern when these complexes are added to PRP is biphasic in the presence of Ca^{2+} and, as is the case with ZC, the second wave of aggregation is associated with release of endogenous ADP and large amounts of vasoactive amines. The second phase is inhibited by AMP and so appears to constitute a true platelet release reaction (Marney, 1971; Marney et al., 1975). Both aggregation and release are markedly diminished by EGTA according to this group of workers, but

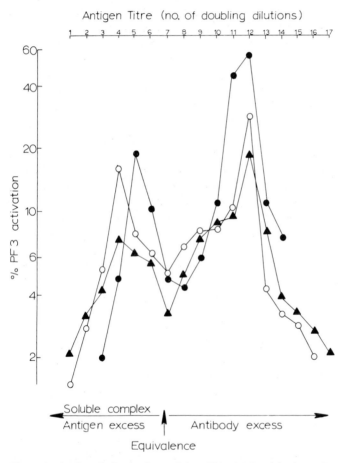

Fig. 1. Activation of platelet factor 3 in rabbit platelet-rich plasma by antigen–antibody complexes. Complexes formed from ovalbumin-antiovalbumin activated PF_3 over a wide range of antigen concentration, from x8 antigen excess to x512 antibody excess, but activation was greatly reduced around equivalence. The different symbols show results from three separate experiments.

only minimally reduced according to Henson (1970), who used Mg^{2+} EGTA. It is not entirely clear why these differences were observed, though in the presence of critical amounts of Mg^{2+} EGTA, the Ca^{2+} concentration is too low to support complement fixation by the classical pathway (Fine et al., 1972). It is important to establish whether the immune complex used for any particular study can fix complement only by the classical pathway or by both pathways. PF3 requires Cl–9 for its activation by soluble complexes in antibody excess, and is generated in heparinized or lightly citrated plasma but not in Mg^{2+} EGTA plasma (Brown, unpublished observations).

3.2.1. Lysis

A large body of experimental evidence supports the view that complement mediated platelet lysis can take place. One complication of the interpretation of results of experiments with immune complexes is the difficulty of distinguishing events associated with the platelet release reaction from complement mediated platelet lysis, both of which may result in the liberation of large amounts of 5-hydroxytryptamine (5HT) ADP, and, in the case of rabbit platelets (though not those of other species), histamine. The generation of soluble complexes unrelated to the platelets in complement-sufficient PRP releases large amounts of cytoplasmic constituents, such as ^{51}Cr-labelled cytoplasmic protein, ^{86}Rb (a cation marker which exchanges with intracellular potassium) and lactic dehydrogenase (LDH) (Henson, 1970a); Siraganian et al., 1968a,b). It also causes major activation of PF3 (Fig. 1). Colloidal or semicolloidal complement activators acting primarily via the alternative pathway (e.g., endotoxins, inulin and zymosan) also release cytoplasmic constituents and activate PF3 in normal rabbit PRP (Brown and Lachmann, 1974; Zimmerman, 1974) but not in C6-deficient PRP or in PRP pretreated either in vitro or in vivo with decomplementing doses of CVF. Direct morphological evidence of platelet lysis by complement activating substances has come from the electron microscopic studies of platelet damage by endotoxin (Spielvogel, 1967) and immune complexes (Henson, 1970a). Lysis appears to be a passive event in that unlike the release reaction, it is not inhibited by metabolic poisons.

One factor that could affect the results of experiments in which immune complexes are allowed to develop in antibody excess in PRP is the platelet concentration. At high platelet concentration the release of ADP and other constituents from some platelets might be sufficient to trigger a sustained release reaction in the whole platelet population, whereas at low platelet concentrations the effect of this would be minimized, thus allowing complement-mediated platelet lysis to dominate the picture. Siraganian et al. (1968b) and Osler and Siraganian (1972), using immune complexes to activate complement, emphasized that platelet aggregation is not a prerequisite for complement-mediated release of platelet constituents. Endotoxin and inulin can also cause platelet lysis and activation of PF3 in vitro without visible agglutination in normal citrated or heparinized PRP, but macroscopically visible agglutination or aggregation of platelets by endotoxin or inulin is often observed, even in C6 deficient rabbit PRP both in vitro and in vivo. This may be the result of several events: (1) immune adherence, (2) aggregation induced by constituents released from platelets and (3) agglutination by immunoconglutinins.

3.2.2. Nonlytic conditions

It has been stressed by Henson (1970a), Siraganian et al. (1973) and Christian and Gordon (1975) that major release of histamine, 5HT and nucleotides from rabbit platelets in plasma by immune complexes or ZC requires complement components beyond C6 and that the reaction accompanies the second wave of platelet aggregation. Endotoxin and inulin injected intravenously cause intense platelet aggregation followed by reversible thrombocytopenia in C6-deficient rabbits. Aggregation in vivo may be amplified by release of constituents from rabbit platelets in C6-deficient plasma and therefore not require the lytic phase of the complement sequence. In studies in vitro Siraganian et al. (1973) and Christian and Gordon (1975) found little or no release of histamine or 5HT in C6-deficient plasma reacted with zymosan, inulin or preformed aggregates. PF3 release was similarly inhibited in C6-deficient rabbit PRP mixed with endotoxin, inulin or zymosan in vitro (Brown and Lachmann, 1973; Brown and Lachmann, 1974; Zimmerman, 1974). CVF-treated rabbit PRP shows no detectable reaction with either particulate or soluble activating agents (Henson and Cochrane, 1969; Brown and Lachmann, 1973; Marney, 1971); there is no aggregation, vasoactive amine release, PF3 activation or lysis.

3.3. Reaction with preformed immune complexes

Antigen and antibody can be reacted together at equivalence in the absence of complement to generate immune complexes which can be washed free of plasma or serum, and, if required, modified to produce soluble complexes in antigenic excess (Barbaro, 1961; Ishizaka and Ishizaka, 1962). When preformed immune complexes are mixed with rabbit PRP their reactivity resembles that of a complement fixing particle like zymosan or EC43, rather than immune complexes forming in antibody excess. This difference of behaviour has led to some confusion when interpreting results, particularly regarding the role of complement in the reaction, though Des Prez and Bryant (1969) recognised that the divalent cation requirements seemed less stringent for preformed complexes than for complexes forming in the reaction mixture since the former were active in the presence of citrate. One view favoured was that the preformed complexes were phagocytized by platelets and that this triggered the platelet release reaction. Electron microscopic evidence for phagocytosis of ferritin-containing complexes by platelets was provided by Movat et al. (1965) and it can be readily demonstrated that immune complexes are trapped in the surface connected canalicular system of the platelet. Whether this is true phagocytosis is, however, questionable, and has been challenged by White (1972) on the basis of evidence that latex spheres lodge in the canalicular system without formation of true phagolysosomes.

More recently it has become clear that preformed immune complexes can activate complement via the alternative pathway (Spiegelberg and Götze, 1972) in a reaction which requires Mg^{2+} ions but a minimal amount of Ca^{2+} ions; this can therefore take place in Mg^{2+} EGTA (Fine et al., 1972). Studies by Siraganian et al. (1973) using immune complexes derived from guinea pig γ-1 and γ-2 antibodies shed further light on this problem. Both complete antibody (7S)γ-1 and F(ab')₂(5S)γ-1 or γ-2 containing immune complexes activate complement exclusively via the alternative pathway in contrast to complete (7S)γ-2 antibody containing complexes which can utilize both alternative and classical pathways. All of these complexes will release histamine from rabbit platelets on prolonged incubation in a reaction which is dependent on Mg^{2+} but not Ca^{2+}. The reaction also requires the lytic phase of the complement sequence since it does not take place in C6-deficient rabbit plasma. Marney et al. (1975) interpret the divalent cation and complement requirement for immune complex damage to rabbit platelets as follows. In short term incubation experiments with immune complexes forming in the reaction mixture in antibody excess the reaction proceeds via the classical pathway and is dependent on Ca^{2+} and Mg^{2+}. Prolonged incubation (up to 60 min) results in the formation of stable complexes which can fix complement via the alternative pathway either as complete IgG containing complexes or as F(ab')₂ containing complexes. Here the reaction is dependent only on Mg^{2+}. For the second wave of aggregation and release, however, Ca^{2+} ions are apparently required. A schematic summary of the reactions of immune adherence positive platelets with complement activating particles is shown in Fig. 2.

3.4. Reaction with soluble complement activators

The most thoroughly investigated soluble activator of the complement system is CVF, the C3b 'analogue' derived from Cobra venom of *Naga* spp. This complement activating and complement consuming protein was first isolated from crude venom by Nelson (1966) and its actions were further characterised by Ballow and Cochrane (1969), Cochrane, Müller-Eberhard and Aiken (1970), and Hunsicker et al. (1973).

An accepted view of its mode of action is that it behaves as an analogue of C3b in the feedback cycle of the alternative pathway and combines with factor B to form a highly stable C3-converting enzyme, CVF-B which has half survival time in vivo of about 35 hours. This enzyme splits C3 into C3b + C3a and activates the lytic phase of the complement sequence (Lachmann, 1976; Müller-Eberhard, 1975).

CVF purified by DEAE chromatography followed by Sephadex G-200 gel filtration (Ballow and Cochrane 1969) decomplements animals within 5–24 h following intravenous or intra-peritoneal injection, reducing C3 levels (as determined immunochemically), to less than 8% and functionally to zero. C5-9 are also

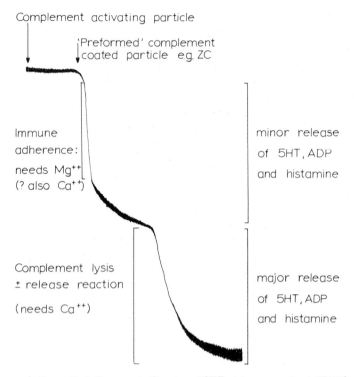

(after Christian and Gordon 1975; Marney et. al. 1975)

Fig. 2. Schematic representation of interactions between immune adherence positive platelets (e.g., from rabbits) and complement activating particles. Two phases of platelet aggregation (as detected photometrically in stirred samples of platelet-rich plasma) are shown, resulting from adding to the PRP either complement activating particles or particles precoated with complement components (e.g., 'activated' Zymosan–ZC). The postulated mechanisms responsible for the aggregation are summarised on the left, and the secretory responses are indicated on the right.

appreciably consumed. This 'fluid phase' activation and consumption of the complement cascade has no effect on platelet counts in rats (Majewski and Brown 1976), in guinea pigs (Dodds and Pickering, 1972) or in dogs (Garner, Chater and Brown, 1974), and causes only a small 'step' in the platelet survival curve in rabbits (Brown, unpublished observations)–quite unlike the profound temporary thrombocytopenia commonly associated with particulate complement activating substances.

At high concentrations CVF slightly prolongs the stypven-Ca^{2+} clotting time of rabbit PRP but at lower doses, still well within the decomplementing range, it has no effect on the clotting time. Washed platelets from rabbits decomplemented with CVF in vivo or from PRP treated with CVF in vitro, will lyse and release PF3 in the normal way when resuspended in normal rabbit PPP and incubated with endotoxin, inulin or zymosan (Brown and Lachmann, 1973).

Dodds and Pickering (1972) demonstrated significant changes in haemostasis in guinea pigs given CVF, though they interpreted some of these changes as being secondary to the observed intravascular haemolysis, which arises from the marked susceptibility of guinea pig red cells to 'fluid phase' activated complement components. However, minor degrees of PF3 activation were observed as well as rather more marked alterations of clot retraction and clot lysis.

Complement can also be activated in the 'fluid phase' by assembling C3 converting enzymes in vivo. Classical pathway activation can be achieved by the intravenous injection of C4oxy2 (a more stable form of the classical pathway C3 convertase) and alternative pathway activation by injecting C3b and activated factor D (Mak, 1975). Both manoeuvres were performed in rats and converted or consumed more than 50% of C3, C6 and C7, causing profound temporary neutropenia without affecting platelet counts.

From the experiments described above it would appear that marked complement activation in the fluid phase, even under conditions which generate the lytic terminal complex of the complement sequence, do not cause major platelet damage in immune adherence positive species; this lends support to the idea that the C3 immune adherence step via a particle or complex, however small, is necessary to activate the lytic phase of the complement sequence in close proximity to the platelet membrane. In this respect platelets are unlike guinea pig red cells or the red cells of patients with paroxysmal nocturnal haemoglobinuria, both of which are highly susceptible to fluid phase complement lysis mediated via CVF (Götze and Müller-Eberhard, 1970).

3.5. Platelet damage by a basophil-dependent reaction

Several investigators independently discovered that rabbit platelets could undergo a platelet release reaction with loss of histamine and 5HT when mixed with leucocytes from a sensitized rabbit in the presence of the sensitizing antigen (Siraganian and Osler, 1969; Barbero and Schoenbechler, 1970; Henson, 1970c).

Henson and Cochrane (1971) showed that the reaction could not be elicited until the immunizing (or sensitizing) antigen had been eliminated from the blood and so presumably did not depend on large quantities of immune complexes. They further showed that the reaction was independent of the complement status of the animal–i.e., took place as effectively with leukocytes obtained from a CVF treated rabbit as from a normal rabbit. The sensitivity could be transferred passively in serum to normal recipient rabbits and both Colwell et al. (1971) and Henson and Cochrane (1971) concluded that the sensitizing agent was probably a 'cytophilic' antibody passively allergizing the leukocytes.

Henson (1970c) had earlier presented tentative evidence that a labile soluble factor was released from the leukocytes in the reaction and that this factor acted on the platelets. This was confirmed by Siraganian and Osler (1971a) who also found that the first step in the reaction, that of leukocyte release, required Ca^{2+} ions and was inhibited by Mg^{2+}. By comparing the amount of histamine release relative to the input of platelets and leukocytes in the reaction mixtures Siraganian and Osler (1971b) were able to conclude that the leukocytes releasing the soluble factor were themselves the histamine rich population, i.e., basophils. The metabolic requirements for release by the leukocytes were virtually identical to those required for IgE mediated granule discharge from basophils (Osler and Siraganian, 1972). Further support for this view that the reaction was mediated by IgE or homocytotropic antibody came from the observation that leukocytes from animals 'hyperimmunized' to the antigen, which might be assumed to have large amounts of circulating IgG antibody, did not generate the platelet releasing factor.

Benveniste et al. (1972) provided direct proof of the requirement for IgE. Rabbits were sensitized to horseradish peroxidase under conditions which gave rise to 'homocytotropic' antibody. The platelet release reaction could be elicited only after several weeks and became fully active only after a booster injection. They confirmed that the sensitivity could be passively transferred by serum and that this could be inhibited by incubation with anti-ε (Epsilon) chain antibody. A platelet activating factor (PAF), almost certainly the soluble factor previously mentioned, was recoverable from leukocytes under conditions optimal for basophil granule discharge and this reaction was also inhibitable by anti-ε chain serum. The requirement for basophils was confirmed by electronmicroscopy of the platelet–leukocyte aggregates. These pictures showed single basophils, partly degranulated, surrounded by a halo of platelets with morphological appearances consistent with a release reaction.

The soluble platelet releasing factor was partially characterized by Benveniste (1974) as ethanol extractable material of low molecular weight (approximately 1100 daltons) with highly basic properties. There are strong similarities between rabbit and human PAF.

Halonen and Pinckard (1975) and Pinckard et al. (1975) reported an anaphylaxis reaction in rabbits, using a neonatal immunization schedule which gives rise to a pure IgE antibody response. Challenge with large doses of antigen resulted in rapid basophil depletion and marked though temporary thrombocytopenia. They suggested that this reaction is the in vivo equivalent of the basophil dependent platelet release reaction.

4. Immunological reactivity of immune adherence negative platelets

Primate platelets (particularly those of man) have been the most studied in this group, though there is one report of the reaction of pig platelets with surface bound IgG (Movat et al., 1965). The early work (summarised in section 2) demonstrated that immune adherence negative platelets reacted with preformed IgG containing immune complexes, with aggregated gammaglobulin, and with a variety of IgG coated surfaces (reviewed in detail by Pfueller and Lüscher, 1972) to generate a platelet release reaction whose aggregation phase could be inhibited by adenosine and AMP. The release of vasoactive amines in this reaction was independent of the calcium ion concentration (Mueller-Eckhardt and Lüscher, 1968b).

4.1. Reaction with aggregated or complexed IgG

Further insight into the nature of primate platelet reactions with immune complexes has come from the work of Pfueller and Lüscher (1972a, 1972b) and Henson and Spiegelberg (1973). Pfueller and Lüscher (1972a) investigated reactions with heat aggregated, bis-diazobenzidine aggregated, and organic solvent precipitated IgG, and demonstrated platelet aggregation and major release of 5HT without a detectable lag phase, when washed human platelets were mixed with IgG modified in these different ways. The reactions were not subclass specific though the weakest reactions were with IgG₃. This seems an interesting observation in relation to the problem of evaluating the role of complement in immune reactions involving human platelets, since IgG₃ is the most active subclass of IgG at fixing complement (Augener et al., 1971). However, in a second report, Pfueller and Lüscher (1972b) showed that structural modifications of IgG, particularly acetylation and acetamidation, destroyed both platelet aggregating activity and complement fixing ability. Henson and Spiegelberg (1973) carried out related experiments with heat or bis-diazobenzidine aggregated myeloma proteins and complexes formed between tetanus toxoid and antibody. There were no major differences in the ability of the IgG subclasses from IgG₁ through IgG₄ to aggregate platelets and release 5HT though a large series of other immunoglobulin aggregates (IgA₁, IgA₂, IgD, IgE, IgM and F(ab′)₂), were unreactive. Only (Fc)n retained some 5HT releasing potential. The demonstration that both F(ab′)₂ and IgA aggregates fail to generate the release reaction is possibly a further point of difference from rabbit platelets (Siraganian et al., 1973) since both types of complex are potentially able to activate the alternative complement pathway and convert C3 (Spiegelberg and Götze, 1972). Fresh serum inhibited the platelet release reaction induced by aggregated IgG₁ and IgG₃ but not that induced by the other two subclasses, IgG₂ and IgG₄. Henson and Spiegelberg (1973) concluded that the inhibiting effect was related to complement fixation by the aggregated IgG.

It seems reasonable to postulate that complement fixation to the exposed Fc regions in the aggregates is blocking interaction with an Fc receptor on the platelet. This interpretation seems equally applicable to the finding that partially purified C1 and purified C1q inhibit the reaction when added to the mixture (Pfueller and Lüscher, 1972a). These platelet release reactions do not require Ca²⁺ and are apparently non-lytic since neither LDH nor ⁵¹Cr is released under the appropriate experimental conditions. The presence of neutrophils does not enhance the release reaction, unlike the reaction seen when rabbit platelets are mixed with neutrophils in the presence of complexed IgG (Henson, 1970b).

4.2. Reaction with zymosan

A distinctive and apparently unique release reaction develops when human platelets are mixed with zymosan particles. The unravelling of the complexities of this reaction is largely due to the work of Zucker and Grant (1974), Zucker et al.

(1974) and Pfueller and Lüscher (1974a), who independently came to similar conclusions regarding its mechanism. Zymosan is unreactive when mixed with washed human platelets but can be 'conditioned' by preincubation in fresh heparinized, citrated, or Mg^{2+}-EGTA plasma at 37°C for varying lengths of time (10–60 min). Zymosan activated in this manner (Pfueller and Lüscher, 1974a; Zucker and Grant, 1974) caused an immediate biphasic release reaction and liberated up to 70% of platelet 5HT. The second phase was inhibitable by AMP, Adenosine or EDTA (Pfueller and Lüscher, 1974a), by aspirin, or by the substitution of thrombasthenic platelets for normal platelets (Zucker and Grant, 1974). This reaction of human platelets with activated zymosan is reminiscent of the biphasic release reaction observed when rabbit platelets or PRP are mixed with preincubated zymosan (Christian and Gordon, 1975; Marney et al., 1975).

A number of factors influence the capacity of fresh plasma to activate zymosan. Generation of activated zymosan in plasma could be inhibited by heating plasma at 50°C for 30 min, incubation conditions which are known to destroy factor B of the alternative pathway and by hydrazine treatment, which destroys C3. Mixing the heated and hydrazine treated plasmas restored the ability to activate zymosan (Zucker and Grant, 1974a). It can be concluded from the above evidence that alternative pathway activity and complement fixation up to the C3 step (but probably not beyond it), are required to activate zymosan, and it can be indirectly concluded that this requires the assembly of the alternative pathway C3-converting enzyme, C3bB on the zymosan particle (Brade et al., 1974) since the zymosan treated plasma (containing 'fluid phase' complement activation and breakdown products) retained no platelet releasing and aggregating activity (Zucker and Grant, 1974a). The reaction with activated zymosan was non-lytic and did not cause loss of LDH; exactly as had been previously demonstrated in the release reaction with aggregated immunoglobulins.

A further critical requirement for the reaction noted by both groups was the presence of fibrinogen in the activating system, since serum could not be substituted for plasma unless approximately 100 μg/ml of fibrinogen was added back. Further proof of the involvement of the alternative pathway in the formation of activated zymosan (ZC) has recently been provided by Zucker et al. (1975). Factor B depleted plasma and C3 depleted or deficient plasma could be reconstituted in their activity by adding back purified factor B or C3 respectively. Properdin is another complement component, whose position in the alternative pathway and the feedback cycle (Lachmann, 1975) is still not entirely clear, though it may be involved in the generation of ZC, since properdin deficient plasma made by adsorbing plasma with zymosan at 17°C for 60 min (Pillemer et al., 1965) lost its ability to activate zymosan. The early part of the classical pathway (Cl–4) does not seem to be a critical requirement since both human and guinea pig C4-deficient plasma generate the platelet releasing activity on zymosan.

Neither CVF (Pfueller and Lüscher, 1974a), endotoxin nor inulin (Pfueller and Lüscher, 1974b; Zucker et al., 1974) cause aggregation and release by human platelets. Similar conclusions about the unreactivity of human platelets with endotoxin were made by Mueller-Eckhardt and Lüscher (1968c) and morphological evidence of the unreactivity of primate platelets has been recorded by Spielvogel (1967). Furthermore, release and activation of PF3 does not occur when endotoxins are mixed with human platelets (Brown and Lachmann, 1973). Nagayama et al. (1971), however, found variable 5HT release from human platelets when testing a wide variety of endotoxins derived from different gram negative organisms.

5. Biological significance of platelet participation in immune reactions

In those species whose platelets are immune adherence positive, intravenous injection of complement-fixing particles or the intravenous generation of complement-fixing immune complexes causes profound though temporary thrombocytopenia with the majority of the platelets returning to the circulation within hours or minutes. Evidence that this temporary sequestration is solely responsible for the local or generalized intravascular coagulation is equivocal (for review see Brown, 1975), since certain substances – notably the endotoxins – invariably cause some degree of intravascular coagulation, but the mechanisms responsible may be partly or wholly unrelated to their capacity to activate and fix complement. In the rat, for example, the immediate complement-dependent thrombocytopenia can be clearly separated from the later non complement-dependent consumption of platelets associated with an endotoxin induced vasculitis (Majewski and Brown, 1976).

Platelets are also prominently involved in certain inflammatory lesions such as the Arthus reaction (Uriahara and Movat, 1964), the local Shwartzman reaction (Taichman, 1971) and the Forssman reaction (Taichman et al., 1972). However, although their presence in the lesions enhances the intensity of inflammation and thrombosis, they do not appear to be an essential component. The real biological role of the immune adherence reaction and the events which follow it can only be conjectured, though one need only go back to the original observations of Levaditi to see that the rate of removal of foreign particles and microorganisms from the circulation may be greatly enhanced by adherence mechanisms. These arguments cannot, however, be applied with the same conviction to the platelets in immune adherence negative species, since in this situation the platelet-aggregating effect seems to be biologically important only after IgG antibody formation has taken place.

Whether platelets are involved to a major degree in acute anaphylaxis in man through the liberation of platelet activating factor is uncertain, since to date the necessary experiments have not been performed in primates. Furthermore, the full evolution of anaphylaxis or acute serum sickness is rarely observed clinically under conditions which allow careful recording of laboratory parameters, and when thrombocytopenia appears late in acute inflammatory reactions it is difficult to determine whether immunological or clotting mechanisms caused platelet consumption. This question is also unresolved at present in relation to the thrombocytopenias associated with lowered complement levels in *Plasmodium malariae* infections (Srichaikul et al., 1975), in dengue haemorrhage shock (Bokisch et al., 1973) and in the Jarisch-Herxheimer reaction of relapsing fever (Bryceson A., personal communication, 1975). Therefore, although platelets undoubtedly participate in several immunological reactions and contribute to the biological consequences, the complex inter-relationships between these reactions and other biological processes (in which platelets are also involved), together with inter-species differences in platelet reactivity, make it difficult to gauge the precise nature and significance of the platelet contribution.

References

Ackroyd, J.F. (1951) Clin. Sci., *10*, 185.
Alper, C.A. and Rosen, F.S. (1974) in Progress in Immunology, II (Brent, L. and Holborow, J., eds), Vol. 1, p. 201, North-Holland, Amsterdam.
Augener, W., Grey, H.M., Cooper, N.R. and Müller-Eberhard, H.J. (1971) Immunochemistry, *8*, 1011.
Aynaud, M. (1911) Compt. Rend. Soc. Biol., *70*, 54.
Ballow, M. and Cochrane, C.G. (1969) J. Immunol., *103*, 944.
Barbero, J.F. (1961) J. Immunol., *86*, 369.
Barbero, J.F. and Schoenbechler, M.J. (1970) J. Immunol., *104*, 1124.
Becker, E.L. and Henson, P.M. (1973) Adv. Immunol., *17*, 93.
Benveniste, J., Henson, P.M. and Cochrane, C.G. (1972) J. Exp. Med., *136*, 1356.
Benveniste, J. (1974) Nature, *249*, 581.
Brade, V., Nicholson, A., Bitter-Suermann, D. and Hadding, U. (1974) J. Immunol., *113*, 1735.
Bokisch, V.A., Top, F.H., Russel, P.K., Dixon, F.J. and Müller-Eberhard, H.J. (1973) New Eng. J. Med., *289*, 996.
Brown, D.L. (1975) Brit. J. Haemat., *30*, 377.
Brown, D.L. and Lachmann, P.J. (1973) Int. Arch. Allerg., *45*, 193.
Brown, D.L. and Lachmann, P.J. (1974) in Advances in the Biosciences, *12* (G. Raspé, ed), p. 300, Pergamon, Vieweg.
Brown, D.L., Lachmann, P.J. and Dacie, J.V. (1970) Clin. Exp. Immunol., *7*, 401.
Christian, F.A. and Gordon, J.L. (1975) Immunology, *29*, 131.
Cochrane, C.G., Müller-Eberhard, H.J. and Aikin, B.S. (1970) J. Immunol., *105*, 55.
Colwell, E.J., Ortaldo, J.R., Schoenbechler, M.J. and Barbaro, J.F. (1971) Int. Arch. Allergy, *41*, 754.
Des Prez, R.M. and Bryant, R.E. (1969) J. Immunol., *102*, 241.
Dodds, W.J. and Pickering, R.J. (1972) Blood, *40*, 400.
Fine, D.P., Marney, S.R., Colley, D.G., Sergent, J.S. and Des Prez, R.M. (1972) J. Immunol., *109*, 807.
Garner, R., Chater, B.V. and Brown, D.L. (1974) Brit. J. Haemat., *28*, 393.
Gitlin, J.D., Rosen, F.S. and Lachmann, P.J. (1975) J. Exp. Med., *141*, 1221.
Gocke, D.J. (1965) J. Immunol., *94*, 247.
Gocke, D.J. and Osler, A.G. (1965) J. Immunol., *94*, 236.
Gotze, O. and Müller-Eberhard, H.J. (1970) J. Exp. Med., *132*, 898.
Govaerts, P. (1923) Compt. Rend. Soc. Biol., *88*, 993.
Grette, K. (1962) Acta Physiol. Scand. (Suppl.), *195*, 1.
Halonen, M. and Pinckard, R.N. (1975) J. Immunol., *115*, 519.
Henson, P.M. (1960) Immunology, *16*, 107.
Henson, P.M. (1970a) J. Immunol., *105*, 476.
Henson, P.M. (1970b) J. Immunol., *105*, 490.
Henson, P.M. (1970c) J. Exp. Med., *131*, 287.
Henson, P.M. and Cochrane, C.G. (1969) J. Exp. Med., *129*, 166.
Henson, P.M. and Cochrane, C.G. (1971) J. Exp. Med., *133*, 554.
Henson, P.M. and Spiegelberg, H.L. (1973) J. Clin. Invest., *52*, 1282.
Humphrey, J.H. and Jacques, R. (1955) J. Physiol., *128*, 9.

Hunsicker, L.G., Ruddy, S. and Austen, K.F. (1973) J. Immunol., *110*, 128.
Ishizake, T. and Ishizake, K. (1962) J. Immunol., *89*, 709.
Jobin, F. and Tremblay, F. (1969) Thrombos. Diathes. Haemorrh., *22*, 450.
Kinsell, L.W., Kopeloff, L.M., Zwemer, R.L. and Kopeloff, N. (1941) J. Immunol., *42*, 35.
Kopeloff, N. and Kopeloff, L.M. (1941) J. Immunol., *40*, 471.
Kritschewsky, I.L. (1927) Klin. Wochschr., *6*, 1103.
Kritschewsky, I.L. and Tscherikower, R.S. (1928) Z. Immunitätsforsch., *57*, 234.
Lachmann, P.J. (1976) in The Immune System: A Course on the Cellular and Molecular Basis of Immunity (Hobart, M.J. and McConnell, I., eds), p. 56, Blackwell Scientific, Oxford.
Lachmann, P.J. and Müller-Eberhard, H.J. (1968) J. Immunol., *100*, 691.
Lamanna, C. (1957) Bact. Rev., *21*, 30.
Levaditi, C. (1901) Ann. Inst. Pasteur, *15*, 894.
Majewski, J.B. and Brown, D.L. (1976) Proc. VI Int. Congr. Nephrol., Karger, Basel (in press).
Mak, L.W. (1975) A study of complement inactivation with reagents derived from human complement components, Ph.D. Thesis, Univ. London.
Mardiney, M.R. and Müller-Eberhard, H.J. (1965) J. Immunol., *94*, 877.
Marney, S.R. (1971) J. Immunol., *106*, 82.
Marney, S.R., Colley, D.G. and Des Prez, R.M. (1975) J. Immunol., *114*, 696.
Martin, A.M.B. (1976) Complement activation pathways. Generation of C3 and C5 convertases. Ph.D. Thesis Univ. London.
Movat, H.Z., Mustard, J.F., Taichman, N.S. and Uriahara, T. (1965) Proc. Soc. Exp. Biol. Med., *120*, 232.
Mueller-Eckhardt, C. and Lüscher, E.F. (1968a) Thrombos. Diathes. Haemorrh., *20*, 155.
Mueller-Eckhardt, C. and Lüscher, E.F. (1968b) Thrombos. Diathes. Haemorrh., *20*, 168.
Müller-Eberhard, H.J. (1975) Ann. Rev. Biochem., *44*, 697.
Mustard, J.F. and Packham, M.A. (1970) Pharmacol. Rev., *22*, 97.
Nagayama, M., Zucker, M.B. and Beller, F.K. (1971) Thrombos. Diathes. Haemorrh., *26*, 467.
Nelson, D.S. (1963) Adv. Immunol., *3*, 131.
Nelson, R.A. (1956) Proc. Roy. Soc. Med., *49*, 55.
Nelson, R.A. (1966) Surv. Ophthal., *11*, 498.
Nicholson, A., Brade, V., Schorlemmer, H.U., Burger, R., Bitter-Suermann, D. and Hadding, U. (1975) J. Immunol., *115*, 1108.
Osler, A.G. and Siraganian, R.P. (1972) Progr. Allergy, *16*, 450.
Pfueller, S.L. and Lüscher, E.F. (1972a) J. Immunol., *109*, 517.
Pfueller, S.L. and Luscher, E.F. (1972b) J. Immunol., *109*, 526.
Pfueller, S.L. and Luscher, E.F. (1972c) Immunochemistry, *9*, 1151.
Pfueller, S.L. and Luscher, E.F. (1974a) J. Immunol., *112*, 1201.
Pfueller, S.L. and Luscher, E.F. (1974b) J. Immunol., *112*, 1211.
Philips, J.K., Snyderman, R. and Mergenhagen, S.E. (1972) J. Immunol., *109*, 334.
Pillemer, L., Blum, L., Lepow, I.H., Ross, O.A., Todd, E.W. and Wardlow, A.C. (1954) Science, *120*, 279.
Pinckard, R.N., Tanigawa, C. and Halonen, M. (1975) J. Immunol., *115*, 525.
Rieckenberg, H. (1917) Z. Immunitatsforsch., *26*, 53.
Rocha e Silva, M. (1950) Ann. New York Acad. Sci., *50*, 1045.
Ruddy, S. and Austen, K.F. (1971) J. Immunol., *107*, 742.
Siquiera, M. and Nelson, R.A. (1961) J. Immunol., *86*, 516.
Siraganian, R.P. and Osler, A.G. (1969) J. Allergy, *43*, 167.
Siraganian, R.P. and Osler, A.G. (1971a) J. Immunol., *106*, 1244.
Srichaikul, T., Puwasatien, P., Karnjanajetanee, J. and Bokisch, V.A. (1975) Lancet *1*, 770.
Siraganian, R.P. and Osler, A.G. (1971b) J. Immunol., *106*, 1252.
Siraganian, R.P., Sandberg, A.L., Alexander, A. and Osler, A.G. (1973) J. Immunol., *110*, 490.
Siraganian, R.P., Secchi, A.C. and Osler, A.G. (1968a) J. Immunol., *101*, 1130.
Siraganian, R.P., Secchi, A.C. and Osler, A.G. (1968b) J. Immunol., *101*, 1148.
Spiegelberg, H.L. and Götze, O. (1972) Fed. Proc., *31*, 655.
Spielvogel, A.R. (1967) J. Exp. Med., *126*, 235.
Srichaukul, T., Puwasatien, P., Karnjanajetanee, J. and Bokisch, V.A. (1975) Lancet *1*, 770.
Stetson, C.A. (1951a) J. Exp. Med., *93*, 489.
Stetson, C.A. (1951b) J. Exp. Med., *94*, 347.
Stormorken, H. (1969) Scand. J. Haemat. (Suppl.) *9*, 3–24.
Swisher, S.N. (1956) J. Clin. Invest., *35*, 738.
Taichman, N.S. (1971) in Inflammation, Immunity and Hypersensitivity, (Movat, H.Z. ed) p. 479, Harper and Row, New York.

Taichman, N.S., Creigton, M., Stephenson, A. and Tsai, C.-C. (1972) Immunology, *22*, 93.
Uriahara, T. and Movat, H.Z. (1969) Lab. Invest., *13*, 1057.
Weiss, H.J. (1975) New Eng. J. Med., *293*, 531.
White, J.G. (1972) Amer. J. Path., *69*, 439.
Zimmerman, T.S. (1974) in Advances in the Biosciences, *12*, (Raspe, G. ed), p. 291, Pergamon, Vieweg.
Zucker, M.B. and Grant, R.A. (1974) J. Immunol., *112*, 1219.
Zucker, M.B., Grant, R.A., Alper, C.A., Goodkofsky, I. and Lepow, I.H. (1974) J. Immunol., *113*, 1744.

CHAPTER 13

Prostaglandin synthesis by platelets and its biological significance

J.B. SMITH and M.J. SILVER

Cardeza Foundation and Department of Pharmacology, Thomas Jefferson University,
1015 Walnut Street, Philadelphia, Pennsylvania 19107, U.S.A.

1. Introduction

During the last five years the number of publications dealing with prostaglandin synthesis by platelets has increased dramatically. In view of the fact that few people have had the opportunity to keep abreast of the rapidly developing knowledge in the field of prostaglandins, we begin this chapter with a brief historical introduction to prostaglandins, then turn to the discovery that, of all tissues studied, seminal vesicles have the greatest capacity for prostaglandin synthesis. Almost all of the early advances in elucidating mechanisms of prostaglandin synthesis were made with preparations of this tissue, and a review of these advances gives insight as to why the existence of prostaglandin endoperoxides was postulated. The importance of their subsequent isolation can then be readily appreciated.

The metabolism of arachidonic acid by platelets has been elucidated in recent years and shows that the platelet transforms prostaglandin precursors differently from seminal vesicles. While the platelet has high levels of the first enzyme involved in prostaglandin biosynthesis by seminal vesicles (fatty acid cyclooxygenase) it has very little of the second (prostaglandin E Isomerase). Of great importance is the fact that prostaglandin endoperoxides are produced by platelets, and these are more potent platelet aggregating agents than ADP. The mechanism by which the endoperoxides induce platelet aggregation is at present the subject of intensive investigation and will be discussed later in this chapter. We will also consider new approaches which research on platelet prostaglandins has brought to the prophylaxis or treatment of haemorrhage and thrombosis. Some of the aspects of earlier advances in this field, which are touched on briefly here, are considered in more detail in another review (Smith and Macfarlane, 1974).

Gordon (ed) Platelets in Biology and Pathology
© *Elsevier/North-Holland Biomedical Press, 1976*

2. Prostaglandins

Two American gynecologists (Kurzrok and Lieb, 1930) made the novel observation that human seminal fluid contracts uterine strips prepared from pregnant subjects. Subsequently, Goldblatt (1933, 1935) and Von Euler (1934, 1936) independently showed that human semen contains substances which are very potent in stimulating smooth muscle and lowering blood pressure. The physico-chemical properties of the active principles in semen were investigated by Von Euler, who showed that they were lipid-soluble acids and therefore differed chemically from other known biologically active substances. He named this lipid-soluble activity 'prostaglandin' because he believed it came from the prostate gland (see Von Euler, 1936).

In the following years, acidic lipids were extracted from several tissues and shown to possess biological activity. 'Prostaglandin' was found in acidic lipid extracts of seminal vesicles of man and sheep, but extracts of the prostate, seminal vesicles and seminal fluid of the Rhesus monkey contained depressor but not smooth muscle-stimulating activity. This activity was named 'vesiglandin' (Von Euler, 1936). Later, 'irin' was extracted from the human iris (Ambache, 1957) and 'Darmstoff' from frog intestine (Vogt, 1949) but in no extract of tissue did the amount of active lipid approach that of the prostaglandin in human semen.

By constructing a time course of the appearance of prostaglandin during ejaculation, Eliasson (1959) demonstrated that the major source of prostaglandin in human semen is the seminal vesicles and not the prostate gland. However, by then, the name prostaglandin was well established. Shortly afterwards Bergström and Sjöval (1960, 1960a) made the important discovery that two prostaglandins could be extracted from sheep seminal vesicles. One prostaglandin, PGE, lowered rabbit blood pressure and was more soluble in ether than the other. The second, PGF, did not lower blood pressure but stimulated the rabbit duodenum and was more soluble in phosphate (spelt with an 'F' in Swedish) buffer. With this discovery came the realization that the different biological activities (prostaglandin, vesiglandin, irin, etc.) found in acidic, lipid extracts of tissues were in fact prostaglandins.

In 1962 and 1963, Bergström and his co-workers at the Karolinska Institute described the structures of several prostaglandins present in extracts of seminal vesicles and pooled human semen (see Bergström, 1967). These all contained 20 carbon atoms and were related to the same hypothetical parent compound, prostanoic acid (Fig. 1). The prostaglandins differed in their degree of oxygenation and amount of unsaturation. Prostaglandin E was resolved into PGE_1, PGE_2, and PGE_3 which had 1, 2, and 3 double bonds in their side chains respectively. Prostaglandin F was shown to consist of $PGF_{1\alpha}$, and $PGF_{2\alpha}$. The structures of PGE_1, PGE_2, $PGF_{1\alpha}$ and $PGF_{2\alpha}$ are shown in Fig. 1. Other prostaglandins found in human semen had an A-type or B-type structure, but they will not be discussed further as it now appears that they were formed chemically during the storage of the semen (Taylor and Kelly, 1974; Jonsson et al., 1975).

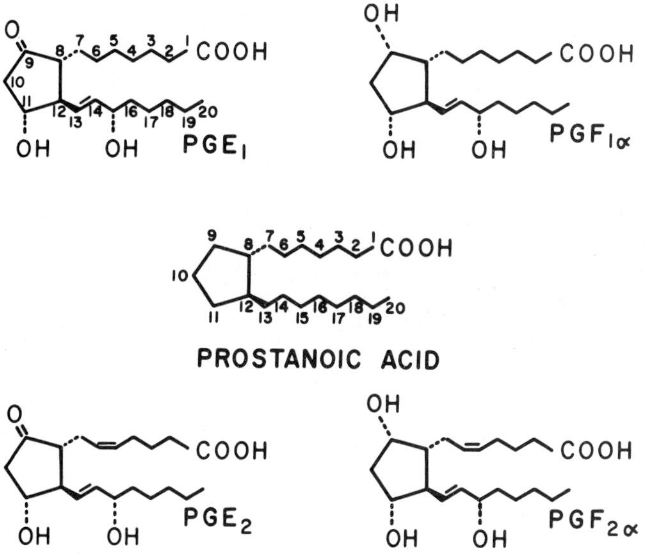

Fig. 1.

3. *Prostaglandin synthesis by seminal vesicles*

Two groups, one working with Bergström (Bergström et al., 1964) and the other with Van Dorp (Van Dorp et al., 1964) simultaneously demonstrated that PGE_2 was formed when arachidonic acid was incubated with cell-free preparations of sheep vesicular glands. This biosynthesis was also demonstrated using a powdered acetone extract of vesicular glands of the bull (Wallach, 1965), and prostaglandin synthetase was later localised in the microsomal fraction of homogenates of the vesicular gland (Samuelsson, 1967; Van Dorp, 1967). Such enzyme preparations became the subject of intensive biochemical investigation during the next ten years.

The precursor of PGE_1 and $PGF_{1\alpha}$ was identified as all-*cis*-8,11,14-eicosatrienoic acid and that of PGE_2 and $PGF_{2\alpha}$ as arachidonic acid (all-*cis*-5,8,11,14-eicosatetraenoic acid) (see Fig. 2). The precursor of PGE_3 was all-*cis*-5,8,11,14,17-eicosapentaenoic acid (see Bergström, 1967). Study of the substrate specificity of the enzyme revealed that eicosapolyenoic acids which have at least two cis-double bonds in positions 11 and 14 are converted into corresponding L-11-hydroxy-12 *trans*, 14 *cis*-eicosapolyenoic acids (Nugteren et al., 1966).

The addition of glutathione was found to enhance greatly the yield of PGE compounds though this was partly at the expense of the corresponding PGF_α (Nugteren et al., 1966a), and other thiol compounds such as cysteine, homocysteine, thioglycolic acid and thiophenol were almost inactive in this respect. On the other hand, the combination of Cu^{2+} and dithiothreitol favored the formation of

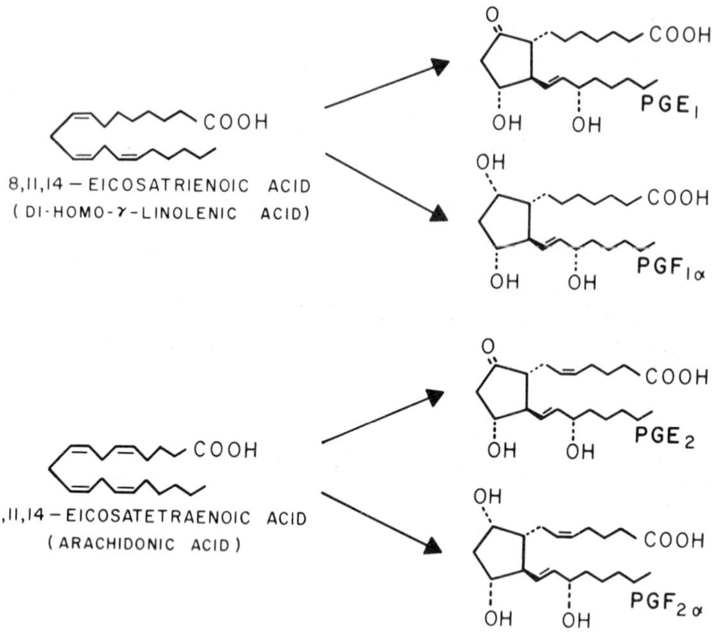

Fig. 2.

PGF_α at the expense of PGE (Lands et al., 1971). Enhancement of biosynthesis was also seen if a moderate amount of antioxidant (5×10^{-4} M) such as hydroquinone or propylgallate, was included in the incubation mixture. A variety of aromatic compounds (L-epinephrine, L-norepinephrine, serotonin, and 5-hydroxyindole-3-acetic acid) could be substituted for hydroquinone, and they appear to act by supplying the reducing equivalents that are required for the biosynthesis of prostaglandins (Takeguchi et al., 1971).

Several products in addition to PGE_1 and $PGF_{1\alpha}$ formed when 8,11,14-eicosatrienoic acid was incubated with sheep vesicular gland homogenates (Nugteren et al., 1966a; Granstrom et al., 1968). Some of these (shown in Fig. 3) include 11-hydroxy-8-cis, 12-trans, 14-*cis*-eicosatrienoic acid (A), 15-hydroxy-8-*cis*, 11-*cis*, 13-*trans*-eicosatrienoic acid (B), 12-hydroxy-8-*trans*-10-*trans*-heptadecadienoic acid (HHD), malondialdehyde (MDA) and 11-dehydro-$PGF_{1\alpha}$ (PGD_1).

3.1. Prostaglandin endoperoxides

Studies using the enzyme from seminal vesicles revealed that all of the oxygen atoms in prostaglandins are derived from molecular oxygen (Nugteren and Van Dorp, 1965; Ryhage and Samuelsson, 1965) and that those at C-9 and C-11 originate from the same molecule of oxygen (Samuelsson, 1965). This led Samuelsson to propose that an intermediate compound in the biosynthesis of PGE and PGF_α should be a cyclic endoperoxide with an oxygen bridge between the 9 and 11 carbon atoms.

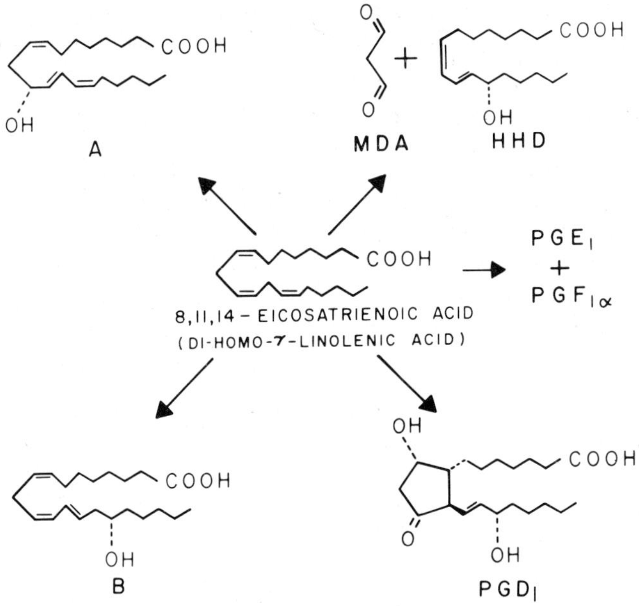

Fig. 3.

The following mechanism was subsequently proposed for prostaglandin biosynthesis (Nugteren et al., 1966a; Hamberg and Samuelsson, 1967a). The first steps (see Fig. 4) involve the abstraction of a hydrogen atom from C-13, followed by isomerism of the 11-*cis* double bond to 12-*trans* and the stereospecific attachment of an oxygen molecule at the C 11-L position.

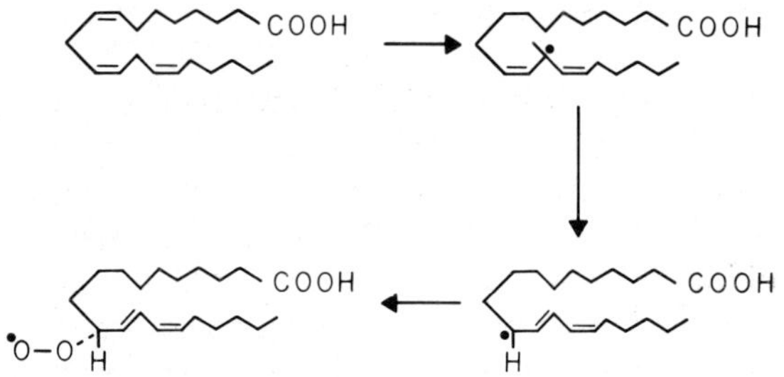

Fig. 4.

Evidence in favour of these steps included the substrate specificity of prostaglandin synthetase (the need for *cis*-double bonds at the 11 and 14 positions) and the isolation of L-11-hydroxy-12-*trans*, 14 *cis*-polyenoic acids as byproducts of prostaglandin biosynthesis. It was also found that 13D-^{3}H, 3-^{14}C-8,11,14-eicosatrienoic acid retained its tritium label during conversion to prostaglandins, whereas, when 13L-^{3}H, 3-^{14}C-8,11,14-eicosatrienoic acid was used as substrate the

PGE$_1$ formed was essentially free of tritium. A kinetic isotope enrichment of the substrate occurred during this latter conversion (^{3}H/^{14}C ratio 2.84 times that at the start), demonstrating that the abstraction of hydrogen at C-13L is an obligatory initiating process in prostaglandin biosynthesis (Hamberg and Samuelsson, 1967a).

The second stage in prostaglandin biosynthesis involves the formation of a cyclic endoperoxide. This could occur in two ways (see Fig. 5): either a second (activated) oxygen molecule might attach at C-15 with concomitant ring closure between C-8 and C-12 and formation of the peroxy bridge between C-9 and C-11 (see Fig. 5a), or firstly the peroxy radical at C-11 might attach at C-9 followed by ring closure and oxygen capture at C-15 (see Fig. 5b).

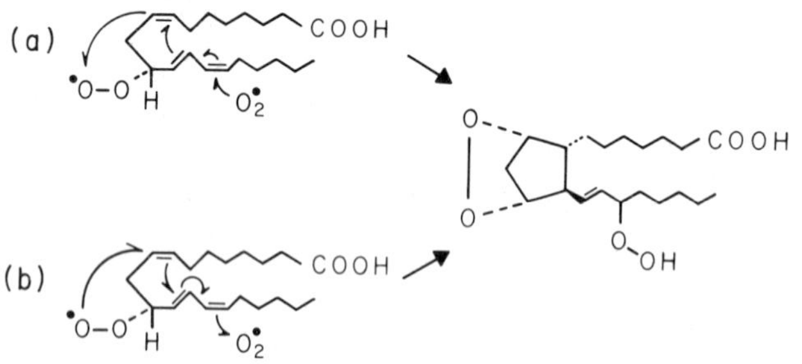

Fig. 5.

Initial evidence for the existence of cyclic endoperoxides was obtained in experiments in which isotopically-labelled precursors were used and the nature of the products was determined. When incubations were conducted without glutathione the major products included 12-hydroxy-8-*trans*, 10-*trans*-heptadecadienoic acid (HHD) and malondialdehyde in roughly equimolar quantities (Nugteren et al., 1966a). Furthermore, when doubly-labelled 8,11,14-eicosatrienoic acid (3-^{14}C and ^{3}H at C-9 or C-11) was used as substrate the fatty acid contained the ^{14}C while the malondialdehyde contained the tritium (see Fig. 6). This was rationalized by postulating a fragmentation reaction of a reverse Diels-Alder type involving the endoperoxide (Hamberg and Samuelsson, 1967a).

When incubations were conducted in the presence of glutathione much more PGE$_1$ was produced, but at the expense of other products. It was suggested (Fig. 7) that this occurred by a glutathione-assisted 1, 2 hydride shift of the endoperoxide (Lands et al., 1971). PGD$_1$ could be produced by a similar mechanism, whereas PGF$_{1\alpha}$ would be produced by reductive cleavage of the endoperoxide.

Identifying the various products formed during biosynthesis gave only presumptive evidence for the existence of cyclic endoperoxides, but a discovery which supported the hypothesis was made in 1973 when it was shown that, during incubations for short times without glutathione, there was a transient accumulation of compounds that could be reduced to PGF$_\alpha$ by mild chemical treatment with sodium dithionite or stannous chloride (Nugteren and Hazelhof, 1973;

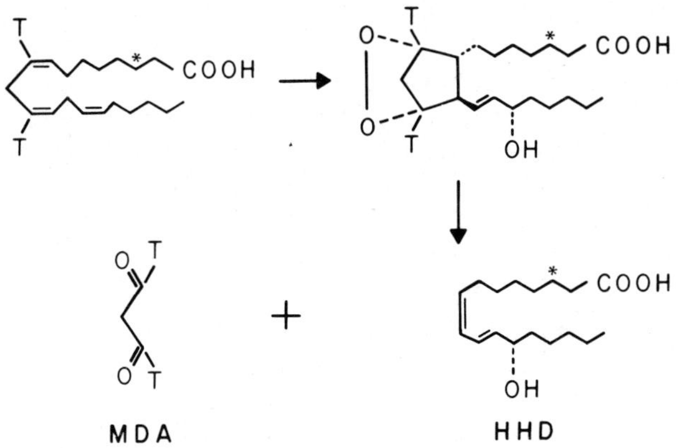

Fig. 6.

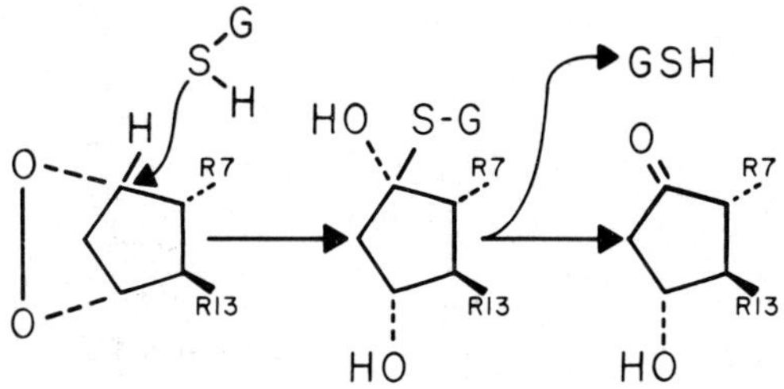

Fig. 7.

Hamberg and Samuelsson, 1973). These compounds were extracted with diethyl ether at $-20°C$ and separated by thin layer chromatography. In addition to the known products of biosynthesis, two compounds were found that were less polar than prostaglandins but more polar than the monohydroxy fatty acids. These intermediates rearranged or decomposed spontaneously in aqueous media to form a mixture of PGE, PGD and monohydroxy fatty acids. One intermediate was a cyclic endoperoxide with a hydroperoxy group at C-15 (PGG) (see Fig. 5) and the other a cyclic endoperoxide with hydroxy group at C-15 (PGH).

Prostaglandin synthetase from seminal vesicle microsomes has been separated by DEAE-cellulose chromatography into two fractions, both of which are required for PGE_1 synthesis. When one fraction was incubated with 8,11,14-eicosatrienoic acid, an unstable compound (presumed to be a cyclic endoperoxide) accumulated. This unstable compound was converted into PGE_1 by the addition of the second enzyme fraction and glutathione. The first fraction is therefore presumed to contain fatty acid cyclooxygenase and the second prostaglandin E isomerase (Miyamoto et al., 1974).

4. Prostaglandin synthesis by other cells and tissues

Apart from human semen and sheep vesicular glands, many human and animal tissues including lungs, renal medulla, iris, brain and thymus contain small amounts of prostaglandins (see Horton, 1972). Prostaglandins are also released from numerous tissues in response to stimuli such as hormones, enzymes and even particulate matter (see Piper and Vane, 1971). Since the tissues always contain less prostaglandin than the amount released, release must result from the stimulation of prostaglandin biosynthesis. Furthermore, since mechanical stimulation of tissues (e.g., stirring) induces prostaglandin formation, it is probable that even the small amounts of prostaglandin found in tissues are the result of inducing biosynthesis during homogenization.

The mechanism by which prostaglandin formation is stimulated is not fully understood, but appears to be related to the distortion or activation of cell membranes. The prostaglandin precursors arachidonic acid and 8,11,14-eicosatrienoic acid do not occur free in cells but are present as esters (phospholipids, triglycerides or cholesterol esters). These ester forms are not substrates of prostaglandin synthetase (Vonkeman and Van Dorp, 1968; Lands and Samuelsson, 1968) and, therefore, it is believed that activation of an enzyme such as phospholipase A (Kunze and Vogt, 1971) is required to liberate the precursor so that biosynthesis can proceed. Prostaglandin synthetase activity has been found in almost every mammalian tissue investigated except red blood cells, but only seminal vesicles have a high biosynthetic capacity: they can apparently convert 75% of substrate into prostaglandins, whereas only 1–2% conversion of added substrate has been found in most other tissues (Christ and Van Dorp, 1972).

5. Prostaglandin synthesis by platelets

5.1. Formation of PGE_2 and $PGF_{2\alpha}$

Platelets do not contain prostaglandins, but small amounts of PGE_2 and $PGF_{2\alpha}$ are formed and released when washed human platelet suspensions are treated with thrombin (Smith and Willis, 1970). These prostaglandins are also formed during the clotting of human and rat blood or platelet-rich plasma (Silver et al., 1972; Orczyk and Behrman, 1972). Smaller amounts of PGE_2 are produced during platelet aggregation induced by collagen, and during the second wave of aggregation induced by adrenaline (Smith et al., 1973).

Erroneously high values were sometimes quoted for levels of prostaglandins in circulating blood because several investigators assayed serum (containing prostaglandins derived from platelets) rather than plasma (see Silver et al., 1973a). The prostaglandin content of plasma increases during storage in proportion to the number of platelets that are present (Jubiz and Frailey, 1974), but the concentration of prostaglandins in normal circulating plasma is probably about 1–10 pmol/l.

The PGE_2 and $PGF_{2\alpha}$ produced by platelets seem to be of little significance in platelet function: $PGF_{2\alpha}$ has no effect on platelets and although added PGE_2 does have effects, the concentrations required are far in excess of those produced during platelet aggregation (see Smith and Macfarlane, 1974).

5.2. Malondialdehyde formation

Malondialdehyde is a metabolite of PGG_2 that is formed when washed platelets are treated with thrombin (Okuma et al., 1971) or during platelet aggregation in platelet-rich plasma in response to ADP, adrenaline or collagen (Smith et al., 1976). The demonstration that both 12-hydroxy-5-*cis*, 8,10 *trans*-heptadecatrienoic acid (HHT) and malondialdehyde are produced in response to thrombin (Hamberg et al., 1974) strongly suggests that the malondialdehyde is derived solely from PGG_2, and since malondialdehyde can easily be measured by incubating it with thiobarbituric acid to form a pink pigment, it serves as a convenient indicator of prostaglandin synthesis by platelets.

5.3. Possible formation of PGE_1 and PGE_3

More than twenty times as much PGE_2 as PGE_1 is formed during the clotting of human blood (Silver et al., 1972). This reflects the fact that, in the phospholipids of normal human platelets, the ratio of 8,11,14-eicosatrienoic acid (the precursor of PGE_1) to arachidonic acid (the precursor of PGE_2) is probably less than 1:30 (Cohen and Derksen, 1969; Marcus et al., 1969). It is interesting that while a similar ratio of these essential fatty acids apparently exists in normal rat platelets, this ratio could be increased to 1:2 by feeding the rats 8,11,14-eicosatrienoic acid (Willis et al., 1974), and this was associated with a diminished responsiveness of the platelets to aggregating agents. Platelets can convert 8,11,14-eicosatrienoic acid into PGE_1 (Silver et al., 1973) and the diminished responsiveness may in part be caused by the formation of this inhibitor of aggregation (Kloeze, 1968).

When platelets were incubated for 2 h with radioactive acetate about 0.01% of the radioactivity behaved as prostaglandins on chromatography, and further analysis suggested that these prostaglandins included a mixture of PGE_1, PGE_2, and PGE_3 (Clausen and Srivastava, 1973). The trace amounts of radioactive prostaglandins were presumably formed by incorporation of radioactive acetate into essential, unsaturated, 18-carbon fatty acids to give 20 carbon fatty acids with 3, 4, or 5 double bonds. Since most of the fatty acids used by platelets for prostaglandin synthesis are released directly from phospholipids, and most of these fatty acids have 4 double bonds, the formation of PGE_1 and PGE_3 by platelets is probably of minor importance under normal conditions.

5.4. Metabolism of arachidonic acid by platelets

5.4.1. Metabolism by washed platelet suspensions

Hamberg and Samuelsson (1974) incubated radioactive arachidonic acid with washed human platelets resuspended in physiological saline solution and found that it was rapidly and almost exclusively converted to three, more polar, oxygenated products. One of the compounds was identified as 12L-hydroxy-5,8,10,14-eicosatetraenoic acid (HETE) which was produced by a previously unrecognized lipoxygenase reaction. A detailed study of the mechanism of this reaction has since been reported (Nugteren, 1975). A second product was 12-hydroxy-5-*cis*-8,10-transheptadecatrienoic acid (HHT) which was formed together with malondialdehyde (see Section 5.2). The third product was a novel hemiacetal compound, 8-(1-hydroxy-3 oxopropyl)-9, 12L-dihydroxy-5,10-heptadecadienoic acid (Hamberg and Samuelsson, 1974), subsequently named thromboxane B_2 (Hamberg et al., 1975). Studies on the mechanism of formation of this compound indicate that it is produced from the prostaglandin endoperoxide PGG_2 via an unstable intermediate compound, thromboxane A_2.

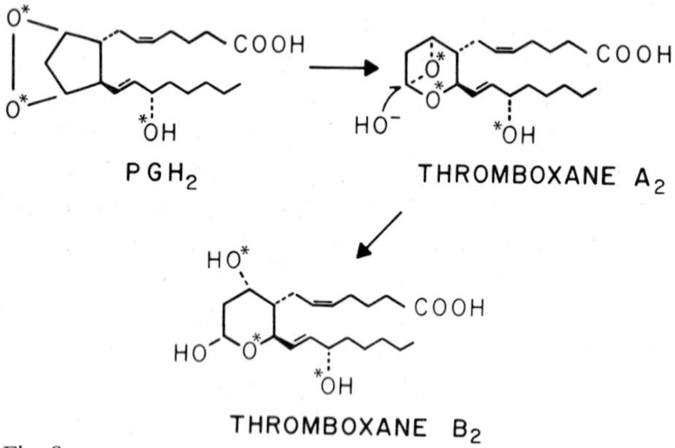

Fig. 8.

Evidence in favour of this pathway includes the following: (a) incubation of arachidonic acid with platelets under $^{18}O_2$ leads to the formation of thromboxane B_2 labelled in the side chain as well as in the nonhemiacetal hydroxy group and the ether oxygen of the oxane ring (Fig. 8); (b) the addition of nucleophilic reagents (CH_3OH; C_2H_5OH; NaN_3) during short incubations of arachidonic acid with platelets results in the formation of two epimeric derivatives of thromboxane B_2 in which the hemiacetal hydroxyl group was replaced by the nucleophile (Fig. 9); (c) addition of CH_3O^2H during short incubations results in the formation of derivatives of thromboxane B_2 lacking deuterium.

Perhaps the most significant point of these studies was the finding that human platelets have a high capacity to convert arachidonic acid to prostaglandin endoperoxides by a pathway involving a cyclooxygenase similar to that found in

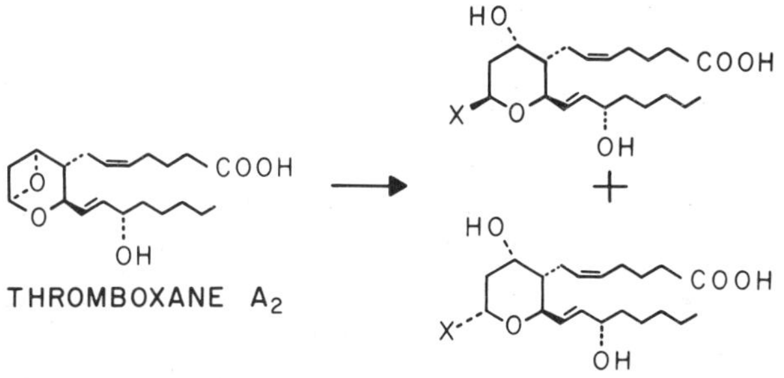

THROMBOXANE A₂

Fig. 9.

seminal vesicles, but in contrast to seminal vesicles (which contain large amounts of prostaglandin E isomerase and hence convert the endoperoxides to PGE) platelets produce predominantly the non-prostanoate compounds HHT and thromboxane B_2.

5.4.2. Metabolism by platelets in plasma

In contrast to the extensive oxidation of arachidonic acid that occurs when it is incubated with washed human platelets resuspended in saline, little or no oxidation of arachidonic acid occurs when it is incubated with platelets in plasma (Bills et al., 1976) or in aqueous medium containing albumin (Nugteren, 1975). This suggests that the affinity of albumin for arachidonic acid is greater than the affinities of the oxidative enzymes in platelets for arachidonic acid. Oxygenation of arachidonic acid does occur in platelet-rich plasma if large amounts are added to give a final concentration around 1 mM (Silver et al. 1973, Smith et al., 1976).

Although arachidonic acid is not normally oxidized in platelet-rich plasma, it is progressively incorporated into platelet phospholipids (Bills et al., 1976), and those phospholipids that accumulate arachidonic acid most avidly (phosphatidyl-choline and phosphatidylinositol) are the same phospholipids that release arachidonic acid for prostaglandin biosynthesis during aggregation. It was suggested that those enzymes involved in the process of arachidonic acid incorporation and release are those of the Lands pathway (Bills et al., 1976).

Several factors probably operate simultaneously to control the fate of arachidonic acid, whether added to platelet-rich plasma or released from platelet phospholipids during aggregation. These include: (1) binding by plasma albumin, (2) incorporation into platelet phospholipids and (3) transformation by platelet lipoxygenase and cyclooxygenase. Plasma albumin has not been considered seriously, heretofore, as an important factor in controlling the metabolism of arachidonic acid by platelets.

6. Induction of platelet aggregation

6.1. In vitro studies

6.1.1. Arachidonic acid

In 1972 it was reported that arachidonic acid caused platelet aggregation when added to stirred, human platelet-rich plasma (Silver et al., 1972a; Smith et al., 1972). Eleven other fatty acids tested under similar conditions were ineffective (Silver et al., 1973). This aggregation was associated with prostaglandin synthesis, inhibited by aspirin and indomethacin, and occurred in the platelets of several mammalian species. Platelets from guinea pigs and rabbits (Silver et al., 1973; Vargaftig and Zirinis, 1973) are very sensitive to the aggregating effects of arachidonic acid. Arachidonic acid at concentrations between 20 and 100 μM causes aggregation in guinea pig or rabbit platelet-rich plasma while concentrations of 0.1 to 1 mM (usually 0.5 mM) are needed to cause aggregation in human platelet-rich plasma. When arachidonic acid is added to platelet-rich plasma in concentrations too low to induce platelet aggregation directly, it enhances aggregation induced by collagen, ADP or epinephrine (Silver et al., 1973).

6.1.2. PGG_2, PGH_2 and thromboxane A_2

Evidence that an intermediate in prostaglandin biosynthesis could cause platelet aggregation was first reported in 1973 (Willis and Kuhn, 1973) and it appeared that this intermediate was a prostaglandin endoperoxide (Willis, 1974). Hamberg et al. (1974a) later demonstrated that adding 10–300 ng/ml of either PGG_2 or PGH_2 (isolated from incubations of arachidonic acid with seminal vesicle microsomes) to suspensions of washed human platelets resulted in rapid platelet aggregation. The relative potency of PGG_2 and PGH_2 was about 3:1, and both the extent and the reversibility of aggregation were concentration-dependent: low concentrations (about 10 ng/ml, or 0.03 μM) gave a small, reversible aggregation, whereas higher concentrations (50–300 ng/ml, or 0.15–1.0 μM) gave a larger aggregation response that was virtually irreversible. Aspirin did not significantly affect the aggregation.

Since the endoperoxides are selectively reduced to $PGF_{2\alpha}$ by treatment with stannous chloride, it is possible to determine whether these intermediates are formed and released during platelet aggregation, and, indeed, very low concentrations of these intermediates (less than 20 ng/ml) are found extracellularly during aggregation induced by thrombin, arachidonic acid, collagen or epinephrine (Hamberg et al., 1974a; Smith et al., 1974). The evidence that PGH_2 is produced during platelet aggregation is now conclusive (Willis et al., 1974a).

When methods were developed for the quantitative determination of HETE, HHT and thromboxane B_2, the three major metabolites of arachidonic acid in human platelets, Hamberg et al. (1974) showed that aggregation of washed platelets (5×10^8/ml) by thrombin is accompanied by release of 1163–2175 ng/ml of HETE, 1129–2430 ng/ml of HHT and 998–2299 ng/ml of thromboxane B_2. From the sum of the amounts of the metabolites of PGG_2, HHT and thromboxane B_2, they calculated that 2477–5480 ng/ml of arachidonic acid was converted into PGG_2, demonstrating that although only very low concentrations of PGG_2 are present at any given time during aggregation, the total amounts of PGG_2 produced and metabolized during aggregation are considerably more. Since the amounts of PGE_2 and $PGF_{2\alpha}$ produced were approximately two orders of magnitude lower than the amounts of the nonprostanoate metabolites of PGG_2, it was clear that the major route by which cyclic endoperoxide intermediates are metabolised in platelets is toward nonprostanoate compounds rather than prostaglandins.

Recent experiments suggest that the endoperoxide intermediates may have to be converted to thromboxane A_2 before they can aggregate platelets (Hamberg et al., 1975): the extent of aggregation induced by mixtures of arachidonic acid and washed platelet suspensions, incubated together for 30 sec, is greater than could be explained by the presence of PGG_2 and PGH_2 alone, and the factor responsible for this increased effect is very unstable, disappearing from incubation mixtures with a $t_{1/2}$ very similar to that of the thromboxane A_2. Since this unstable factor is also produced by incubating PGG_2 with platelet suspensions it could be thromboxane A_2, but since in aqueous medium the endoperoxides PGG_2 and PGH_2 have a longer $t_{1/2}$ (5 min) than thromboxane A_2 (31 sec) they would have been present at all times (albeit in low concentrations) when the biological activity of thromboxane A_2 was tested. It has therefore not yet been established whether all the biological activity of PGG_2 can be attributed to thromboxane A_2, but doubtless this evidence will soon be forthcoming.

6.1.3. Synthetic prostaglandins

Several prostaglandins that induce platelet aggregation have been synthesized recently, the first of which was 11-deoxy-15-methyl-15 RS-PGE$_2$ (Wy-17,186) (Fenichel et al., 1975). Its structure is shown in Fig. 10. This compound causes aggregation in human platelet-rich plasma at a concentration of about 5 μM. The aggregation induced by any concentration of Wy-17,186 so far tested is not inhibited by aspirin or indomethacin, but release of platelet serotonin induced by Wy-17,186 is partially inhibited by these drugs (Smith et al., 1975). Aggregation of washed human platelets by Wy-17,186 is enhanced by either fibrinogen or ADP (Smith et al., 1976).

Two other compounds closer in structure to PGH_2 have been found to aggregate platelets in nanomolar concentrations. Their structures are shown in Fig. 11 and they are designated U-46619 and U-44069 (Bundy, 1975 and 1975a).

An azo analogue of PGH_2 whose structure is shown in Fig. 12 is apparently 7.9

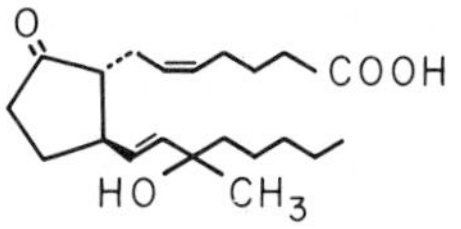

WY–17,186
Fig. 10.

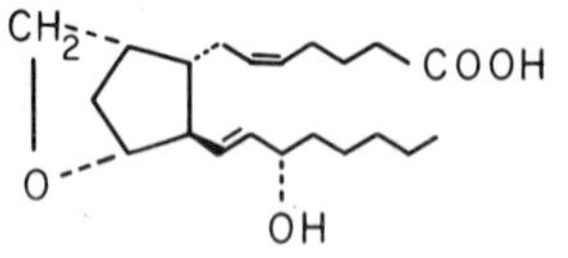

Fig. 11.

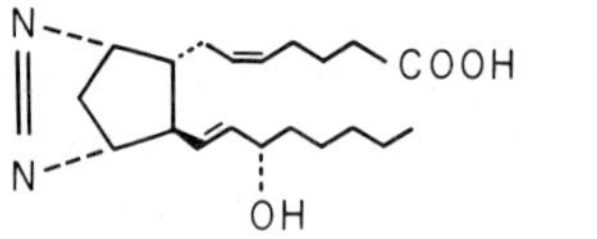

AZO ANALOG OF PGH₂

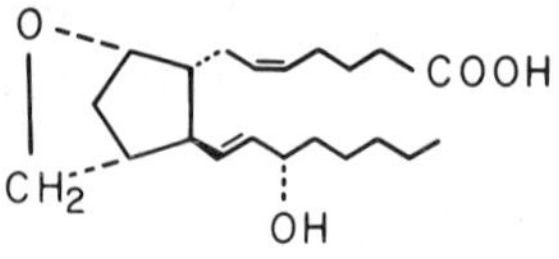

Fig. 12.

times as potent as PGG_2 in causing platelet aggregation and 6 times as potent in inducing the release of $[^{14}C]$serotonin from platelets (Corey et al., 1975). It causes irreversible aggregation of platelets in human PRP at a concentration of 0.1 μM.

Platelet aggregation induced by these stable synthetic prostaglandins is not inhibited by aspirin or indomethacin so they appear to mimic the action of the unstable endoperoxides PGG_2 and PGH_2 and should be of value in elucidating the mechanism of action of the latter.

6.2. In vivo studies

6.2.1. Arachidonic acid

When arachidonic acid was injected into the ear veins of rabbits at a dose of 1.4 mg/kg, the animals died within 3 min (Silver et al., 1974). Death was preceded by acute respiratory distress and platelet aggregates were found in the heart, blood, and in vessels of the pulmonary microcirculation but not those of other organs. The other prostaglandin precursors, 8,11,14-eicosatrienoic acid, 5,8,11,14,17-eicosapentaneoic acid, and other closely related fatty acids had no such effects, even at doses four times the LD_{50} of arachidonic acid. When rabbits were pretreated with aspirin (13 mg/kg intraperitoneally) and then challenged with arachidonic acid they were completely protected from its lethal effects, indicating that the platelet aggregation occurred as a result of prostaglandin synthesis. Rabbits were not protected from death by the anticoagulant heparin and fibrin strands were not detected in the pulmonary platelet aggregates, indicating that the phenomenon is independent of blood coagulation. This rabbit model of pulmonary platelet thrombosis would appear to be an effective system for screening potential anti-thrombotic drugs, and furthermore, it may mimic certain cases of sudden death in which the principal finding at autopsy is platelet aggregates in small vessels of the pulmonary microcirculation (Pirkle and Carstens, 1974).

Injections of sodium arachidonate into the carotid artery of heparinized rats cause unilateral, irreversible, cerebrovascular occlusion (Furlow and Bass, 1975), and this model may help to elucidate mechanisms of ischemic cerebrovascular disease and to develop a rationale for treatment. The intravascular injection of arachidonate may also prove generally useful in clarifying the role of platelet aggregation in thrombotic events in other organs such as the heart and kidneys.

6.2.2. Synthetic prostaglandins

Several synthetic prostaglandins that induce platelet aggregation (see above) cause sudden death in rabbits at concentrations lower than those required for arachidonic acid (Silver, M.J., Kocsis, J.J., Smith, J.B., Ingerman, C., unpublished observations). All eleven rabbits that received an ear vein injection of 100 μg/kg U46619 exhibited symptoms of acute respiratory distress and died within two minutes. Six out of 7 rabbits injected with 70 μg/kg died, which suggests that this compound is at least 14 times as potent as arachidonic acid in this test. In contrast to the effect of aspirin against intravenous arachidonic acid-induced, rabbits pretreated with aspirin were not protected from the lethal effects of U46619. Other synthetic prostaglandins were less effective in the rabbit ear vein model system. U44069 killed only 2 out of 5 rabbits at 100 μg/kg while Wy-17, 186 killed 9 out of 10 rabbits at 400 μg/kg. Considerably higher doses of all of these compounds were necessary to kill mice by tail vein injection.

7. Inhibition of platelet aggregation

7.1. Aspirin and indomethacin

It has been known for some time that aspirin inhibits platelet aggregation, prolongs the bleeding time in normal humans (Weiss et al., 1968), and can cause serious bleeding problems in some patients (Kaneshiro et al., 1969). It can therefore be regarded as an anti-haemostatic agent and, indeed, is presently being investigated clinically as an anti-thrombotic agent (Mustard and Packham, 1975). Although this drug has been widely used for over 50 years as an anti-inflammatory agent, its mechanism of action remained unknown until recently. In 1971 Smith and Willis showed that aspirin and indomethacin inhibited the synthesis of prostaglandins by washed platelets in response to thrombin, which established the mechanism responsible for aspirin's anti-haemostatic action and, along with the findings that it inhibited prostaglandin synthesis in other tissues (Ferreira et al., 1971; Vane, 1971), helped to elucidate its mechanism of action as an anti-inflammatory agent. Inhibition of both platelet aggregation (O'Brien et al., 1968) and prostaglandin synthesis (Silver et al., 1972a; Kocis et al., 1973) persists for several days after ingestion of aspirin, whereas the inhibitory effects of indomethacin in vivo on platelet aggregation and prostaglandin synthesis persist for less than 24 h.

The biological effects of aspirin and indomethacin on platelet function result from inhibition of the platelet release reaction (Weiss et al., 1968; Zucker and Peterson, 1971), and recent biochemical studies have established that aspirin acetylates, and so permanently inhibits, the cyclooxygenase which converts arachidonic acid to PGG_2 and PGH_2 (Roth and Majerus, 1975). Indomethacin also inhibits this enzyme, but its relatively short duration of action in vivo suggests that it does not permanently affect the cyclooxygenase, but rather inhibits platelet cyclooxygenase activity only as long as effective concentrations remain in the bloodstream. This inhibition of cyclooxygenase is associated with diminished production of the metabolites of PGG_2 (i.e., HHT, malondialdehyde, and thromboxane B_2) and increased production of HETE (Hamberg and Samuelsson, 1974; Bills et al., 1976). In summary, we can conclude that aspirin and indomethacin inhibit the synthesis of short-lived intermediates which are the most potent inducers of aggregation and release presently known, but do not interfere with the biological activity of these substances.

7.2. Other inhibitors of prostaglandin synthesis

Several substances are potent inhibitors of cyclooxygenase activity (see Flower, 1974) and many of these (for example, β-naphthol) also inhibit platelet aggregation. (Silver et al., 1973). Furosemide also inhibits both platelet aggregation and prostaglandin synthesis (Ingerman et al., 1975), and adenosine at low concentrations (2 μM) prevents platelet aggregation by arachidonic acid (Silver et al., 1973) but it is not yet known whether this agent inhibits prostaglandin synthesis or works via another mechanism.

7.3. Analogues of arachidonic acid and other fatty acids

5,8,11,14-eicosatetraynoic acid is an analogue of arachidonic acid containing 4 triple bonds rather than 4 double bonds. It inhibits prostaglandin synthesis (Ahern and Downing, 1970) and also inhibits both arachidonic acid- and collagen-induced platelet aggregation (Silver et al., 1973; Willis et al., 1974b). 8,11,14-eicosatrienoic acid and 5,8,11,14,17-eicosapentaenoic acid are prostaglandin precursors which differ from arachidonic acid in having respectively one less or one more double bond, and these fatty acids inhibit platelet aggregation induced by arachidonic acid or collagen as well as the second wave of aggregation induced by 2 μM ADP. Two other closely related fatty acids 11,14,17-eicosatrienoic acid and 4,7,10,13,16,19 docosahexaenoic acid also inhibit arachidonic acid-induced aggregation (Silver et al., 1973).

7.4. Albumin

This plasma protein inhibits platelet aggregation induced by arachidonic acid (Silver et al., 1973; Vargaftig and Zirinis, 1973), and its inhibitory potency is greatly increased when it is pre-incubated with the arachidonic acid. Albumin also inhibits collagen-induced aggregation and the second wave of ADP-induced aggregation (Silver et al., 1973).

8. Control of arachidonic acid metabolism by platelets

8.1. Role of plasma albumin

When trace amounts of [^{14}C]arachidonic acid are incubated with platelet-rich plasma, the only metabolism seen is the incorporation of arachidonic acid into the platelet phospholipids (Bills et al., 1975, 1976), but when similar amounts of radioactive arachidonic acid are incubated with washed platelets, oxidation products of arachidonic acid (i.e., the products of cyclooxygenase and lipoxygenase) are generated. This can be significantly reduced by including 0.25% to 1% albumin in the incubation mixture (Nugteren, 1974; Bills, T.K., Smith, J.B. and Silver, M.J., unpublished results). It therefore follows that the arachidonic acid in normal circulating plasma, being bound to albumin, is not available to platelet cyclooxygenase or lipoxygenase. On the other hand, when blood vessels are damaged and haemostatic or thrombotic processes are initiated, arachidonic acid can be released from phosphatidylcholine and phosphatidylinositol *within* the platelet, and thus be protected from binding by plasma albumin and hence available for metabolism. It is also possible that enough arachidonic acid might be released from nearby tissues to overcome temporarily the binding capacity of plasma albumin. Arachidonic acid that escaped binding would be transformed by platelet lipoxygenase and cyclooxygenase to active products including PGG$_2$.

8.2. Contribution to the inflammatory process

Inflammation has been defined as a local reaction to injury of the microcirculation and its contents (Spector and Willoughby, 1968). Injury to small blood vessels can also initiate adherence of platelets to damaged tissue and platelet aggregation; this is associated with the formation of the inflammatory agent PGE$_2$ by the platelets. This prostaglandin increases vascular permeability and its actions are discussed in detail elsewhere (Willis et al., 1972; Silver et al., 1974a). HETE, a substance formed by platelet lipoxygenase, has recently been shown to be chemotactic for polymorphonuclear leukocytes (Turner et al., 1975), further emphasizing the importance of the metabolism of arachidonic acid by platelets in inflammatory processes. One hitherto unrecognised effect of non-steroidal antiinflammatory agents may be that when the cyclooxygenase pathway is blocked not only is the production of PGE$_2$ inhibited but more arachidonic acid becomes available for the lipooxygenase pathway and therefore more HETE is produced, which could result in increased leukocyte infiltration.

8.3. Opportunities for potential anti-thrombotic action

Although the relationship between prostaglandin synthesis and platelet function has been under investigation for only a few years, important contributions have already been made in elucidating the role of prostaglandin synthesis in haemostasis and thrombosis. The original observations that washed human platelets formed and released prostaglandin E_2 and $F_{2\alpha}$ in response to thrombin, and that aspirin and indomethacin inhibited the production of these prostaglandins by platelets, led to the demonstration that platelet prostaglandin synthesis occurred during blood clotting, and during the aggregation of platelets in platelet-rich plasma in response to agents such as ADP, adrenaline, collagen and thrombin. In this context, it should be noted that since heparin inhibits the formation of thrombin it will prevent any thrombin-induced prostaglandin synthesis, and as aspirin also inhibits platelet prostaglandin synthesis it can be appreciated why both heparin and aspirin can bring relief to patients suffering from thrombophlebitis.

An important finding was that arachidonic acid caused platelets to aggregate, undergo the release reaction and form prostaglandins, and that all these events were inhibited by aspirin, which indicated that arachidonic acid-induced aggregation and release depended on prostaglandin synthesis. At that time it appeared paradoxical that PGE_2 and $PGF_{2\alpha}$, the end products of prostaglandin synthesis, did not induce platelet aggregation, and that other substances later found to be formed in conjunction with prostaglandin synthesis (such as thromboxane B_2, MDA, HHT, and HETE) apparently also did not induce platelet aggregation. It therefore seemed likely that intermediates formed during platelet prostaglandin synthesis were responsible for platelet aggregation and the release reaction induced by arachidonic acid, and indeed it was later shown that PGG_2 and PGH_2, short-lived intermediates in prostaglandin synthesis, can induce platelet aggregation. Possibly even more important is the observation that thromboxane A_2, an intermediate in the formation of thromboxane B_2, apparently is a powerful inducer of the release reaction and platelet aggregation.

The precise roles of arachidonic acid and its metabolic products in platelet function are presently being investigated. Prostaglandins are not detectable during the platelet shape-change and primary aggregation induced by ADP or adrenaline, and these platelet reactions are not inhibited by aspirin, which suggests that they are independent of prostaglandin formation. On the other hand, prostaglandins are produced during aggregation and the release reaction induced by collagen, and since these effects of collagen are inhibited by aspirin, it seems likely that they are mediated by prostaglandin endoperoxides, or thromboxane A_2, or both. Recently, it has been shown that thromboxane A_2 and release-inducing activity persist in plasma (Smith et al., 1976b), which suggests that thromboxane A_2 is a release-inducing agent. Prostaglandins are also produced during the release reaction induced by thrombin, but this release is little affected by aspirin unless a very low concentration of thrombin is used, which suggests that one or more of the initial products of thrombin action (i.e., arachidonic acid, lysolecithin or lysophosphatidylinositol), produced either in the presence or absence of aspirin, are mediators of the thrombin-induced release reaction. Alternatively, thrombin could well be capable of inducing release by another mechanism independent of arachidonic acid or phospholipid metabolism.

Understanding something of the role of prostaglandin synthesis in platelet aggregation has provided a rationale for designing drugs to be used in thrombotic conditions such as myocardial infarction, stroke and pulmonary embolism. Potential sites of drug action include the following:

(1) Inhibition of phospholipase activity. The formation of thrombotic substances like PGG_2, PGH_2 and thromboxane A_2 by platelets requires the prior release of arachidonic acid from platelet phospholipids. Therefore, an inhibitor of the phospholipase(s) responsible for releasing arachidonic acid from platelets in vivo could inhibit platelet aggregation and thrombosis. Unfortunately, however, no such agent is presently known.

(2) Inhibition of the cyclooxygenase pathway in platelets. Aspirin, which acts in this way, is currently under extensive clinical trial as a prophylactic for the prevention of myocardial infarction.

(3) Inhibition of the thrombotic effects of PGG_2, PGH_2, or thromboxane A_2. Such inhibitors could be tested for anti-thrombotic activity in vivo in rabbits injected intravenously with either arachidonic acid or the synthetic prostaglandins which mimic the endoperoxides (see Section 6.2). No such agents are presently known but an intensive search for them is already underway.

(4) Substitution of 8,11,14-eicosatrienoic acid for arachidonic acid. This fatty acid can be incorporated into the phospholipids of human platelets, and when such platelets were treated with thrombin, 8,11,14-eicosatrienoic acid was released specifically from phosphatidylinositol and products were formed that have been tentatively identified as coming from the lipoxygenase and cyclooxygenase pathways (Bills, T.K., Smith, J.B., Silver, M.J., unpublished results). Normally, human platelets contain relatively large amounts of arachidonic acid in their phospholipids and only tiny amounts of 8,11,14-eicosatrienoic acid. Individuals having large amounts of the latter fatty acid in their phospholipids should have diminished tendency toward thrombosis for several reasons: (1) The pool of platelet arachidonic acid would be diminished, and so less PGG_2, PGH_2 and thromboxane A_2 would be formed; (2) 8,11,14-eicosatrienoic acid released from phosphatidylinositol would compete with released arachidonic acid for the platelet cyclooxygenase and (3) one of the products formed from 8,11,14-eicosatrienoic acid by platelets is PGE_1, a potent inhibitor of platelet aggregation. Feeding 8,11,14-eicosatrienoic acid to animals can result in a high ratio of this fatty acid to arachidonic acid in the platelets (Willis et al., 1974; Danon et al., 1975) and this is apparently associated with a diminished sensitivity of the platelets to the effects of aggregating agents. If similar results can be achieved in man without undesirable side effects, this may prove to be an exciting new approach to the problem of thrombosis.

8.4. Pathological implications of abnormal metabolism

It is possible that abnormalities in the metabolism of arachidonic acid by platelets could disturb the haemostatic mechanism, resulting in bleeding or thrombosis.

There have been two reports of apparently defective cyclooxygenase activity in the platelets of patients with bleeding problems not related to a defect in blood coagulation. Willis and Weiss (1973) found several patients whose platelets apparently produced less PGE_2 and $PGF_{2\alpha}$ in response to thrombin or collagen than those of normal individuals, which suggests, but does not prove, that there is a defect in cyclooxygenase activity. Malmsten et al. (1975) reported one case in which 0.2 mM arachidonic acid did not induce platelet aggregation in platelet-rich plasma whereas 0.6 μM PGG_2 did. Also, only primary aggregation was seen in response to ADP and adrenaline and practically no aggregation in response to collagen. Only trace amounts of radioactive thromboxane B_2 and HHT were produced from [^{14}C]arachidonic acid by washed platelets from the patient whereas transformation into HETE was increased. This appears to be more convincing evidence for a cyclooxygenase deficiency, but it must be remembered that it is difficult to prove that a cyclooxygenase deficiency exists in platelets because, in spite of the fact that the patient denies having taken any drug, it is still possible that he may have taken one of the many preparations, sold over-the-counter, which contain aspirin and which the patient does not consider to be a drug. So far there have been no other reports of defective haemostasis or of thrombosis due to abnormal metabolism of arachidonic acid or failure of the platelets to aggregate in response to PGG_2, PGH_2 or thromboxane A_2, but this may be a fruitful area for future clinical investigation. In particular, we should consider the possibility that certain pathological conditions might produce a sudden, local release of large amounts of arachidonic acid, which could cause platelet aggregation, leading to the obstruction of the microcirculation of vital organs such as lungs, brain, heart or kidney and resulting in a disabling illness or sudden death (Silver et al., 1973, 1974, 1975a; Pirkle and Carstens, 1974).

9. Summary

(1) Studies on the metabolism of arachidonic acid by human platelets and its relationship to platelet aggregation in vitro have indicated that intermediates in prostaglandin biosynthesis are vitally important in haemostasis and thrombosis, and have helped to elucidate the mechanisms of platelet aggregation and the release reaction.

(2) Studies in animals have provided a model system for studying thrombosis in vivo and for testing potential antithrombotic agents.

(3) Defects in the metabolism of arachidonic acid by platelets may be responsible for some bleeding disorders (intrinsic or drug-related) and the sudden local release of large amounts of arachidonic acid could be an important factor in thrombosis.

(4) Finally, these studies have provided a new rationale for designing potential anti-thrombotic drugs.

References

Ahern, G.D. and Downing, D.T. (1970) Biochim. Biophys. Acta, *210*, 456.
Ambache, N. (1957) J. Physiol., *135*, 114.
Bergström, S. (1967) Science, *157*, 382.
Bergström, S., Danielsson, H. and Samuelsson, B. (1964) Biochim. Biophys. Acta, *90*, 207.
Bergström, S. and Sjövall, J. (1960) Acta Chem. Scand., *14*, 1693.
Bergström, S. and Sjövall, J. (1960a) Acta Chem. Scand., *14*, 1701.
Bills, T.K. and Silver, M.J. (1975) Fed. Proc. 34, No. 3, Abstr. 3228.
Bills, T.K., Smith, J.B. and Silver, M.J. (1976) Biochim. Biophys. Acta *424*, 303.
Bundy, G.L. Oral Presentation at International Conference on Prostaglandins. Florence, Italy, May, 1975.
Bundy, G.L. (1975a) Tetrahedron Lett., 24, 1957.
Christ, E.J. and Van Dorp, D.A. (1972) Biochim. Biophys. Acta, *270*, 537.
Clausen, J. and Srivastava, K.C. (1973) Lipids, *7*, 246.
Cohen, P. and Derksen, A. (1969) Brit. J. Haemat., *17*, 359.
Corey, E.J., Nicolaou, K.C., Machida, Y., Malmsten, C.L. and Samuelsson, B. (1975) Proc. Natl. Acad. Sci. U.S.A., *72*, 3355.
Danon, A., Heimberg, M. and Oates, J.A. (1975) Biochim. Biophys. Acta, *388*, 318.
Eliasson, R. (1959) Acta Physiol. Scand. 46 (Suppl. 158) 1.
Fenichel, R.L., Stokes, D.D. and Alburn, H.E. (1975) Nature, *253*, 537.
Ferreira, S.H., Moncada, S. and Vane, J.R. (1971) Nature, *231*, 237.
Flower, R.J. (1974) Pharmacol. Reviews, *26*, 33.
Furlow, T.W., Jr. and Bass, N.H. (1975) Science, *187*, 658.
Goldblatt, M.W. (1933) J. Soc. Chem. Ind. (Lond.), *52*, 1056.
Goldblatt, M.W. (1935) J. Physiol. (Lond.), 84, *208*.
Granström, E., Lands, W.E.M. and Samuelsson, B. (1968) J. Biol. Chem., *243*, 4104.
Hamberg, M., and Samuelsson, B. (1967) J. Biol. Chem., *242*, 5336.
Hamberg, M. and Samuelsson, B. (1967a) J. Biol. Chem., *242*, 5344.
Hamberg, M. and Samuelsson, B. (1973) Proc. Natl. Acad. Sci. U.S.A., *70*, 899.
Hamberg, M. and Samuelsson, B. (1974) Proc. Natl. Acad. Sci. U.S.A., *71*, 3400.
Hamberg, M., Svensson, J. and Samuelsson, B. (1974) Proc. Natl. Acad. Sci. U.S.A., *71*, 3824.
Hamberg, M., Svensson, J., Wakabayashi, T. and Samuelsson, B. (1974a) Proc. Natl. Acad. Sci. U.S.A., *71*, 345.
Hamberg, M., Svensson, J. and Samuelsson, B. (1975) Proc. Natl. Acad. Sci. U.S.A., *72*, 2994.
Horton, E.W. (1972) Prostaglandins, 197 pp, Springer Verlag, New York.
Ingerman, C., Smith, J.B. and Silver, M.J. (1975) Proc. 18th Annual Meeting Am. Soc. Hemat. Abst. No. 444.
Jonsson, H.T., Middleditch, B.S. and Desiderio, D.M. (1975) Science, *187*, 1094.
Jubiz, W. and Frailey, J. (1974) Prostaglandins, *7*, 339.
Kaneshiro, M.M., Mielke, C.H., Casper, C.K. and Rapaport, S.I. (1969) New Eng. J. Med., *281*, 1039.
Kloeze, J. (1967) in Prostaglandins (Bergström, S. and Samuelsson, B., eds), p. 243, Almquist and Wiksell, Stockholm.
Kocsis, J.J., Hernandovich, J., Silver, M.J., Smith, J.B. and Ingerman, C. (1973) Prostaglandins, *3*, 141.
Kunze, H. and Vogt, W. (1971) Ann. N.Y. Acad. Sci., *180*, 123.
Kurzrok, R. and Lieb, C.C. (1930) Proc. Soc. Exp. Biol. Med., *28*, 268.
Lands, W., Lee, R. and Smith, W. (1971) Ann. N.Y. Acad. Sci., *180*, 107.
Lands, W.E. and Samuelsson, B. (1968) Biochim. Biophys. Acta, *164*, 426.
Malmsten, C., Hamberg, M., Svensson, J. and Samuelsson, B. (1975) Proc. Natl. Acad. Sci. U.S.A., *72*, 1446.
Marcus, A.J., Ullman, H.L. and Safier, L.B. (1969) J. Lipid Res., *10*, 108.
Miyamoto, T., Yamamoto, S. and Hayaishi, O. (1974) Proc. Natl. Acad. Sci. U.S.A., *71*, 3645.
Mustard, J.F. and Packham, M.A. (1975) Drugs, *9*, 19.
Nugteren, D.H. (1975) Biochim. Biophys. Acta, *380*, 299.
Nugteren, D.H. and Van Dorp, D.A. (1965) Biochim. Biophys. Acta, *98*, 654.
Nugteren, D.H., Van Dorp, D.A., Bergström, S., Hamberg, M. and Samuelsson, B. (1966) Nature, *212*, 38.
Nugteren, D.H., Beerthuis, R.K. and Van Dorp, D.A. (1966a) Rec. Trav. Chim. Pays-Bas, *85*, 405.

Nugteren, D.H. and Hazelhof, E. (1973) Biochim. Biophys. Acta, *326*, 448.
Okuma, M., Steiner, M. and Baldini, M. (1971) J. Lab. Clin. Med., *77*, 728.
Orczyk, G.P. and Behrman, H.R. (1972) Prostaglandins, *1*, 3.
Piper, P. and Vane, J. (1971) Ann. N.Y. Acad. Sci., *180*, 363.
Pirkle, H. and Carstens, P. (1974) Science, *185*, 1062.
Roth, G.J. and Majerus, P.W. (1975) J. Clin. Invest., *56*, 624.
Ryhage, R. and Samuelsson, B. (1965) Biochem. Biophys. Res. Commun., *19*, 279.
Samuelsson, B. (1965) J. Am. Chem. Soc., *87*, 3011.
Samuelsson, B. (1965) Pharmacol., *3*, 59.
Silver, M.J., Smith, J.B., Ingerman, C. and Kocsis, J.J. (1972) Prostaglandins, *1*, 429.
Silver, M.J., Hernandovich, J., Ingerman, C., Kocsis, J.J. and Smith, J.B. (1972a) in Platelets and
    Thrombosis (Sherry, S. and Scriabine, A., eds), p. 91, University Park Press, Baltimore.
Silver, M.J., Smith, J.B., Ingerman, C. and Kocsis, J.J. (1973) Prostaglandins, *4*, 863.
Silver, M.J., Smith, J.B., Ingerman, C. and Kocsis, J.J. (1973a) Prostaglandins in Blood: Measurement,
    Sources and Effects, in Progress in Hematology (Brown, E., ed), Vol. 8, p. 235, Grune and Stratton,
    New York.
Silver, M.J., Hoch, W., Kocsis, J.J., Ingerman, C. and Smith, J.B. (1974) Science, *183*, 1085.
Silver, M.J., Smith, J.B. and Ingerman, C.M. (1974a) Agents Actions, *4*, 233.
Silver, M.J., Hoch, W.S., Kocsis, J.J., Ingerman, C. and Smith, J.B. (1975) Science, *190*, 491.
Smith, J.B. and Willis, A.L. (1970) Brit. J. Pharmac., *40*, 545 P.
Smith, J.B. and Willis, A.L. (1971) Nature, *231*, 235.
Smith, J.B., Silver, M.J., Ingerman, C. and Kocsis, J.J. (1972) in Platelets and Thrombosis (Sherry, S. and
    Scriabine, A., eds), p. 81, University Park Press, Baltimore.
Smith, J.B., Ingerman, C. Kocsis, J.J. and Silver, M.J. (1973) J. Clin. Invest., *52*, 965.
Smith, J.B., Ingerman, C., Kocsis, J.J. and Silver, M.J. (1974) J. Clin. Invest., *53*, 1468.
Smith, J.B. and Macfarlane, D.E. (1974) Platelets in Prostaglandins (Ramwell, P., ed), Vol. 2, p. 293,
    Plenum Press, New York.
Smith, J.B., Ingerman, C., Mills, D.C.B. and Silver, M.J. (1975) Proc. 18th Annual Meeting Am. Soc.
    Hematol. Abstr. No. 463.
Smith, J.B., Ingerman, C. and Silver, M.J. (1976) J. Lab. Clin. Med. *88*, 167.
Smith, J.B., Ingerman, C. and Silver, M.J. (1976a) Adv. Prostagl. Thromb. Res., *2*, 747.
Smith, J.B., Ingerman, C. and Silver, M.J. (1976b) J. Clin. Invest. In press.
Spector, W.G. and Willoughby, D.A. (1968) The Pharmacology of Inflammation, Grune and Stratton,
    New York.
Stuart, M.J., Murphy, S. and Oski, F.A. (1975) New Eng. J. Med., *292*, 1310.
Takeguchi, C., Kohno, E. and Sin, C.J. (1971) Biochemistry, *10*, 2372.
Taylor, P.L. and Kelley, R.W. (1974) Nature, *250*, 665.
Turner, S.R., Tainer, J.A. and Lynn, W.S. (1975) Nature, *257*, 680.
Van Dorp, D.A. (1967) Prog. Biochem. Pharmacol., *3*, 71.
Van Dorp, D.A., Beerthuis, R.K., Nugteren, D.H. and Vonkeman, H. (1964) Biochim. Biophys. Acta, *90*,
    204.
Vane, J.R. (1971) Nature, *231*, 232.
Vargaftig, B.B. and Zirinis, P. (1973) Nature, *244*, 114.
Vogt, W. (1949) Naumyn-Schmiedenberg Arch. Pharmakol., *206*, 1.
Von Euler, U.S. (1934) Naumyn-Schmiedenberg Arch. Pharmakol., *175*, 78.
Von Euler, U.S. (1936) J. Physiol (London), *88*, 213.
Vonkeman, H. and Van Dorp, D.A. (1968) Biochim. Biophys. Acta, *164*, 430.
Wallach, D.P. (1965) Life Sci., *4*, 361.
Weiss, H.J., Aledort, L.M. and Kochwa, S. (1968) J. Clin. Invest., *47*, 2169.
Willis, A.L. (1974) Prostaglandins, *5*, 1.
Willis, A.L., Davison, P., Ramwell, P.W., Brocklehurst, W.E. and Smith, J.B. (1972) in Prostaglandins in
    Cellular Biology (Ramwell, P.W. and Phariss, B.B., eds), p. 227, Plenum Press, New York.
Willis, A.L. and Kuhn, D.C. (1973) Prostaglandins, *4*, 127.
Willis, A.L. and Weiss, H.J. (1973) Prostaglandins, *4*, 783.
Willis, A.L., Comai, K., Kuhn, D.C. and Paulsrud, J. (1974) Prostaglandins, *8*, 509.
Willis, A.L., Vane, F.M., Kuhn, D.C., Scott, C.G. and Petrin, M. (1974a) Prostaglandins, *8*, 453.
Willis, A.L., Kuhn, D.C. and Weiss, H.G. (1974b) Science, *183*, 327.
Zucker, M.B. and Peterson, J. (1970) J. Lab. Clin. Med., *76*, 66.

CHAPTER 14

Proteinases in platelets

H.P. EHRLICH and J.L. GORDON

Tissue Physiology Department, Strangeways Research Laboratory, Worts Causeway, Cambridge, CB1 4RN, England, and University Department of Pathology, Tennis Court Road, Cambridge CB2 1QP, England

1. Introduction

1.1. Platelet proteinases previously described

The presence of lysosomal granules in blood platelets is well established, and since lysosomes characteristically contain numerous hydrolytic enzymes (including proteinases) one might have expected that the proteinases in platelets would already have been well defined. In fact, although there have been several studies of platelet lysosomal enzymes, these have been chiefly concerned with the glycosidases and phosphatase activities (for review, see Gordon, 1975), and there have been few attempts to characterise the proteinases of platelet lysosomes. Nachman and Ferris (1968), found that human platelets contained enzymes capable of degrading haemoglobin, casein and fibrinogen. On the basis of heat lability and lack of inhibition by trypsin inhibitors they concluded that the proteolytic activity was not attributable to plasmin. They found evidence of proteolytic activity in both neutral and acid conditions, and concluded that the degradation of haemoglobin at pH 3.5 was attributable to lysomal carboxypeptidase A ('cathepsin A'), because the synthetic substrate N-carbobenzoxy-α-L-glutamyl-L-tyrosine was also hydrolyzed. There was no hydrolysis of N-acetyl-tyrosine-ethyl-ester, suggesting that dipeptidyl peptidase I ('cathepsin C'), was absent, and since the activity was not potentiated by cysteine or inhibited by iodoacetamide there was no cathepsin B present. On the basis of the lack of sulphydryl dependence, these authors also concluded that cathepsin E was absent, but cathepsin E is not generally regarded as being a sulphydryl dependent enzyme (see Section 2.1). They also concluded that there was no cathepsin D present because there was little evidence of proteolytic activity at pH 2.8, but the pH optimum for cathepsin D activity is usually around 4, and in our recent studies using a specific antiserum against human cathepsin D, we found significant activity in platelet extracts (see Section 4). Nachman and Ferris (1968), themselves emphasized that since their studies were performed on a platelet extract which had been extensively dialyzed against distilled water, lyophilysed, and defatted with chloroform and methanol, their results probably do not accurately reflect the proteolytic activities which may be present in intact platelets.

Several peptidases from platelets have been described by Kocholaty (1962), and Haschen (1975). Some of these may be the same activities which have been studied by other workers in a different context–for example, those which increase vascular permeability, release histamine from mast cells, and split complement components to liberate leukocyte chemotactic factors (Packham et al., 1968; Nachman et al., 1972; Weksler and Coupal, 1973). It may be of some biological significance that Haschen (1975), found platelets to contain greater exopeptidase activity than any other blood cells.

Other proteolytic enzymes which have been reported to be present in human platelets include an elastase (Robert et al., 1970; Legrand et al., 1970; 1973; 1975) and a collagenase (Chesney et al., 1974). The elastolytic enzyme hydrolysed both ^{125}I-labelled elastin and N-acetyl-L-alanyl-L-alanine methyl ester (AcAla$_3$OMe) with a pH optimum around 8.6. Legrand et al. (1973), did not establish the subcellular localization of this enzyme, and, indeed, some recent work from our own laboratory suggests that it may not have originated from platelets at all (see Section 4). The collagenase extracted from platelets was capable of hydrolyzing purified collagen, and Chesney et al. (1974), suggested that the enzyme might be present partly in lysosomal granules and partly in the platelet plasma membrane. They found no activity in platelets under normal conditions but could demonstrate collagenase both in platelets and in the extracellular fluid after the addition of platelet stimulating agents. Collagenase activity could apparently be liberated when the platelets were treated with a concentration of ADP which was too low to release any of the platelet 5HT or lysosomal glycosidases. These observations are difficult to explain satisfactorily, and further work is needed to clarify the significance of this. Also, some caution is necessary in estimating the amounts of collagenase activity present in platelets, since contamination of the platelet preparation with a small number of leukocytes may lead to large errors (see Sections 4 and 5).

1.2. Potential biological roles of platelet proteinases

If elastolytic activity could be released in biologically significant amounts when platelets are stimulated in vivo (for example, by contact with subendothelial collagen–see Chapters 2, 3 and 9), it is conceivable that the elastin in the vascular walls could be attacked by the enzyme. Indeed, Legrand et al. (1973), suggested that platelet elastase could be at least partly responsible for the degradation of arterial elastic tissue which is a characteristic feature of atherosclerosis, although Robert et al. (1974), later showed that arterial tissue itself contained elastase activity. Robert et al. (1970), found that after elastin had been treated with 'platelet' elastase it was then susceptible to further digestion by other proteolytic enzymes, suggesting that a range of platelet proteinases might contribute to the destruction of vascular integrity after the initial effects of elastase. By the same token, it is possible that platelet elastase released into the pulmonary vasculature could contribute to the development of emphysema. However, before these hypotheses can be seriously entertained, it will be necessary to demonstrate conclusively that elastolytic activity can be released from blood platelets in biologically significant amounts by biologically relevant stimuli. This has not yet been done.

It is also possible that platelet collagenase could degrade vascular collagen, and Chesney et al. (1974), suggested that because the enzyme can destroy the platelet aggregating activity of collagen, platelet collagenase may function in a negative feedback system to limit platelet aggregation (and hence thrombus formation). Again, before such a hypothesis can be accepted, it is important to examine critically the data regarding the amount of collagenase activity which can be released from platelets. In addition, platelet collagenase is inhibited by normal human plasma, although the factors responsible for this inhibition have not been fully characterized (Chesney et al., 1974). Accordingly, the levels of enzyme activity measured in a plasma-free system may bear little relation to those which could operate in vivo.

The role of the cathepsins in platelets, as in other cells, has not yet been unequivocally established. It is possible that they act as 'helper' enzymes in the degradation of connective tissue; structural proteins such as collagen and elastin are not usually susceptible to degradation by acid-acting cathepsins (except for cathepsin B_1), but when these proteins have been exposed to elastase or collagenase, further degradation by these cathepsins is possible. However, because acid proteinases act at subphysiological pH values, their site of activity must be either intracellular (in phagocytic vacuoles) or in the immediate pericellular environment, where local pH values may be kept low enough to allow the cathepsins to act. Since platelets do exhibit phagocytic activity, and can ingest connective tissue particles (Mustard and Packham, 1968), the concept of their acid proteinases acting intracellularly to degrade such particles seems reasonable. Also, when platelets adhere to subendothelial components of the vascular wall they can spread out (thus achieving an intimate contact with the components) and degranulate, releasing the contents of their lysosomal granules (see Chapter 2). This situation could permit a pericellular action of platelet cathepsins.

2. *Characterisation of proteinases*

A detailed discussion of the characteristics and classification of proteinases is beyond the scope of this chapter; for a comprehensive treatment of the subject the interested reader should consult the companion volume in this series, entitled 'Proteinases of mammalian cells and tissues' (ed. Barrett, 1977), and the monograph on 'Proteases and biological control' (eds. Reish et al., 1975). The following outline merely summarises certain points relevant to the enzymes investigated during this study.

Proteinases are, by definition, enzymes which hydrolyse the bond between amino acid residues in the peptide linkage of proteins. There are 'exopeptidases' which hydrolyse amino acid residues adjacent to the carboxy or amino terminals of the polypeptide chain, and 'endopeptidases' which cleave interior bonds, thus splitting large polypeptide chains into smaller peptide units. The proteinases mainly discussed in this chapter are cathepsins D and E, and elastase.

Cathepsin D (EC 3.4.23.5) is a carboxy endopeptidase found in the lysosomes of most cells. There are no satisfactory synthetic substrates for this proteinase, but several protein substrates have been used to characterise the enzyme's activity. The most widely used substrate is denatured haemoglobin, and, on this, the pH optimum for cathepsin D is about 3.5, although the pH optimum on proteoglycan is around 4.5, and that on casein is around pH 5.0. These discrepancies probably arise because the acid pH differentially affects the substrates, altering their susceptibilities to attack by the enzyme. Cathepsin D is normally stable at neutral pH, but is irreversibly inhibited in the presence of reducing agents such as dithiothreitol (Barrett, 1967). It is not affected by DFP, iodacetate, cysteine or EDTA, but is inhibited by pepstatin (Dingle et al., 1972).

The molecular weight of cathepsin D ranges from 50,000 (Barrett, 1967) to 37,000 (Kregar et al., 1967) based upon gel chromatography. Yago and Bowers (1975) found a new cathepsin D-like enzyme in rat lymphocytes that is a carboxy proteinase, inhibited by pepstatin, with a pH optimum on haemoglobin of 3.6. Although the molecular weight of this enzyme was 95,000 (based upon gel chromatography), it became 45,000 after treatment with dithiothreitol. The enzyme was searched for in human and rabbit lymphoid tissues but not found, although it is apparently present in several tissues of rat and mouse.

Cathepsin E (also EC 3.4.23.5) is, like cathepsin D, a carboxy endopeptidase with pepsin-like activity, inhibited by pepstatin but unaffected by DFP, iodoacetate, EDTA or thiol reagents (Turk et al., 1968). It differs from cathepsin D in being strongly anionic (therefore binding tightly to DEAE ion exchange resin), with a molecular weight around twice as large and a lower pH optimum (around 3.0). Its tissue distribution is also much more restricted–its presence has been confirmed only in rabbit bone marrow, spleen, and polymorphonuclear leukocytes (Lapresle, 1971). In this context, it should be remembered that blood platelets are formed in the bone marrow, and are present in large numbers in the spleen.

The elastase which was first characterised was that from the pancreas (EN 3.4.21.11; pancreatopeptidase E), which is synthesised as a zymogen (proenzyme) and, when activated, degrades elastin at neutral pH. Another elastase (EN 3.4.2.1.–) is present in human polymorphonuclear leukocytes, and this is identical to the elastase from spleen which has been recently characterised by Barrett and Starkey (1976). This enzyme, which has a molecular weight around 28,000, is a serine proteinase with a pH optimum of 7.5 to 8.0, which still retains 50% of its maximal activity at pH 6.0 (Vissel and Blout, 1972). As well as hydrolysing elastin, it splits the synthetic substrate Z-benzyloxy carboxy-L-alanine-2-naphthol ester (Janoff, 1970). Its activity is not affected by EDTA, cysteine or iodacetate (Janoff, 1972) but it is inhibited by α-1 proteinase inhibitor (Ohlsson, 1971), peptide chloromethyl ketones (Tuhy and Powers, 1975) and soybean trypsin inhibitor (Janoff, 1972).

3. Acid proteinases in rabbit platelets

We investigated the acid proteinases in rabbit platelets and characterized the enzymes present in terms of their molecular weight, pH optimum, substrate specificity, susceptibility to inhibitors, and ion exchange properties. The results of these studies and of immuno-identification experiments indicate that the two major acid proteinases in rabbit platelets are cathepsins D and E.

3.1. Measurement of enzyme activity

Proteolytic activity was routinely assayed using denatured bovine haemoglobin as substrate. After incubation at 45°C the reaction was terminated by adding trichloroacetic acid and the mixture filtered. Absorbance of the filtrate was read at 280 nm and one unit of enzymatic activity is defined as a 1.0 change in optical density after one hour incubation at 45°C.

When a more sensitive assay of enzymatic activity was required, the degradation of ^{35}S-labelled proteoglycan was measured. Bovine nasal cartilage was incubated with ^{35}S-labelled sodium sulphate and the proteoglycan extracted with 4 M guanidinium chloride. After purifying the labelled proteoglycan by ethanol precipitation, it was incorporated into a polyacrylamide matrix in bead form. Samples to be tested were incubated for 4 h at 37°C with a 1.25% w/v slurry of beads containing ^{35}S-labelled proteoglycan in a roller rack at 5 rev/min. Proteolytic activity cleaves the polypeptide backbone of the proteoglycan and the fragments thus released escape from the beads. After terminating the reaction with 1% v/v sodium dodecylsulphate and hydrochloric acid, the mixture was centrifuged and the radioactivity in the supernatant was counted; this represents a highly sensitive measure of proteinase activity (Dingle, J.T., Barrett, A.J., Blow, A.M.J. and Martin P.E.N., in preparation).

Platelet samples for the measurement of proteinase activity were obtained by centrifuging citrated platelet-rich plasma, decanting the supernatant, and homogenizing the platelet pellet in 0.1% v/v Trition X-100 using a miniature glass homogenizer with null-clearance teflon pestle. Particular care was taken to ensure that contamination of the preparations by leukocytes was lower than 1 cell per 10^4 platelets (see Section 4).

3.2. pH Dependence

Samples of platelet homogenate (0.3 ml; each corresponding to 6×10^7 cells) were incubated with polyacrylamide beads containing ^{35}S-labelled proteoglycan and release of radioactivity was measured in the presence of buffers ranging from pH 2.0 to 8.0. One main peak of enzyme activity was found, with a pH optimum around 4.0. The peak obtained was not entirely symmetrical, having a slight shoulder on the lower pH side (Fig. 1). When samples of platelet homogenate were tested using bovine serum albumin or denatured bovine haemoglobin as substrates, the pH optimum for enzymic activity against both substrates was 3.0, with

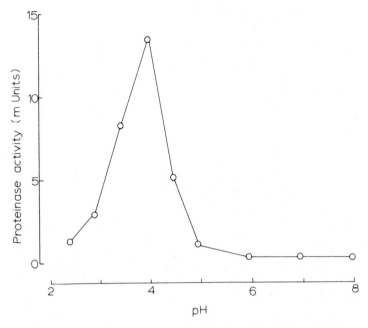

Fig. 1. pH-dependence of proteinase activity in rabbit platelets. Rabbit platelets (2×10^9 cells), were homogenized in 10 ml of 0.1% Triton X-100. Proteolytic activity in 0.3 ml samples was measured using ^{35}S-labelled proteoglycan in polyacrylamide beads. Each point represents the mean of triplicate determinations. Buffers used (1.0 M concentration) were: pH 2.0–3.5, sodium formate; pH 4.0–6.0, sodium acetate; pH 6.5–8.0, Tris–HCl. Proteolytic activity is expressed in milliunits, based on a standard curve obtained with purified rabbit cathepsin D.

a smaller peak at pH 4.0 (Fig. 2). When these experiments were repeated in the presence of 10 mM EDTA and 5 mM cysteine there was no change in the amount of enzyme activity or the positions of the peaks.

To investigate the identity of the proteinase activity, further samples of platelet homogenate were assayed using ^{35}S-labelled proteoglycan in polyacrylamide beads at pH 4.0 in the presence of antibodies to rabbit cathepsin D. Anti-rabbit cathepsin D antiserum was raised in sheep and an IgG-rich fraction was extracted by precipitation with 50% ammonium sulphate and mixed with Sepharose 4B previously activated by cyanogen bromide (March et al., 1974). The final preparation contained 1 mg of IgG protein adsorbed per gram of sepharose. Control sepharose beads were also prepared using the same method but substituting normal sheep serum for the sheep anti-rabbit cathepsin D antiserum. By coupling the IgG to sepharose, any possible problems associated with antibody excess were obviated. To check the potency of the sepharose-coupled IgG, purified cathepsin D from rabbit liver was assayed (using denatured bovine haemoglobin as substrate) after exposure to sepharose with normal sheep IgG or with anti-cathepsin D IgG attached: cathepsin D activity in the supernatant was reduced by over 95% after adsorption by beads with antibody, but only by about 5% after adsorption by beads with normal IgG (Table 1).

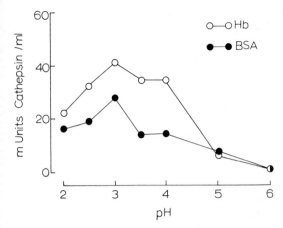

Fig. 2. pH-dependence of rabbit platelet proteinase activity, using denatured bovine haemoglobin (Hb), and bovine serum albumim (BSA), as substrates. Platelets were homogenised as described in Fig. 1, and proteolytic activity in samples corresponding to 1.5×10^8 cells were measured using the haemoglobin assay described in the text. Where appropriate, 8% BSA was substituted for haemoglobin. Each point represents the mean of triplicate determinations, and activity is expressed in milliunits, based on a standard curve obtained with purified rabbit cathepsin D.

TABLE 1
Immunoadsorption of cathepsin D

	mU cathepsin D
Cathepsin D alone; no beads	70
Cathepsin D plus beads with immunoglobin from normal sheep	66
Cathepsin D plus beads with sheep anti-rabbit cathepsin D immunoglobin	3

Pure cathepsin D isolated from rabbit liver was diluted with 0.15 M NaCl containing 0.1% Brij. A 0.1 ml slurry of sepharose beads with covalently-linked immunoglobins was incubated with 0.9 ml of diluted enzyme preparation containing 70 mU cathepsin D. A 0.5 ml aliquot of the supernatant was assayed using haemoglobin as substrate following a 30 min incubation with immunoadsorbent at 23°C.

When a similar experiment was performed using samples of platelet homogenate, and proteolytic activity was measured at pH 4.0 with ^{35}S-labelled proteoglycan as substrate, activity was reduced by about 70% in the presence of sepharose-coupled antibody to rabbit cathepsin D (Table 2).

3.3. Molecular weight

A Sephadex G-100 column was calibrated with standards of known molecular weights–bovine serum albumin (67,000); egg albumin (43,000); carbonic anhydrase (30,000); and lysozyme (14,700). Samples of platelet homogenate were passed through this column and the ability of the fractions eluted to degrade ^{35}S-labelled proteoglycan at pH 4.0 or denatured bovine haemoglobin at pH 3.0 was deter-

TABLE 2

Immunoadsorption of proteolytic activity in rabbit platelet homogenate

	mU proteolytic activity
Platelet homogenate alone	6.0
Platelet homogenate plus sepharose beads with normal sheep immunoglobulin	5.5
Platelet homogenate plus sepharose beads with sheep anti-rabbit cathepsin D	1.5

Proteolytic activity in samples of homogenized rabbit platelets (each equivalent to 10^7 cells) was measured at pH 4.0 using ^{35}S-labelled proteoglycan as a substrate. Activity below is expressed in mU from a cathepsin D standard curve.

mined. Two peaks of enzyme activity were found with molecular weights of approximately 60,000 (peak I) and 33,000 (peak II). When purified rabbit cathepsin D was passed through the same column, the enzyme activity eluted at the same point as peak II of the platelet homogenate and we therefore tentatively identified the enzyme activity of peak II as cathepsin D. However, since the platelet homogenate contained numerous other substances which might bind to cathepsin D and thus alter its position of elution from the column, we prepared radiolabelled cathepsin D and incubated this with a sample of platelet homogenate for 16 h at 4°C before passing the mixture through a G-100 column. The purified cathepsin D from rabbit liver (a gift from Dr. A.J. Barrett) was labelled with ^{125}Iodine by the technique of Bolton and Hunter (1973). The labelled material was tested on an immunodiffusion plate against an antibody to cathepsin D, and when the plate was subjected to autoradiography, the radioactive lines on the photographic plate were superimposed on the stained immunodiffusion lines (Fig. 3), thus confirming that

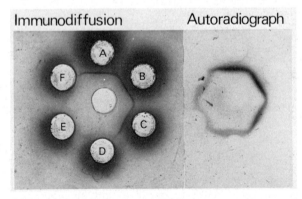

Fig. 3. Immunological identity of radiolabelled rabbit cathepsin D. Purified cathepsin D was labelled with ^{125}I (see text), and subjected to Ouchterlony analysis as shown. The central well contains iodinated cathepsin D, and the peripheral wells contain dilutions of an antiserum raised in sheep to rabbit cathepsin D. A, undiluted; B, 1:2; C, 1:4; D, 1:8; E, 1:16; F, 1:32: An autoradiograph was prepared from the Ouchterlony plate, which confirmed that the immunoprecipitin lines contained the radioactive label.

the radio-labelled material represented cathepsin D activity. When the mixture of radio-labelled cathepsin D and platelet homogenate was added to the G-100 column the radioactivity appeared as a single peak which corresponded with peak II (Fig. 4). This strongly supported our earlier conclusion that peak II of the platelet homogenate was indeed cathepsin D. Note that the activity of peak II shown in Fig. 4 is exaggerated because the radiolabelled cathepsin D in the mixture had significant enzymic activity. Immunodiffusion analysis of peak II from another sample of platelet homogenate, using an antibody to rabbit cathepsin D, confirmed that the material in peak II was immunologically identical to rabbit cathepsin D.

When peak I from the G-100 column (fractions 22 to 25: Fig. 4) was assayed using ^{35}S-labelled proteoglycan, the pH optimum for enzymic activity was 3.5 (Fig. 5); purified rabbit cathepsin D tested under the same conditions gave a pH optimum of 4.3 and when peak II of the homogenate (fractions 30 to 33) was similarly tested, the pH optimum was 4.5.

Although our earlier experiments indicated that cathepsin D did not readily associate with other components of the platelet homogenate to form a complex with a higher molecular weight than the native enzyme, we wished to check the

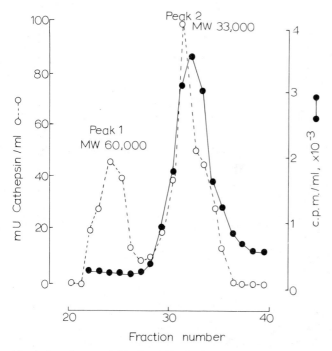

Fig. 4. Proteinase activities in rabbit platelets, separated by gel chromatography. A sample (2.0 ml), of rabbit platelet homogenate containing 2.5×10^9 cells was applied to a Sephadex G 100 column with 8×10^4 counts/min of labelled cathepsin D. The column was eluted with 0.2 M NaCl and 0.1% Brij, and 50 drop fractions were collected for proteinase assay and for measurement of radioactivity. For details of homogenisation and proteinase assay, see text and legend to Fig. 1.

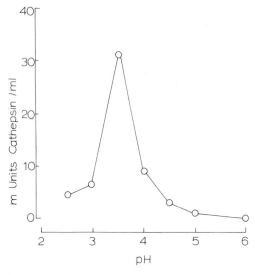

Fig. 5. pH-dependence of proteinase activity from the 60,000 mol. wt fraction of a rabbit platelet homogenate. The proteolytic activity of peak I from a Sephadex G-100 column separation of homogenised rabbit platelets (see Fig. 4), was measured using ^{35}S-labelled proteoglycan (see Fig. 1). Fractions 22 to 25 from the column were pooled, and 0.3 ml samples used to assay proteolytic activity. Each point is the mean of triplicate determinations.

possibility that the peaks of enzyme activity which we observed might represent enzymes of lower molecular weight present in a multimeric form (c.f. Yago and Bowers, 1975). Accordingly, a sample of platelet homogenate was incubated for 16 h at 4°C with 5 mM dithiothreitol, then passed through a G-100 column equilibrated in 5 mM dithiothreitol. To check whether this procedure affected the position at which cathepsin D eluted, purified radiolabelled cathepsin D was added to the platelet homogenate before incubation. The same two peaks of enzyme activity were seen, and the positions at which these peaks and purified cathepsin D eluted were unchanged (Fig. 6). The level of activity in peak II was greatly reduced after treatment with dithiothreitol, although the activity in peak I was little affected; this is consistent with the previous observation that cathepsin D activity is inhibited by incubation with dithiothreitol (Barrett, 1967).

3.4. Ion exchange chromatography

Ion exchange chromatography was performed using Whatman DE 52 resin in a 1 × 4 cm column equilibrated with starting buffer (50 mM Tris; pH 7.6). A sample of platelet homogenate was dialyzed into starting buffer and applied to the top of the column. The column was subsequently eluted by a linear salt gradient made from 50 ml starting buffer and 50 ml eluting buffer (50 mM Tris, pH 7.6, containing 1.0 M NaCl) at 23°C. Two main peaks of enzyme activity were seen: one peak (peak II) was followed by possibly two small subsidiary peaks, and appeared before the salt gradient was started, whereas the other peak eluted at approxi-

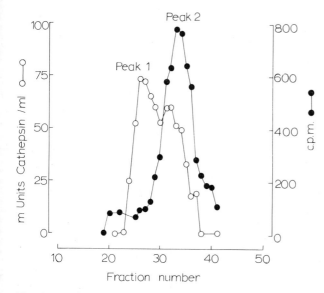

Fig. 6. Proteinase activities in homogenised rabbit platelets after incubation with dithiothreitol. A sample of homogenised platelets (2×10^9 cells), was incubated for 16 h with 5 mM dithiothreitol and 2×10^4 counts/min of ^{125}I-labelled cathepsin D, then applied to a Sephadex G-100 column. Experimental details are as for Fig. 4, except that the eluting buffer contained 5 mM dithiothreitol.

mately 0.4 M NaCl (Fig. 7). The enzyme activity of fractions eluted from the column was assayed using ^{35}S-labelled proteoglycan.

The proteolytic activity of the peak II (and of the subsidiary peaks beside it) was abolished in the presence of antibody to cathepsin D, suggesting that these

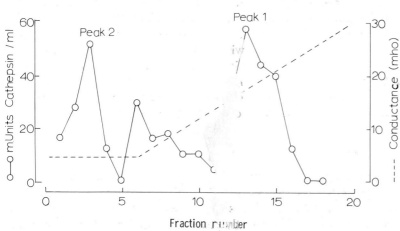

Fig. 7. Proteinase activities in homogenised rabbit platelets, separated by ion exchange chromatography. A sample of homogenised platelets ($8 \times$ cells) was dialyzed against 50 mM Tris buffer (pH 7.6), and applied to a DE-52 column and eluted with a linear salt gradient made from 50 ml Tris–HCl (50 mM, pH 7.6) and 50 ml eluting buffer (Tris–HCl with 1.0 M NaCl). Fractions were assayed for proteolytic activity using ^{35}S-labelled proteoglycan.

peaks might be isoenzymes of cathepsin D (Barrett, 1970). The proteolytic activity of peak I (eluting at 0.4 M NaCl) was unaffected by this antibody, and we concluded that this peak represented the same enzymatic activity as peak I of the G-100 column.

3.5. Substrate and inhibitor specificity

Both the main enzyme activities of rabbit platelet homogenates (obtained either from a G-100 column or from a DE 52 column) were more effective against haemoglobin than against albumin, and the ratio of activities against the two substrates was roughly similar for each enzyme. Rabbit platelet homogenates failed to degrade the synthetic substrate benzoyl-D,L-arginine-2-naphthylamide, which is hydrolysed by cathepsin B (EC 3.4.22.1.).

The proteolytic activity of peak I and peak II eluted from the G-100 column was determined in the presence of several different inhibitors. The activity of both enzymes was abolished by pepstatin (10 μg/ml) but was unaffected by chloromercuribenzoate (10 mM); EDTA (10 mM); cysteine (5 mM); iodoacetate (10 mM); or ovoinhibitor (10 μg/ml). Activity of peak II was abolished in the presence of Sepharose-coupled antibody to purified rabbit cathepsin D, whereas this antibody had no significant effect on the activity of peak I. Normal sheep serum coupled to sepharose did not affect the activity of either enzyme. The values obtained for enzymic activity in this set of experiments are shown in Table 3.

When a similar experiment with antibody to cathepsin D was performed using peaks I and II from the DE 52 column, the activity of peak II was abolished by the antibody, while that of peak I was unaffected (Table 4). On the basis of the data from all our experiments with rabbit platelets, we concluded that there were two main acid proteinases present: cathepsin D (mol. wt. approximately 33,000) and cathepsin E (mol. wt. approximately 60,000). We found no evidence of other

TABLE 3
Effects of potential inhibitors on platelet acid proteinases eluted from Sephadex G-100 column

	Proteinase activity (mU)	
Additions	Peak I (cathepsin E)	Peak II (cathepsin D)
None	12	17
10 μg/ml pepstatin	0	0
10 mM-parachloromercuribenzoate	13	17
10 mM EDTA	12	13
5 mM cysteine	11	17
10 mM iodoacetate	12	16
10 μg/ml ovoinhibitor (Matsushima, 1958)	12	15
Normal sheep immunoglobin coupled to sepharose	13	15
Sheep anti-rabbit cathepsin D antibody coupled to sepharose	15	< 1

TABLE 4

Effects of antiserum to cathepsin D on rabbit platelet proteinases separated by ion-exchange chromatography

	Cathepsin activity (mU)	
	Peak I*	Peak II*
Column fraction adsorbed by normal sheep immunoglobulin coupled to sepharose	10	14
Column fraction adsorbed by anti-rabbit cathepsin D coupled to sepharose	11	< 1

Proteolytic activity was measured using ^{35}S-labelled proteoglycan.
*   See Fig. 7.

acid proteinases; in particular, we concluded that cathepsin B was probably absent because iodoacetate and cysteine had no effect, and the relevant synthetic substrate was not degraded. We observed no degradation of ^{35}S-labelled proteoglycan by platelet homogenates at neutral pH, but it should be emphasized that we did not attempt to remove any inhibitors which might have been present in the homogenate, and it is possible that the absence of neutral proteinase and cathepsin B activity could have been due to endogenous inhibitors.

4. Proteinases in human platelets

The characteristics of the proteinase activities which we observed in human platelets were essentially similar to those of the rabbit platelet. When the pH dependence of proteinase activity from a human platelet homogenate was investigated using ^{35}S-labelled cartilage proteoglycan as substrate, two peaks of activity were revealed with pH optima around 3.0 and 4.5 (Fig. 8). The activity at pH 4.5 was greatly reduced after adsorption by Sepharose beads with antibodies to human cathepsin D whereas the activity at pH 3.0 was little affected.

We concluded that there is probably no cathepsin B in human platelets since the homogenates failed to degrade the synthetic substrate benzoyl-D,L-arginine-2-naphthylamide, and since the acid proteinase activity of our platelet homogenates was not inhibited by iodoacetate or potentiated by cysteine, but we did not test for the presence of cathepsin B inhibitors.

When the proteinases in human platelets were separated by ion exchange chromatography using a DE 52 column and elution by a linear salt gradient, the main peak (peak II) of activity (measured using ^{35}S-labelled proteoglycan) eluted at just under 0.1 M NaCl, with a minor peak (peak I) eluting at a little over 0.3 M NaCl. When the activity in fractions 1 to 10 from this column (i.e., the main peak) was tested after adsorption by Sepharose-coupled antibodies to human cathepsin D, the activity was virtually abolished, but the inhibitory effect of the antibody became progressively less as fractions from 10-20 were tested. When samples of

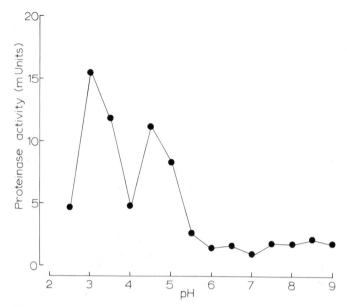

Fig. 8. pH-dependence of proteinase activity in human platelets. Release of ^{35}S-labelled proteoglycan from polyacrylamide beads was used to assay proteolytic activity in 0.3 ml samples of platelet homogenate (2×10^9 cells in 10 ml 0.1% Triton X-100). Buffers used were: pH 2.5–3.5, sodium formate; pH 4.0–6.0, sodium acetate; pH 6.5–8.5, Tris–HCl. Each point represents the mean of three determinations and the proteolytic activity is expressed as percent release of the total radioactivity contained in the polyacrylamide beads.

human platelet homogenate were subjected to immunodiffusion analysis using a monospecific antibody to cathepsin D an immuno-precipitin line was observed, and a similar line was produced when peak II (fractions 1–10) from the DE 52 column was tested. No precipitin line was observed when peak I (fractions 18–20) from the DE 52 column was tested.

When samples of platelet homogenates were eluted from a Sephadex G-100 column, one main peak of enzymatic activity was observed with a molecular weight of approximately 33,000 (peak II) and a smaller peak eluted with an apparent molecular weight of 60,000 (peak I). Before the homogenate was added to the G-100 column it was mixed with ^{125}I-labelled human cathepsin D, as previously described for rabbit platelets (see Section 3.3), and this cathepsin D co-chromatographed with peak II of the platelet homogenate (Fig. 10). When a similar experiment was performed with a sample of platelet homogenate pre-incubated for 16 h at 4°C with 5 mM dithiothreitol (as for rabbit platelets; see Section 3.3), there was no change in the position of either peak.

When the pH dependence of the enzyme activities from the G-100 column was determined, the pH optimum for peak I (fractions 16–20), was 3.5 to 4.0 and that for peak II (fractions 26–32), was pH 4.5 to 5.0. The activity of both peaks was inhibited by pepstatin, but ovoinhibitor, cysteine, EDTA, and soybean trypsin inhibitor had no effect on the activity of either peak. We conclude that the major

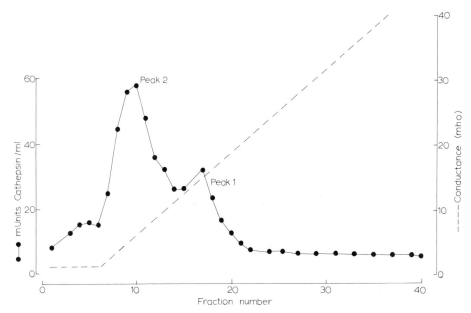

Fig. 9. Proteinase activity in human platelets, separated by ion exchange chromatography on a column of 5.0 ml DE-52 resin packed in 50 mM Tris–HCl (pH 7.5). A sample of homogenised platelets (3×10^9 cells) was dialysed into 50 mM Tris–HCl (pH 7.5), applied to the column, and eluted with a linear salt gradient made from a starting buffer of 50 ml Tris–HCl (50 mM; pH 7.5) and an eluting buffer of 50 ml Tris–HCl (50 mM; pH 7.5) and 1.0 M NaCl. Fractions of 2.5 ml were collected, and duplicate 0.3 ml volumes assayed for proteolytic activity at pH 4.0, using labelled proteoglycan in polyacrylamide beads.

acid proteinase present in human platelets is cathepsin D and that there is also a smaller amount of cathepsin E present. The cathepsin D from human and rabbit platelets is unlike the enzyme recently found in rodent lymphoid tissue (Yago and Bowers, 1975).

Neutral proteinase activity has previously been reported in extracts of human platelets (Nachman and Ferris, 1968), and it was suggested that part of this activity represents an elastase (Robert et al., 1970; Legrand et al., 1970; 1973; 1975). Because of these observations we investigated human platelet homogenates for possible elastase activity using three assay methods; an elastin plate, tritiated elastin (Takahashi et al., 1973), and the synthetic substrate Z-ala-2-O-Nap (a gift from Dr. Graham Knight of Strangeways Research Laboratory). Immunodiffusion analysis was also performed using a monospecific antiserum to human spleen elastase (a gift from Dr. A.J. Barrett). Details of these methods are given in Table 5.

In our initial experiments we used platelet preparations from blood donations supplied by the Blood Transfusion Service of Addenbrooke's Hospital, Cambridge, to ensure that we had sufficient platelet material for all our investigations. Platelet homogenates were prepared 24–48 h after collection of the blood. In all cases we found evidence of elastase activity against tritiated elastin, the elastin plate, and the synthetic substrate; precipitin lines were also produced on the

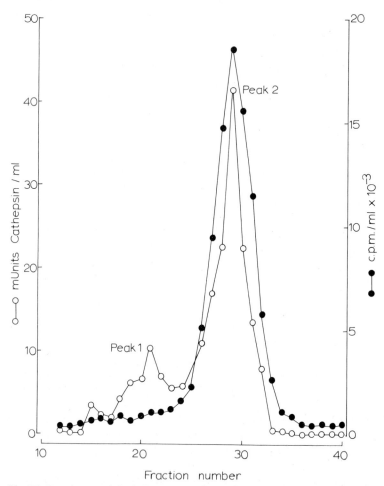

Fig. 10. Proteinase activity in human platelets, separated by gel chromatography on a Sephadex G-100 column packed in 50 mM sodium acetate (pH 5.5), with 0.2 M sodium chloride and 0.1% Brij. A cell pellet containing 2×10^9 platelets was homogenized in 2.0 ml of 0.1% Triton X-100 containing 4.2×10^5 counts/min of ^{125}I-labelled purified human cathepsin D and incubated at 4°C overnight. Fractions of 3.0 ml were collected for proteinase assay (using bovine haemoglobin as substrate) and for measurement of radioactivity.

immunodiffusion plates. When samples of these platelet homogenates were separated by ion exchange chromatography on a DE 52 column the elastase activity eluted at approximately 0.1 M NaCl and we also found two separate inhibitors of neutral proteinase activity in the homogenate; one inhibitor eluted with the elastase, and the other eluted at approximately 0.3 M NaCl. Both these inhibitors were active against trypsin. The amount of elastase activity that we observed in platelet homogenates from different donors varied considerably from sample to sample, even when corrections for differences in platelet count were made. Microscopic investigation of the platelet suspensions before they were homogenized revealed relatively few polymorphonuclear leukocytes (about 1

TABLE 5
Methods used to assess elastase activity

Elastin plate	Labelled elastin	Synthetic substrate	Immunodiffusion
Powered elastin (1% w/v) was added to 0.15% agarose in 50 ml Tris–HCl (pH 8.0) with 5 mM CaCl$_2$ and 0.25 mg/ml sodium dodecyl sulphate. Plates were poured at 50°C and gelled at 20°C, then 20 µl samples were added to 2 mm diameter wells and the plates incubated at 40°C for at least 24 h. The opaque elastin–agarose became translucent when the elastin was digested.	Powdered elastin was acetylated with [³H]acetic anhydride, then dispersed at 2 mg/ml in Tris–HCl (50 mM, pH 8.0) with 5 mM CaCl$_2$, 0.4 M NaCl and 0.1% Brij. Samples being tested were roller-mixed at 37°C with the [³H]elastin suspension, and elastase activity was measured as ³H in the supernatant after stopping the reaction with ice-cold soybean trypsin inhibitor (final concentration 0.2 mg/ml) and centrifuging (1500 × g; 5 min; 4°C). Method based on that of Takahashi et al. (1973).	Test samples (0.5 ml) were diluted with 1.5 ml Tris–HCl and incubated for 10 min at 50°C with 20 µl of Z-benzyloxycarboxy-L-alamine-2-naphthyl ester (5 mg/ml in DMSO). After stopping the reaction with 1 ml of soybean trypsin inhibitor (1 mg/ml in 1 M K$_2$HPO$_4$, pH 7.8) the enzyme product was coupled with 1 ml Fast Garnet (600 mg/ml in 4% Brij) and the absorbance read at 520 nm (Starkey and Barrett, 1976).	Agarose immunodiffusion plates contained 10 mM phosphate buffer (pH 7.5) 1 M NaCl and 0.1 sodium azide. Test samples were added to central wells and peripheral wells contained dilutions of a monospecific antiserum raised in rabbits to human spleen elastase (cf. Fig. 3).

In each case, standards were included which contained known amounts of purified elastase from human spleen, and thus the elastase activity in the test samples was determined.

cell per 10^4 platelets). This is the level of leukocyte contamination usually encountered when using conventional centrifugation methods to separate platelets from whole blood.

To investigate the possibility that the elastase activity previously reported from platelets (and found in our own experiments) might be derived wholly or in part from leukocytes, we repeated our studies using platelet homogenates prepared from blood samples immediately after venepuncture, with particular care taken to exclude leukocytes (contamination less than 1 cell per 10^8 platelets). This was achieved by successive centrifugations of platelet-rich plasma, or by separating the leukocytes through a layer of Ficoll (23% w/v). The platelet count of platelet-rich plasma prepared in this way was always about 20% lower than that prepared in a conventional manner, but we felt that this loss was justified by the extremely low levels of leukocyte contamination which we achieved. When platelet homogenates were prepared from these samples no elastase activity could be detected using any of the assay methods. Also, no immunoprecipitin lines were found on immunodiffusion analysis using the antibody to human spleen elastase, although leukocyte homogenates gave a strong positive response (Barrett, Ehrlich, Gordon and Starkey, unpublished observations). It therefore seems possible that previous reports of elastase in platelets might be due to contamination of the preparations by leukocytes.

It has also been reported that the elastase in 'platelet' preparations is present mainly as an inactive zymogen which can be activated by treatment with trypsin and that the elastase and proelastase can be separated by binding the former to an elastin affinity column (Legrand et al., 1975). We found no elastase activity in our purified platelet homogenates even after trypsin treatment, and although we believe that the elastase in the experiments of Legrand et al. (1975), was not in fact derived from platelets, the increase in activity which they observed following trypsin treatment could be explained at least in part by trypsin neutralizing an inhibitor of elastase, like those found in our platelet preparations. Elastase bound to an inhibitor could behave like a proenzyme, both on an affinity column and in response to trypsin. If trypsin is acting by competing for an inhibitor, the trypsin activity will be reduced as the elastase activity increases; if it is acting on an elastase zymogen, then the trypsin activity should not fall. This experiment remains to be done.

5. Discussion

The major proteinases in both human and rabbit platelets are cathepsins D and E. The ratio of cathepsin D to E in rabbit platelets varied from sample to sample, but in human platelets the amount of cathepsin D was always much greater than cathepsin E. The presence of cathepsin E has previously been confirmed only in rabbit polymorphonuclear leukocytes, spleen and bone marrow; an early report of cathepsin E in human spleen (McMaster and Webb, 1963) was not confirmed (Lapresle, 1971).

We found no neutral proteinase activity in crude homogenates of human or rabbit platelets, but because there were at least two inhibitors of neutral proteinases in our human platelet homogenates, it is possible that there was neutral proteinase activity in human or in rabbit platelets which was obscured by the effects of inhibitors. Further work is necessary to clarify this point. We did, however, investigate carefully the possible presence of a specific elastase or a specific collagenase in human platelets, checking for the presence of inhibitors in the fractions of the homogenate which we tested for enzyme activity. Using three different assay methods for elastase we could find no activity in human platelets, and immunoidentification experiments using a specific antiserum failed to reveal any elastase. Also, we could detect no collagenase activity (E.D. Harris and J.L. Gordon, unpublished observations) using tritiated fibrillar collagen as a substrate (Werb and Burleigh, 1974). These findings require confirmation, but at the very least they indicate that caution is necessary in any speculations regarding the potential biological roles of neutral proteinases from platelets. It is important to emphasize that the levels of collagenase previously reported in platelets are low (Chesney et al., 1974) and since 1 ml of platelet-rich plasma may contain over 10^4 leukocytes, the collagenase in these leukocytes might account for all the enzyme activity in the sample. Similar calculations led us to the conclusion that 'platelet' elastase might also be derived in fact from leukocytes, but a definitive answer to these questions awaits further experimental work – not only using highly purified platelet and leukocyte preparations, but also investigating the possibility that platelet–leukocyte interaction might facilitate the extracellular release of proteinases.

Since platelets undoubtedly contain substantial amounts of acid proteinases, it is quite probable that these play some important role, as yet undefined, in physiology or pathology. However because these enzymes are maximally effective at acid pH, we must assume that they act either intracellularly (by being discharged into phagocytic vacuoles) or in the immediate pericellular environment where the pH may be maintained sufficiently low to allow the enzymes to act. Since there is increasing interest in the potential role of blood platelets in several aspects of the inflammatory process (including the degradation of connective tissue components) the biological significance of platelet proteinases merits further investigation.

Acknowledgement

This study was supported by a research grant (to J.L.G.) from the Arthritis and Rheumatism Council.

References

Barrett, A.J. (1967) Biochem. J., *104*, 601.
Barrett, A.J. (1970) Biochem. J., *117*, 601.
Barrett, A.J. (1972) in Lysosomes: A Laboratory Handbook, (Dingle, J.T., ed), p. 46, North-Holland, Amsterdam.
Bolton, A.E. and Hunter, W.M. (1973) Biochem. J., *133*, 529.

Chesney, C. McI., Harper, E. and Colman, R.W. (1974) J. clin. Invest., *53*, 1647.
Dingle, J.T., Barrett, A.J., Poole, A.R. and Stovin, P. (1972) Biochem. J., *127*, 443.
Gordon, J.L. (1975) in Lysosomes in Biology and Pathology, (Dingle, J.T. and Dean, R.T., eds), Vol. 4, p. 3, North-Holland, Amsterdam.
Gross, J. and Lapière, C.M. (1960) Proc. Natl. Acad. Sci. U.S.A., *48*, 1014.
Harris, E.D. (1972) J. clin. Invest., *51*, 2973.
Harris, E.D. and Krane, S.M. (1974) N. Engl. J. Med., *291*, 557.
Haschen, R.J. (1975) in Lysosomes in Biology and Pathology, (Dingle, J.T. and Dean, R.T., eds), Vol. 4, p. 251, North-Holland, Amsterdam.
Hook, C.W., Brown, S.I., Iwang, W. and Nakanishi, I. (1971) Invest. Ophthalmol., *10*, 496.
Janoff, A. (1970) Lab. Invest., *22*, 228.
Janoff, A. (1972) Am. J. Path., *68*, 579.
Kocholaty, W. (1962) Thrombos. Diathes. Haemorrh., *7*, 295.
Lapresle, C. (1971) in Tissue proteinases (Barrett, A.J. and Dingle, J.T., eds), p. 135, North-Holland, Amsterdam.
Lapresle, C. and Webb, J. (1962) Biochem. J., *84*, 855.
Legrand, Y., Robert, B., Szigeti, M., Pignaud, G., Caen, J. and Robert, L. (1970) Atherosclerosis, *12*, 451.
Legrand, Y., Caen, J., Booyse, F.M., Rafelson, M.E., Robert, B. and Robert, L. (1973) Biochim. Biophys. Acta, *309*, 406.
Legrand, Y., Pignaud, G., Caen, J.P., Robert, B. and Robert, L. (1975) Biochem. Biophys. Res. Comm., *63*, 224.
March, S.C., Parikh, I. and Cuatrecasas, P. (1974) Anal. Biochem., *60*, 149.
Matsushima, K. (1958) Science, *127*, 1178.
McMaster, P.B. and Webb, T. (1963) Ann. Inst. Pasteur., *104*, 90.
Mustard, J.F. and Packham, M.A. (1968) Ser. Haemat. I, *2*, 168.
Nachman, R.L. and Ferris, B. (1968) J. clin. Invest., *47*, 2530.
Nachman, R.L., Weksler, B.B. and Ferris, B. (1972) J. clin. Invest., *51*, 549.
Ohlsson, K. (1971) Scand. J. clin. Lab. Invest., *28*, 251.
Packham, M.A., Nishizawa, E.E. and Mustard, J.F. (1968) Biochem. Pharmac., Suppl., *17*, 171.
Robert, B., Szigeti, M., Robert, L., Legrand, Y., Pignaud, G. and Caen, J. (1970) Nature, *227*, 1248.
Robert, B., Deronette, J.-C. and Robert, L. (1974) C.R. Acad. Sci. Paris, *278*, 3251.
Starkey, P.M. and Barrett, A.J. (1976) Biochem. J., *155*, 255.
Takahashi, S., Sufter, S. and Yang, F.C. (1973) Biochim. Biophys. Acta, *327*, 138.
Tuhy, P.M. and Powers, J.C. (1975) FEBS Lett., *50*, 359.
Turk, V., Kregar, I. and Leber, D. (1968) Enzymologia, *34*, 89.
Uriel, J. (1963) N.Y. Acad. Sci., *103*, 956.
Vissel, L. and Blout, E.R. (1972) Biochim. Biophys. Acta, *268*, 257.
Weksler, B.B. and Coupal, C.D. (1973) J. exp. Med., *137*, 1419.
Werb, Z. and Burleigh, M.C. (1974) Biochem. J., *137*, 373.
Woessner, J.F. (1973) Clin. Orthopaed., *96*, 310.
Yago, N. and Bowers, W.E. (1975) J. Biol. Chem., *250*, 4749.

CHAPTER 15

Trophic stimulation by platelets

R. ROSS, J. GLOMSET and L. HARKER

*Departments of Pathology, Medicine and Biochemistry, University of Washington School of Medicine,
Seattle, Washington 98195, U.S.A.*

1. Introduction

Proliferation of diploid cells in culture is widely recognized to be dependent upon the presence of whole blood serum which contains factors that are required to initiate DNA synthesis and cell division. Many investigators have studied this problem and have succeeded in isolating a number of fractions from serum that can be shown to play various roles in these phenomena (Holley and Kiernan, 1974; Shodell and Rubin, 1970; Temin, 1971, 1972). One of the principal mitogens of serum is clearly derived from the thrombocyte during the process of adherence, aggregation and release (Ross, 1974; Rutherford and Ross, 1976). This chapter will present a brief review of the role played by this factor in the growth of cells in culture. It will also provide data to demonstrate that platelet factor(s) play a role in stimulating cell proliferation in vivo, particularly in relation to the pathogenesis of the proliferative lesions of atherosclerosis.

2. Platelet mitogens and growth control in cell culture

In 1971, Balk (1971) studied the regulation of the proliferation of chick embryo fibroblasts and found that these cells would not grow in the presence of plasma derived serum but would grow in the presence of whole blood serum containing adequate levels of calcium. He postulated that thrombocytes might provide regulatory substances in whole blood serum that were missing in cell-free plasma derived serum, but did not pursue this idea further.

In a series of studies of the growth of primate arterial smooth muscle cells in culture, Ross et al. (1974, 1976) noted that when these cells are grown in the presence of serum derived from cell-free plasma, they remain in a quiescent state in which very little cell proliferation occurs. The mitogenic activity present in whole blood serum, and missing in serum made from plasma, is derived from platelets, as evidenced by the appearance of mitogenic activity in serum derived

Gordon (ed) Platelets in Biology and Pathology
© *Elsevier/North-Holland Biomedical Press, 1976*

from a mixture of cell-free plasma and purified platelets. Furthermore, the activity restored by addition of thrombocytes to cell-free plasma is also present in constituents released from platelets, as can be shown by adding a supernatant, derived from the exposure of gel-washed platelets to purified bovine thrombin in vitro, to serum derived from cell-free plasma (Fig. 1). Under these circumstances, platelets represent the principal source of the mitogenic activity of whole blood serum. In other studies, the effectiveness of neutrophils and lymphocytes to restore the mitogenic capacity of serum was examined. Neither of these cells was capable of restoring the activity.

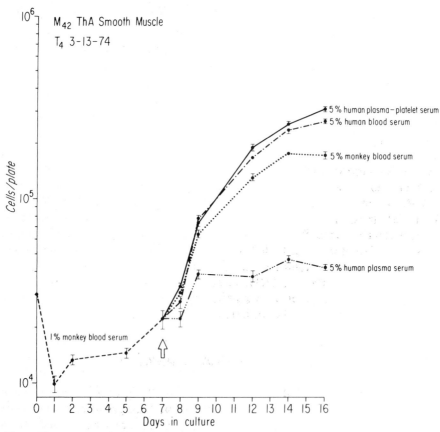

Fig. 1. The response of primate arterial smooth muscle to monkey blood serum, human blood serum, human plasma serum, and human plasma serum containing added platelet factor(s). Equal numbers (3×10^4) of arterial smooth muscle cells were added to a large series of 35 mm Petri dishes and incubated in medium containing 1% serum pooled from several *Macaca nemestrina*. After seven days (arrow), the dishes were separated into four groups. The groups were grown in medium containing: 5% dialyzed human cell-free plasma-serum; 5% dialyzed monkey whole blood serum; 5% dialyzed human whole blood serum (containing 3.95×10^8 platelets per ml); or 5% dialyzed plasma serum which had been exposed during the process of recalcification and serum formation to an equivalent number of purified platelets derived from the same pool of human blood. This experiment demonstrates that 5% cell-free plasma derived serum has little to no proliferative effect unless allowed to clot in the presence of platelets.

Kohler and Lipton (1974) have also studied platelets as a potential source of mitogenic activity for 3T3 cells in culture. In a similar set of experiments, they found that when platelets are lysed by repeated freezing and thawing, a component in the supernatant of the centrifuged-lysed platelets is capable of restoring the mitogenic capacity to plasma serum. Their observations also suggested that platelets are a source of mitogenic factor(s) in whole blood serum that may be important for a variety of cell types. The platelet factor is also required for the growth of diploid skin fibroblasts in cell culture as shown by experiments similar to those described for arterial smooth muscle (Rutherford and Ross, 1976).

Rutherford and Ross (1976) further characterized the mitogenic activity derived from platelets by demonstrating that fibroblasts or arterial smooth muscle cells grown in the presence of serum derived from cell-free plasma had a cell turnover of approximately 3% under these circumstances. Addition of the platelet factor to such medium recruited a relatively large percentage (approximately 25%) of the cells from 'G-0' into the G-1 phase of the cell cycle and committed these cells to DNA synthesis and mitosis. It was also shown that exposure of the cells to platelet factor for a period as short as one hour recruited the cells into the cycle. Once the cells were exposed to the platelet factor, it was possible to wash them carefully and replace them in medium containing cell-free plasma derived serum without interrupting the cell cycle.

The isolation and characterization of the platelet factor is currently underway. It appears to be a heat stable, non dialyzable, possibly basic protein.

Although growth stimulation in culture is a fundamental biological phenomenon, the question of in vivo relevance remained unanswered. Therefore, a series of experiments were performed to evaluate the significance of platelet activity in vivo.

3. Stimuli decreasing platelet survival

3.1. Homocystinemia

Individuals with the hereditary disease, homocystinuria, develop arteriosclerosis at a young age. Until recently, the mechanism has not been well understood. Harker and his colleagues (1974, 1976), noted that many of these patients demonstrated a decrease in platelet survival. This decrease in survival correlated with plasma homocystine concentrations.

To understand better the significance of decreased platelet survival observed in homocystinurics, this phenomenon was reproduced in the baboon by continuously infusing homocystine at a rate that exceeded its clearance. It was possible to maintain plasma levels of homocystine that were comparable with the concentrations observed in severely homocystinuric patients.

After six days of chronic homocystinemia, the baboons demonstrated a reduction in platelet survival that paralleled that previously observed in the homocystinurics. Examination of the aorta and iliac arteries of these homocystinemic baboons after perfusion fixation in vivo with silver nitrate demonstrated that approximately 10% of the endothelial cells were missing in contrast to the control animals which showed no loss of endothelium (Harker et al., 1976). These observations suggested a relation between the loss of endothelium and the decreased platelet survival, suggesting that the decrease in survival might be due to adherence and aggregation of platelets at sites of endothelial injury where desquamation and exposure of the subendothelial connective tissue might have occurred. To test this idea further, a series of baboons were made homocystinemic for three months and then compared with a group of control animals. After three months, all of the homocystinemic baboons continued to show decreased platelet survival and patchy endothelial cell loss as in the acute studies. This loss of endothelium was associated with a marked increase in [^{3}H]thymidine incorporation in vitro by an isolated segment of the carotid artery from the same animal. All of the animals, however, developed eccentric intimal smooth muscle proliferative lesions in the large caliber arteries. The lesions were histologically identical to the fibromusculoelastic lesions of atherosclerosis (Natl. Heart and Lung Inst., 1971), or to early fibrous plaques, and often contained lipid-laden foam cells deep within the lesions. In addition to the proliferation of intimal smooth muscle cells, a large amount of newly formed connective tissue matrix surrounded the cells. The control animals not only demonstrated normal platelet survival and no loss of endothelium, but no proliferative lesions as well.

To determine whether or not the decreased platelet survival was related to the presence of the smooth muscle proliferative lesions, an additional series of baboons was made homocystinemic and simultaneously given the antiplatelet drug, dipyridamole. In contrast to the untreated experimental group, the homocystinemic-dipyridamole treated animals demonstrated normal platelet survival and no proliferative lesions, although the amount of endothelial cell loss was not reduced. These observations suggested that platelet adherence, aggregation and release are required for the proliferative smooth muscle response to occur in vivo since inhibition of platelet function prevented this response.

3.2. Chronic endothelial injury

The importance of platelets in stimulating smooth muscle proliferation in vivo has been confirmed in three other experimental approaches. Moore et al. (Moore et al., 1976), were able to produce preatherosclerotic and atherosclerotic lesions in rabbits by the use of a chronic indwelling catheter. When the animals were made severely thrombocytopenic by antiplatelet serum, no proliferative lesions were produced at the sites of catheter-induced injury. Friedman et al. (1975) have also been able to prevent balloon catheter induced smooth muscle proliferation in rabbit arteries (Stemerman and Ross, 1972), by use of antiplatelet serum induced thrombocytopenia. Finally, in pigs affected with Von Willebrand's disease, a genetic defect of altered platelet–surface interaction, there is a reduced frequency of atherosclerosis in adult animals (Bowie et al., 1975).

Thus, platelet adherence, aggregation, and release at sites of exposed suben-dothelial connective tissue are apparently important in the induction of the smooth muscle proliferative response seen in the lesions of atherosclerosis.

3.3. Hypercholesterolemia

Ross and Harker (1976) have further examined the role of chronic hypercholes-terolemia in atherogenesis. Many individuals who are chronically hypercholes-terolemic have shortened platelet survival, and more than half of the patients with symptomatic coronary atherosclerosis show a decrease in platelet survival that becomes prolonged toward normal by saphenous vein-aorta-coronary bypass procedures, or by dipyridamole therapy (Ritchie and Harker, 1976). It has, however, been unclear as to whether there is an intrinsic defect in the platelets in hypercholesterolemia or whether the decreased platelet survival is a manifestation of endothelial cell injury. To answer this question, Ross and Harker (1976) examined a series of subhuman primates that were made hypercholesterolemic for 3 to 18 months by diet. All of the animals showed a statistically significant decrease in platelet survival and approximately 5%–7% loss of endothelium from the thoracic and abdominal aorta and iliac arteries associated with the long term development of atherosclerotic lesions. Experiments were performed in which ^{51}Cr-labelled platelets obtained from normolcholesterolemic monkeys were trans-fused into hypercholesterolemic animals and vice versa. After infusion of normocholesterolemic platelets into the hypercholesterolemic animals, the normal platelets showed decreased levels of survival similar to that observed in the chronic hypercholesterolemic monkeys. In contrast, ^{51}Cr-labelled platelets derived from hypercholesterolemic monkeys showed normal levels of platelet survival when infused into normocholesterolemic animals. These observations support the concept that decreased platelet survival observed in chronic hypercholesterolemia is not due to an intrinsic defect in the platelets, but rather to a loss of endothelium. Apparently, some form of 'injury' is sustained by the endothelial cells during chronic hypercholesterolemia that results in endothelial desquamation and de-creased platelet survival.

4. Summary

In vitro and in vivo studies demonstrate that platelets have an important role not only in hemostasis and thrombosis but in the proliferative response of connective tissue cells, at least in the smooth muscle cell response of atherogenesis and in other responses to injury such as wound repair. In vitro studies of the growth promotion of smooth muscle cells and fibroblasts in culture demonstrate that one of the principal mitogenic components present in whole blood serum and missing in platelet-poor plasma serum is derived from the main physiological response of platelets – adhesion, aggregation and release upon exposure to thrombin. In the absence of the platelet mitogenic factor, cells remain quiescent in the 'G-0' phase of the cell cycle. Exposure to the platelet factor recruits a large percentage of these cells into G-1 which is followed by DNA synthesis and mitosis. This platelet derived factor is probably ubiquitous to all sera derived from whole blood, and may be the principal mitogen in serum. It is, therefore, of general importance in the growth response of cells in culture. The intimal smooth muscle proliferative lesions observed in homocystinemia and in chronic hypercholesterolemia have been correlated with a decrease in platelet survival in both instances. This decreased platelet survival is associated with a loss of 5%–10% of the endothelial cells of the aorta and iliac arteries and with intimal smooth muscle proliferation. Inhibition of platelet function in homocystinemia or after mechanical injury to the endothelium prevents the smooth muscle proliferative response.

These studies in primates, and platelet survival studies in man, suggest a principal role for platelets in cell proliferation and a possible therapeutic capacity of some antiplatelet drugs in the pharmacologic inhibition of atherogenesis.

Acknowledgment

These studies were supported in part by grants from the U.S. Public Health Service, Nos. HL-18645 and HL-11775, and the Regional Primate Center of the University of Washington, No. RR-00166.

References

Balk, S. (1971) Proc. Natl. Acad. Sci. U.S.A., 68, 271.
Bowie, E.J.W., Fuster, V., Owen, C.A. and Brown, A.L. (1975) Thrombos. Diathes. Haemorrh., 34, 599.
Friedman, R.J., Stemerman, M.B., Spaet, T.H., Moore, S., Gauldie, J. (1976) Fed. Proc., 35, 207.
Harker, L.A., Ross, R., Slichter, S.J. and Scott, C.R. (1976) J. Clin. Invest. (in press).
Harker, L.A., Slichter, S.J., Scott, C.R. and Ross, R. (1974) New Eng. J. Med., 291, 537.
Holley, R.W. and Kiernan, J.A. (1974) Proc. Natl. Acad. Sci. U.S.A., 71, 2908.
Kohler, N. and Lipton, A. (1974) Exp. Cell Res., 87, 297.
National Heart and Lung Institute Task Force on Arteriosclerosis, Arteriosclerosis (National Institutes of Health, Bethesda, Md., Department of Health, Education, and Welfare Publ. No. (NIH) 72–219, June, 1971) Vol. 2.
Moore, S., Friedman, R.J., Singal, D.P., Gauldie, J. and Blajchman, M. (1976) Thromb. Diathes. Haemorrh. (in press).
Ritchie, J.L. and Harker, L.A. (1976) Submitted for publication.
Ross, R., Glomset, J., Kariya, B. and Harker, L. (1974) Proc. Natl. Acad. Sci. (U.S.A.), 71, 1207.
Ross, R. and Harker, L. (1976) Science, in press.
Rutherford, B.R. and Ross, R. (1976) J. Cell Biol., 69, 196.
Shodell, M. and Rubin, H. (1970) In Vitro, 6, 66.
Stemerman, M.B. and Ross, R. (1972) J. Exp. Med., 136, 769.
Temin, H.M. (1971) J. Cell Physiol., 78, 161.
Temin, H.M., Pierson, Jr., P.W. and Dulak, N.C. (1972) in Growth, Nutrition and Metabolism of Cells in Culture (Cristafalo, V. and Rothblat, G., eds), p. 50, Academic Press, New York.

Index